New Paradigms in Hepatology Research

New Paradigms in Hepatology Research

Editor: Amy McMahon

FOSTER ACADEMICS

www.fosteracademics.com

www.fosteracademics.com

FOSTER ACADEMICS

Cataloging-in-Publication Data

New paradigms in hepatology research / edited by Amy McMahon
p. cm.
Includes bibliographical references and index.
ISBN 978-1-64646-595-8
1. Hepatology. 2. Hepatology--Research. 3. Liver--Diseases.
4. Gastroenterology. I. McMahon, Amy.
RC845 .N49 2023
616.362--dc23

Foster Academics,
118-35 Queens Blvd., Suite 400,
Forest Hills, NY 11375, USA

ISBN 978-1-64646-595-8 (Hardback)

Contents

Preface

Hepatology refers to the branch of medicine that studies and manages disorders of the gallbladder, pancreas, liver and biliary tree. It was previously considered as a subspecialty of gastroenterology, but it is now becoming recognized as a separate field of study. Clinical research in hepatology is focused on developing novel medications, such as improvements to well-established liver transplantation procedures, antiviral medicines and developing new strategies for sustenance of failing liver. The application of molecular biology methods has helped to shed light on the vulnerability to various liver problems, as well as the mechanisms of liver diseases with hereditary and viral origins. This book aims to shed light on some of the unexplored aspects of hepatology and the recent researches in this field. Those in search of information to further their knowledge will be greatly assisted by it.

This book unites the global concepts and researches in an organized manner for a comprehensive understanding of the subject. It is a ripe text for all researchers, students, scientists or anyone else who is interested in acquiring a better knowledge of this dynamic field.

I extend my sincere thanks to the contributors for such eloquent research chapters. Finally, I thank my family for being a source of support and help.

Editor

1

Investigating effect of *Helicobacter pylori* treatment on improvement of non-alcoholic fatty liver parameters

Amir Mohammad Kazemifar[1], Ali Akbar Shafikhani[2], Elaheh Haji Noormohammadi[3], Zahra Azarion[3] and Aliakbar Hajia ghamohammadi[4*]

Abstract

Background and objective: The correlation between the eradication of *Helicobacter pylori* (HP) and non-alcoholic fatty liver disease (NAFLD) is a controversial one. The aim of this study is to investigate the effect of *Helicobacter pylori* treatment on liver function tests and lipid profiles and to compare its effects with exercise therapy and diet alone.

Method: This was a double-blind randomized clinical trial conducted at Qazvin University of Medical Sciences. One hundred patients with NAFLD having a positive test for urea breath testing were randomly assigned into one of the intervention and comparison groups. The diet and physical activity program were given to two groups of patients for 8 weeks, three sessions per week. In addition to the above therapy, the patients in the intervention group also received HP treatment for 2weeks. The data corresponding to anthropometric and clinical features before and after the intervention were collected in both groups and compared using appropriate statistical methods.

Results: After the treatment interventions, the variables of weight, BMI, blood glucose, triglyceride, AST, ALT, total cholesterol, and LDL-C were significantly decreased in both groups ($p < .05$). In the between-group comparisons, only ALT was significantly lower in the intervention group (HP) ($p < .05$).

Conclusion: Findings of this study showed that the eradication of *Helicobacter pylori* could significantly improve the ALT index, but it had no additional effect on changes in metabolic indicators.

Trial registration: Registration number: IRCT2015042020951N2
Name of trial registry: The study of treatment of *Helicobacter pylori* in improvement of non-alcoholic fatty liver disease
The date of registration: 2015-05-12
Where the full trial protocol can be accessed: https://fa.irct.ir/trial/18489

Keywords: Non-alcoholic fatty liver disease, Helicobacter pylori, Alanine transaminase, Aspartate aminotransferases

Background

Non-alcoholic fatty liver disease (NAFLD) is a type of liver injury caused by metabolic stress and hereditary sensitivity. Generally, this disease is considered to be the liver manifestation of the metabolic syndrome [1, 2]. NAFLD includes non-alcoholic fatty liver (NAFL), non-alcoholic steatohepatitis (NASH), and non-alcoholic steatohepatitis associated with hepatic cirrhosis and hepatocellular carcinoma. The incidence of NAFLD complications is rapidly increasing in the world [2, 3]; therefore, the economic and clinical burden of this disease is significant. Recently, except for the known risk factors such as obesity, type 2 diabetes, hypertension, and dyslipidemia, the role of the pathogenesis of *Helicobacter pylori* (HP) is also discussed in the disease and may be associated with NAFLD [4, 5].

HP is a Gram-negative bacterium that is selectively placed in the gastric mucosa. This bacterium is the cause of most cases of gastric ulcers and leads to development of some

* Correspondence: ahmohammadi@qums.ac.ir
[4]Gastroenterologist Metabolic Diseases Research Center, Qazvin University of Medical Sciences, Qazvin, Iran

gastro-intestinal cancers. However, this microbe does not cause cancer in all people [6, 7]; nearly 15% of patients with long-term infections might have one or more complications. According to estimates, about 25–50% of people in the developed countries and 70–90% of people in the developing countries are infected with this bacterium. The higher the age, the greater the chance of infection would be [7–9].

Recently, the HP infection has been implicated in non-digestive diseases, cardiovascular diseases, type 2 diabetes, and iron deficiency anemia [6, 10, 11]. In previous theories, Taylor et al. pointed out these cases and said that the HP species can cause damage to liver cells with the production of liver toxins [12]. Recently, HP infection has been reported as one of the risk factors for the development of non-alcoholic fatty liver disease [13]. However, recent findings have been focused on the correlation between HP infection and NAFLD, and their results are contradictory. On the one hand, Polyzos et al. showed that the eradication of HP infection might provide specific therapeutic approaches to NAFLD treatment. On the other hand, Jamali et al. presented contradictory results [14].

This study aimed to evaluate the effect of HP eradication on the liver function tests and lipid profiles and to compare its effects with diet and exercise therapy. Given the relatively high prevalence of HP infection in Iranian patients [15] and high prevalence of fatty liver [16], it could be significantly important to establish a correlation between the two abovementioned factors and eradicate it in the fatty liver treatment in Iran.

Method

The present research was a clinical trial with the pre- and post-test design, which was carried out at Velayat Hospital, Qazvin University of Medical Sciences. The statistical population of this research was the patients who were investigated for evaluating high levels of aspartate aminotransferase (AST) and alanine aminotransferase (ALT) (above 40 units per liter). From among the patients visiting Velayat Hospital, Qazvin Province, 105 NAFLD patients who had a positive urea breath test were selected randomly. Then, the participants were divided into two groups of intervention and comparison with a one-to-one ratio using a computer block method. This study was approved by the Ethics Committee of Qazvin University of Medical Sciences, and the participation of individuals was subject to a written consent.

The inclusion criteria were the age of above 12 years old, positive results for HP antibodies (in serological tests), and evidence of fatty liver in ultrasonography. It should be noted that the use of any therapeutic strategy for HP and any factors affecting aminotransferase were classified as the exclusion criteria.

The patients in both groups received lifestyle changes as the standard treatment. The lifestyle changes in both groups included moderate to intense exercises such as walking, running, swimming, and cycling for 45–60 min at least 3 days per week in all the patients for 8 weeks. Furthermore, the participants were asked to follow a certain diet. The diet included the reduced starchy, glucose, and oil. A nutritionist who was unaware of the study protocol implemented the treatment and examined the daily calorie intake of people during the study period. In addition to the above treatment, the intervention group underwent a standard treatment of clarithromycin, amoxicillin, and omeprazole for 2 weeks in order to eradicate the HP infection.

All the patients underwent anthropometric tests including height, weight, and body mass index (weight per kg divided by height per m^2). Weight and height were measured in straight and upright postures while wearing light underwear and no shoes. The waist circumference of the participants was measured in cm in the intermediate region of the lower margin of the ribs and anterior superior iliac crest. A radiologist who was unaware of the clinical data of the patients and data allocation performed the liver ultrasound. The fatty liver was diagnosed by echo with a 3.5-MHz probe. All the patients were examined by the physician, and the necessary tests (routine fasting blood biochemistry) such as fasting blood glucose, high-density lipoprotein (HDL) cholesterol, and low-density lipoprotein (LDL) cholesterol were carried out. The blood pressure was measured periodically using a 2-mmHg graded sphygmomanometer after 5 min of resting. The blood samples were taken after 12 h of fasting, and then, the blood tests were run. Fasting blood glucose was measured by glucose oxidase method [17, 18], lipid profiles (total triglyceride and cholesterol), and HDL using immunocolorimetric assay and LDL by Friedewald formula [19]. In order to measure ALT and AST, the enzymatic methods were used [20]. The laboratory researchers were unaware of the intervention or allocation of the comparison group. All of the indicators were compared in the base and post-intervention modes (1 month later).

Statistical analysis

In this research, the descriptive statistics was used to show the central and dispersion indicators, and Kolmogorov-Smirnov test was employed for evaluating the normality of the data distribution. A paired t-test was used to assess the within-group difference in the anthropometric and biochemical variables. Additionally, to investigate the effect of the intervention on biochemical and demographic variables, the independent t-test was used for difference in the scores. All the statistical analyses were performed using SPSS V.23, and a p value of < 0.05 was considered significant.

Results

From 105 patients, 100 patients with the mean age of 37.63 ± 10.33 years old were included. Five patients were excluded due to unwillingness to continue the study. Table 1 shows the baseline characteristics of the participants in both groups. There was no significant difference between the two groups in terms of age, sex, and fatty liver level.

Table 2 shows anthropometric measurements between the treatment groups. Regarding the within-group analysis, both treatment groups were significantly improved in terms of variables such as weight, BMI, and waist circumference ($p < .05$). Between-group analysis regarding the variables of weight, BMI, and waist circumference showed no significant difference between the two groups ($p > .05$).

Table 3 shows the comparison of laboratory parameters between the treatment groups. The within-group analysis showed a significant reduction in the intervention and comparison groups regarding the variables of blood glucose, total cholesterol, triglyceride, HDL, LDL, AST, and ALT ($p < 0.05$). In the intervention group, the between-group statistical analysis on the ALT variable showed a significant reduction ($p < .05$). No significant relationship was observed between the two groups in terms of other variables. In this study, no adverse side-effects occurred following the HP treatment. Moreover, there was no need to reduce or stop the treatment dose.

Discussion

This study was designed to answer the uncertainties regarding the effectiveness of HP treatment in non-alcoholic fatty liver patients. The results showed that the ALT indicator was reduced more in the intervention group (HP treatment) than the comparison group. This indicator is highly important in the liver injury, so it can be argued that the eradication of HP has a significant effect on the improvement of patient's fatty liver. These results were consistent with Polyzos et al.'s findings. In a research, they showed that treatment of HP infection was effective in the improvement of fatty liver [21]. In contrast to the present study, Jamali et al. in Tehran [14] and Okushin et al. in Japan showed that the eradication of HP had no positive effect on the fatty liver of the patients [22]. Probably, one of the most important factors involved in different results is the eradication method of HP, duration of dietary intervention, nature of exercise, intensity and volume of aerobic exercise, and individual differences. In the present study, contrary to Jamali et al. [14], the diet therapy was considered for 8 weeks. Afterwards, in the intervention group, the eradication of HP was performed for 2 weeks. This strategy could have led to different results. Studies on this topic have shown that significant changes in serum aminotransferase level of the patients with NASH followed by diet therapy require interventions for more than 8 weeks [23]; this could be a reasonable justification for differences between studies.

Results of the present study demonstrated a significant decrease in body weight index, waist circumference, and BMI in two groups, while no significant difference was found between two groups of intervention and comparison with regard to these indicators. One of the reasons for the improvement of these indicators in both groups could be the calorie intake restriction or aerobic exercises. Studies on this field have shown that the most prevalent treatment for obesity and fatty liver is daily calorie restriction. Since weight loss through daily calorie restriction is often limited and reversible, in addition to calorie intervention, exercise was also given to two therapy groups. Slancy et al. said that aerobic exercises can lead to reduced abdominal and visceral fat [24], so it is thought that simultaneous exercise and diet can be effective in weight loss in both groups.

In the present study, a significant decrease was seen in the variables of triglyceride, total cholesterol, LDL, and HDL in both groups, while no significant difference was observed between the two groups. These findings were consistent with the study by Park et al., who showed exercise could lead to a significant change in all lipid indicators [25].

Since no significant difference was seen between the intervention and comparison groups, it can be argued that exercise leads to significant changes in lipid indicators in both groups.

A significant improvement was found in the blood glucose index in both groups, whereas the difference between the two groups was not considerable. Sigal et al. also showed that exercise programs can considerably reduce blood glucose [26].

Table 1 Baseline characteristics of participants in two treatment groups

Variable	Intervention group	Comparison group	*p* value
Age (year)	36.88 ± 11.50	38.38 ± 9.06	0.47
Sex			
Male	23 (46%)	21 (42%)	0.68
Female	27 (54%)	29 (58%)	
Fatty liver level			
Grade 1	25 (50%)	29 (58%)	0.72
Grade 2	20 (40%)	17 (34%)	
Grade 3	4 (8%)	5 (10%)	

Table 2 Comparison of anthropometric measurements between treatment groups during the study

Variable	Pre-test	Post-test	*p* value	Within-group *p* value
Weight (kg)				
Intervention group	86.44 ± 10.78	82.52 ± 11.51	0.24	$p < .001$
Comparison group	83.04 ± 9.65	79.66 ± 10.17		$p < .001$
p value	0.1	0.19		... ...
BMI (kg/m^2)				
Intervention group	27.46 ± 4.79	26.40 ± 4.04	0.52	$p = .012$
Comparison group	26.32 ± 3.51	25.58 ± 2.82		$p = .013$
p value	0.17	0.243		... ...
Waist circumference (cm)				
Intervention group	102.50 ± 6.27	100.2 ± 5.67	0.96	$p < .001$
Comparison group	100.32 ± 8.22	98.04 ± 9.40		$p < .001$
p value	0.14	0.17		... ...

One of the limitations of this study was that liver biopsy was not applied to determine histological response. In this study, the diagnosis of non-alcoholic fatty liver was based on ultrasonography, while the liver biopsy is the standard golden method for the diagnosis of non-fatty liver.

Conclusions

Findings of this study showed that the eradication of HP could considerably improve the ALT index. In the case of changes in the metabolic indicators, the HP had no additional effect. Since the lifestyle modification was applied in two groups, achieving an ideal

Table 3 Comparison of laboratory parameters between treatment groups during the study

Variable	Group	Pre-test	Post-test	*p* value	Within-group *p* value
Blood glucose (mg/dl)	Intervention group	112.56 ± 8.31	109.54 ± 8.69	0.23	$p = .005$
	Comparison group	112.9 ± 8.65	107.70 ± 10.81		$p = .001$
	Between-group *p* value	0.84	0.35		
Total cholesterol (mg/dl)	Intervention group	209.48 ± 14.42	180.68 ± 14.51	0.71	$p < .001$
	Comparison group	206.28 ± 6.61	180.12 ± 7.50		$p < .001$
	Between-group *p* value	0.157	0.809		
Triglyceride (mg/dl)	Intervention group	148.22 ± 18.52	110.06 ± 19.35	0.73	$p < .001$
	Comparison group	145.98 ± 19.88	106 ± 13.96		$p < .001$
	Between-group *p* value	0.56	0.23		
HDL (mg/dl)	Intervention group	46.46 ± 4.01	48.98 ± 4.32	0.48	$p < .001$
	Comparison group	46.50 ± 6.90	49.58 ± 6.63		$p < .001$
	Between-group *p* value	0.97	0.59		
LDL (mg/dl)	Intervention group	133.94 ± 4.85	111.42 ± 6.37	0.1	$p < .001$
	Comparison group	132.52 ± 3.44	111.26 ± 10.67		$p < .001$
	Between-group *p* value	0.09	0.92		
AST (mg/dl)	Intervention group	44.14 ± 16.67	37.72 ± 8.45	0.06	$p = .026$
	Comparison group	43.52 ± 11.52	41.06 ± 8.42		$p = .036$
	Between-group *p* value	0.83	0.051		
ALT (mg/dl)	Intervention group	64.02 ± 22.26	48.12 ± 11.52	0.012	$p < .001$
	Comparison group	59.60 ± 19.07	53.52 ± 14.02		$p < .001$
	Between-group *p* value	0.28	0.038		

LDL low-density lipoprotein, *HDL* high-density lipoproteins, *ALT* alanine aminotransferase, *AST* aspartate aminotransferase

body weight could result in the sustained biochemical improvement. Given the limitations expressed in the diagnosis of the disease, for future studies, it is recommended to use biopsy and magnetic resonance elastography (MRE) to diagnose and MRE to follow up.

Abbreviations

ALT: Alanine aminotransferase; AST: Aspartate aminotransferase; HDL: High-density lipoprotein; HP: Helicobacter pylori; LDL: Low-density lipoprotein; NAFL: Non-alcoholic fatty liver; NAFLD: Non-alcoholic fatty liver disease; NASH: Non-alcoholic steatohepatitis

Acknowledgements

The researchers would like to acknowledge and appreciate the contributions of all clinical residents of the Qazvin University of Medical Sciences who helped in conducting the present study.

Authors' contributions

All authors read and approved the final manuscript. AK did the design, data gathering, and manuscript preparation. AS did the data gathering, analysis, and manuscript preparation. EH did the data gathering and manuscript preparation. ZA did the data gathering and manuscript preparation. AH did the design, data gathering, analysis, and manuscript preparation.

Competing interests

The authors declare that they have no competing interests.

Author details

[1]Clinical Toxicology, Metabolic Diseases Research Center, Qazvin University of Medical Sciences, Qazvin, Iran. [2]Department of Occupational Health Engineering, Shahid Beheshti University of Medical Sciences, Tehran, Iran. [3]Department of Internal Medicine, Metabolic Disease Research Center, Qazvin University of Medical Sciences, Qazvin, Iran. [4]Gastroenterologist Metabolic Diseases Research Center, Qazvin University of Medical Sciences, Qazvin, Iran.

References

1. Benedict M, Zhang X (2017) Non-alcoholic fatty liver disease: an expanded review. World J Hepatol 9(16):715
2. Neuschwander-Tetri BA (2017) Non-alcoholic fatty liver disease. BMC Med 15(1):45
3. Engin AB, Engin A (2017) Obesity and lipotoxicity: Springer
4. Cai O, Huang Z, Li M, Zhang C, Xi F, Tan S (2018) Association between Helicobacter pylori infection and nonalcoholic fatty liver disease: a single-center clinical study. Gastroenterol Res Pract 2018:8040262 Pubmed Central PMCID: PMC5828541. Epub 2018/03/13. eng
5. Kang S, Kim D (2016) PTH-112 association between Helicobacter pylori infection and nonalcoholic fatty liver disease in the United States. BMJ Publishing Group 65: A273–A274
6. Malfertheiner P, Megraud F, O'Morain CA, Gisbert JP, Kuipers EJ, Axon AT et al (2017) Management of Helicobacter pylori infection-the Maastricht V/Florence consensus report. Gut 66(1):6–30 PubMed PMID: 27707777. Epub 2016/11/02. eng
7. Burucoa C, Axon A (2017) Epidemiology of Helicobacter pylori infection. Helicobacter 22(Suppl 1):e12403 PubMed PMID: 28891138. Epub 2017/09/12. eng
8. Eusebi LH, Zagari RM, Bazzoli F (2014) Epidemiology of Helicobacter pylori infection. Helicobacter 19(Suppl 1):1–5 PubMed PMID: 25167938. Epub 2014/08/30. eng
9. Leja M, Axon A, Brenner H (2016) Epidemiology of Helicobacter pylori infection. Helicobacter 21(Suppl 1):3–7 PubMed PMID: 27531531. Epub 2016/08/18. eng
10. Franceschi F, Gasbarrini A, Polyzos SA, Kountouras J (2015) Extragastric diseases and Helicobacter pylori. Helicobacter 20(Suppl 1):40–46 PubMed PMID: 26372824. Epub 2015/09/16. eng
11. Nasif WA, Mukhtar MH, Nour Eldein MM, Ashgar SS (2016) Oxidative DNA damage and oxidized low density lipoprotein in Type II diabetes mellitus among patients with Helicobacter pylori infection. Diabetol Metab Syndr 8: 34 PubMed PMID: 27148410. eng
12. Taylor NS, Fox JG, Yan L (1995) In-vitro hepatotoxic factor in Helicobacter hepaticus, H. pylori and other Helicobacter species. J Med Microbiol 42(1): 48–52 PubMed PMID: 7739025. Epub 1995/01/01. eng
13. Takuma Y (2011) Helicobacter pylori infection and liver diseases. Gan To Kagaku Ryoho 38(3):362–364 PubMed PMID: 21403438. Epub 2011/03/16. jpn
14. Jamali R, Mofid A, Vahedi H, Farzaneh R, Dowlatshahi S (2013) The effect of helicobacter pylori eradication on liver fat content in subjects with non-alcoholic Fatty liver disease: a randomized open-label clinical trial. Hepat Mon 13(12):e14679 PubMed PMID: 24358044. eng
15. Hashemi MR, Rahnavardi M, Bikdeli B, Dehghani ZM (2006) H pylori infection among 1000 southern Iranian dyspeptic patients. World J Gastroenterol 12(34):5479–5482 PubMed PMID: 17006984. Epub 09/14. eng
16. Lankarani KB, Ghaffarpasand F, Mahmoodi M, Lotfi M, Zamiri N, Heydari ST et al (2013) Non alcoholic fatty liver disease in southern Iran: a population based study. Hepat Mon 13(5):e9248 PubMed PMID: 23922564. eng
17. Ambade VN, Sharma YV, Somani BL (1998) Methods for estimation of blood glucose : a comparative evaluation. Med J Armed Forces India 54(2):131 PubMed PMID: 28775446. Pubmed Central PMCID: PMC5531325. Epub 1998/04/01. eng
18. Jia KK, Zhang J (2010) Evaluation of five routine glucose methods on an Olympus AU5400 analyzer using the CDC hexokinase reference method. Clin Chem Lab Med 48(3):361–364 PubMed PMID: 20170396. Epub 2010/02/23. eng
19. Knopfholz J, Disserol CC, Pierin AJ, Schirr FL, Streisky L, Takito LL et al (2014) Validation of the friedewald formula in patients with metabolic syndrome. Cholesterol 2014:261878 PubMed PMID: 24672715. Pubmed Central PMCID: PMC3941209. Epub 2014/03/29. eng
20. Jamali R, Khonsari M, Merat S, Khoshnia M, Jafari E, Bahram Kalhori A et al (2008) Persistent alanine aminotransferase elevation among the general Iranian population: prevalence and causes. World J Gastroenterol 14(18):2867–2871 PubMed PMID: 18473412. Pubmed Central PMCID: PMC2710729. Epub 2008/05/14. eng
21. Polyzos SA, Nikolopoulos P, Stogianni A, Romiopoulos I, Katsinelos P, Kountouras J (2014) Effect of Helicobacter pylori eradication on hepatic steatosis, NAFLD fibrosis score and HSENSI in patients with nonalcoholic steatohepatitis: a MR imaging-based pilot open-label study. Arq Gastroenterol 51(3):261–268 PubMed PMID: 25296089. Epub 2014/10/09. eng
22. Okushin K, Takahashi Y, Yamamichi N, Shimamoto T, Enooku K, Fujinaga H et al (2015) Helicobacter pylori infection is not associated with fatty liver disease including non-alcoholic fatty liver disease: a large-scale cross-sectional study in Japan. BMC Gastroenterol 15:25 PubMed PMID: 25880912. Pubmed Central PMCID: PMC4349671. Epub 2015/04/17. eng
23. Della Pepa G, Vetrani C, Lombardi G, Bozzetto L, Annuzzi G, Rivellese AA (2017) Isocaloric dietary changes and non-alcoholic fatty liver disease in high cardiometabolic risk individuals. Nutrients 9(10):1065
24. Slentz CA, Bateman LA, Willis LH, Shields AT, Tanner CJ, Piner LW et al (2011) Effects of aerobic vs. resistance training on visceral and liver fat stores, liver enzymes, and insulin resistance by HOMA in overweight adults from STRRIDE AT/RT. Am J Physiol Endocrinol Metab 301(5):E1033–E1039 PubMed PMID: 21846904. Pubmed Central PMCID: PMC3214001. Epub 2011/08/19. eng
25. Park SK, Park JH, Kwon YC, Kim HS, Yoon MS, Park HT (2003) The effect of combined aerobic and resistance exercise training on abdominal fat in obese middle-aged women. J Physiol Anthropol Appl Hum Sci 22(3):129–135 PubMed PMID: 12808225. Epub 2003/06/17. eng
26. Sigal RJ, Kenny GP, Boule NG, Wells GA, Prud'homme D, Fortier M et al (2007) Effects of aerobic training, resistance training, or both on glycemic control in type 2 diabetes: a randomized trial. Ann Intern Med 147(6):357–369 PubMed PMID: 17876019. Epub 2007/09/19. eng

2

Hepatic sclerosing hemangioma mimics hepatic malignancies: a case report and multidisciplinary approach

Dina M. Sweed[1*], Zeinab A. Fayed[1], Enas M. Sweed[2], Ahmed El-Sherif[3] and Mohamed Mohamady[1]

Abstract

Background: Hepatic sclerosing hemangiomas (HSH) are rare benign vascular tumors that mimic radiologically hepatic malignancies. HSH is characterized by extensive fibrosis and hyalinosis as a result of degeneration and thrombosis. Pre-operative diagnosis is very difficult and most of the cases undergo surgical resections.

Case presentation: A 65 years old, hepatitis C virus-infected female presented by an accidentally discovered hepatic focal lesion. Magnetic resonance imaging (MRI) showed a T2 hyperintense mass displaying peripheral enhancement in porto-venous phase. The patient had a simultaneous typical hepatic hemangioma and multiple vertebral bodies' hemangiomata. Tissue-guided biopsy revealed a densely sclerotic stroma containing vascular spaces with occasional obliteration of the lumen. Immunohistochemical staining was performed for Pan CK, CD34, SMA, VEGF, and c-Kit which confirmed the vascular nature of neoplasm and the involuting phase of hemangioma development. The patient was reassured and recommended for a regular radiological follow-up to reassess the lesion size.

Conclusion: The definitive preoperative diagnosis of HSH is still problematic. However, the awareness of surgeons by this entity, peripheral enhancement in porto-venous phase on dynamic MRI, the presence of simultaneous typical hepatic hemangioma in the absence of cancer history could raise suspicion for HSH. Liver biopsy is still the gold standard in approaching the accurate diagnosis.

Keywords: Biopsy, Hemangioma, MRI, Sclerosing

Background

Hepatic hemangioma is the most common benign tumor occurring in the liver. Hemangioma is a vascular tumor that passes through three stages of development: angiogenesis, regression, and involution [1]. The diagnosis is generally secured on radiologic examination with magnetic resonance imaging (MRI) is the most sensitive and specific imaging tool [2]. However, the sclerosing variant of hepatic hemangioma is extremely rare and mimics radiologically hepatic malignancies which necessitate surgical intervention [3, 4]. Here, we report a case of hepatic sclerosing hemangioma (HSH) that simulates liver metastasis radiologically and give a short brief on the pathogenesis of this rare variant.

* Correspondence: dr.dinasweed@yahoo.com
[1]Pathology Department, National Liver Institute, Menoufia University, Al Menoufia, Egypt

Case presentation

A 65-year-old female presented to a medical physician when hepatic focal lesion during routine examination for hepatitis C virus (HCV) infection was accidentally discovered. The patient was diabetic, hypertensive, and obese. There was no past or present history of cancer. She was HCV positive. Serum alpha-fetoprotein (AFP) level was 6.1 IU/mL, CA19–9 42.6 U/L, and CEA 2.7 ng/mL. Laboratory investigations were normal apart of slight anemia (hemoglobin 12 g/dL). Clinical and radiological findings established the primary hepatic origin of the lesion with no extrahepatic masses. Imaging showed a left hepatic lobe segment II focal lesion measured 3.5 × 3 cm surrounded by focal intrahepatic biliary radicles dilatation (IHBRD) on a background of non-cirrhotic liver. The mass showed a rather well defined hyperintense in axial fat suppression T2 with peripheral enhancement in porto-venous phase and hypointense with filling defect in the hepatocyte (late) phase of dynamic MRI. A simultaneous left hepatic lobe segment IVb focal lesion measuring 1.5 cm showed a rather well defined hyperintense with discontinuous peripheral nodular enhancement in arterial phase with central fill in in the delayed phase (Fig. 1). Osseous vertebral bodies' hemangiomata were accidentally discovered. The radiological features were in favor of hepatic metastasis or intrahepatic cholangiocarcinoma (IHCC). However, the rare possibility of HSH could not be ruled out for liver-guided biopsy.

Histopathological examination showed thin-walled vascular spaces lined by bland-looking endothelial cells within a hypocellular stroma demonstrating varying degrees of fibrosis and sclerosis. Some blood vessels were obliterated. Focal area of the classic cavernous hemangioma was evident. The dense sclerotic stroma was demarcated by masson trichrome (MT) stain. The adjacent liver tissue showed features of chronic hepatitis consistent with HCV infection. Immunohistochemical studies (IHC) for CD34 confirmed the vascular nature of neoplastic cells. The negative staining for cytokeratin (CK) marker ruled out the rare possibility of biliary hamartoma. In an attempt to define the phase of development of hemangioma, a panel of IHC stain was performed. Vascular spaces showed immunopositivity for smooth muscle actin (SMA) and negativity for vascular endothelial growth factor (VEGF). Additionally, c-Kit IHC highlighted degenerated mast cells granules (Fig. 2). The patient was reassured and discharged on a regular radiological follow up to re-evaluate the mass size.

Discussion

Hepatic sclerosing/sclerosed hemangioma (HSH) is a rare benign vascular tumor showing degenerative changes, fibrosis, and sclerosis as a result of thrombosis of the blood vessels [5]. It was first described by Shepherd and Lee as a possible cause of solitary necrotic hepatic nodules [6]. Berry reported another two cases of accidentally discovered HSH in a study of 1000 autopsy specimens [7]. In 1994, the objective basis for the development of HSH was postulated, and the lesion was recognized as a mimicker of hepatic malignancy [1]. Yugawa et al. reported the characterization of 41 cases of HSH [8]. However, after a thorough search for the terms of sclerosing, sclerosed, or hyalinized, we recognized 77 cases in the literatures including the present case. The clinico-radiological and histopathological features were summarized in Table 1. The median age was in sixth or seventh decades with female predominance. Nine cases raised on top of chronic liver disease; HBV or HCV, non-alcoholic fatty liver disease (NAFLD), or mixed HBV and alcoholic liver disease. In addition, seven cases had metabolic syndrome; diabetes mellitus, obesity, or hyperlipidemia. The present case was female, diabetic, and obese accidentally discovered HCV infection. The majority

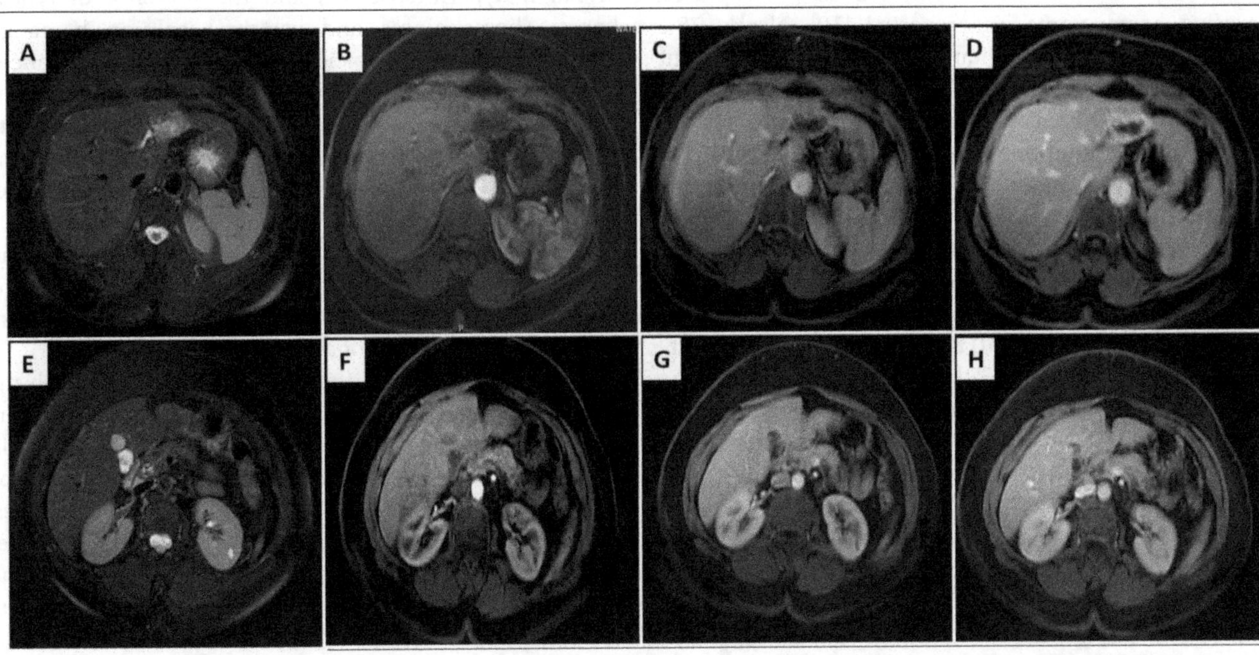

Fig. 1 **a** Axial fat suppression T2 showed a rather well-defined hyperintense left hepatic lobe segment II focal lesion surrounded by focal intrahepatic biliary radicles dilatation on background of non-cirrhotic liver. **b** Inconscipous enhacenemt in arterial phase **c** Mild ring enhancement in porto-venous and **d** Obvious ring enhacement in delayed phase of dynamic MRI. **e** Axial T2 fat suppression of the typical hemangioma showwd a rather well-defined bright left hepatic lobe segment IVb focal lesion, **f** Discontinuous peripheral nodular enhancement in arterial phase, **g** Centripetal fillin in porto-venous and **h** Closed iris sign in delayed equilibrium phase

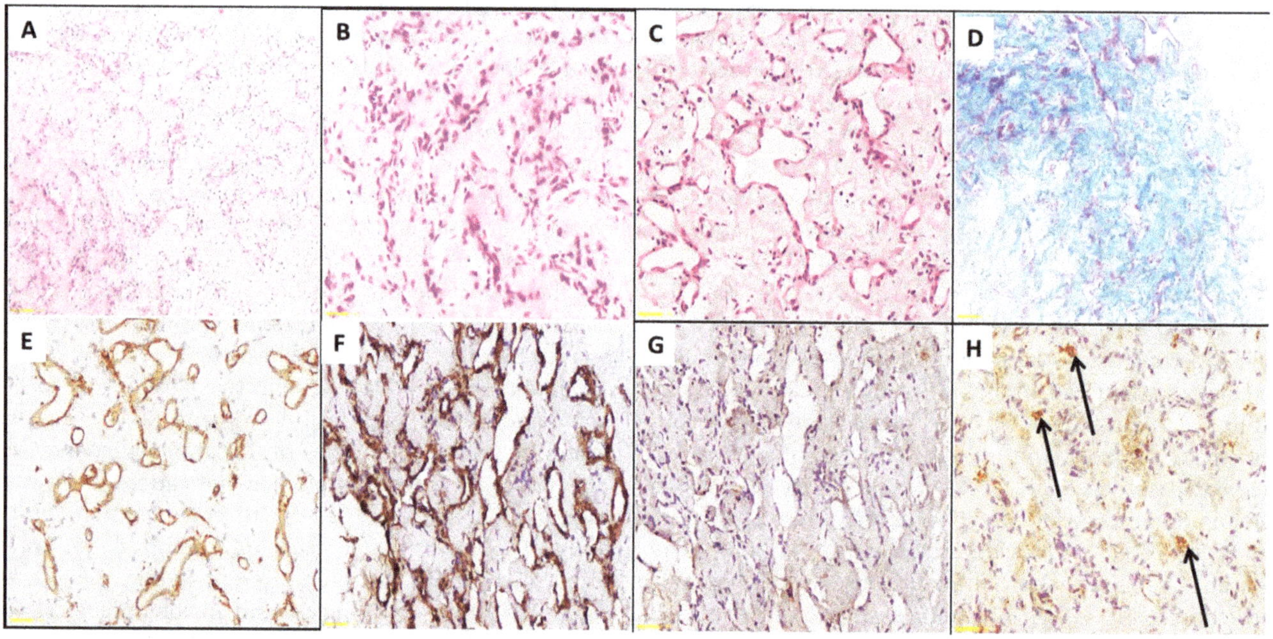

Fig. 2 **a** A case of HSH showed proliferated, focally obliterated blood vessels surrounded by dense sclerotic stroma (H&E 100×). **b** Higher power view (H&E 200×). **c** Area of cavernous hemangioma (H&E 200×). **d** Dense sclerotic stroma (MT 100×). **e** Vascular spaces were positive for CD34 (IHC 200×). **f** Smooth muscle proliferation was positive for SMA (IHC 200×). **g** Endothelial cells and fibroblasts were negative for VEGF (IHC 200×). **h** Degenerated masts cells were positive for C-Kit (IHC 200×)

of HSH was discovered during abdominal imaging or for abdominal pain [9]. However, only one case of ruptured sclerosing hemangioma was reported [10]. Nearly 78% and 60% of cases were solitary and located in the right lobe of the liver, respectively.

Typical hepatic hemangioma has a diagnostic peripheral nodular discontinuous enhancement following a blood pool on computed tomography (CT) with the MRI has the highest sensitivity and specificity [2]. However, the preoperative radiological diagnosis of HSH is very difficult and mimics hepatic malignancies; 23 cases, 9 cases, and 7 cases were misdiagnosed as metastasis, hepatocellular carcinoma (HCC), and IHCC, respectively. In the present case, the liver was non-cirrhotic with the lesion did not follow the typical pathological enhancement pattern of HCC, homogenous arterial enhancement, washout of contrast in porto-venous, and hypointense in hepatocyte phase of dynamic MRI study. The presence of focal IHBRD was in favor of IHCC but the absence of delayed enhancement made this diagnosis unlikely. Additionally, IHBRD may occur as a consequence of all intra- or extra-hepatic lesions with mass effect especially around segment IV [11]. The obvious peripheral enhancement of the lesion in the porto-venous phase favored metastatic process that should be considered at the top of differential diagnosis. However, the patient had no past or present history of any cancer. The awareness of radiologist for the radiological features of HSH, hyperintense T2, and the presence of typical hepatic hemangioma and vertebral column hemangiomata raised the suspicious of HSH. With advanced radiological imaging, Miyata et al. postulated that apparent diffusion coefficient (ADC) mean to differentiate HSH from other liver malignancies as, in particular, the higher ADC mean value of using diffusion-weighted sequences (DW-MRI). They reported the ADC mean value of HSH was $1.94 \times 10{-}3$ mm2/s, which was higher than the value of common malignant liver tumors [4]. In the present case, liver biopsy and pathological review were advised to elucidate the nature of the lesion.

Tissue pathology was the standard tool to establish the diagnosis. Tissue was obtained at autopsy in 5 cases, surgical resection specimen in 37 cases and liver biopsy in 13 cases. Only two cases were proofed radiological to be HSH on regular follow up [12, 13]. In the present cases, liver core biopsy was obtained and assessed by two independent liver pathologists. In routine hematoxylin and eosin stain, dense acellular fibrous tissue with few dispersed blood vessels lined by flattened endothelial cells was evident. There was no evidence of cytological atypia, mitosis, or necrosis. Perivascular smooth muscle proliferation was occasionally seen. MT stain established dense fibrous stroma. IHC staining was not essential except in the area of dense sclerosis to rule out the rare

Table 1 Review of literature for hepatic sclerosing hemangioma (HSH) cases

Variables	No (%)
Median age	65.5 years
Gender (M:F ratio)	31/45
Site	
Right	36 (60%)
Left	19 (31.7%)
Both lobes	5 (8.3%)
Focality	
Solitary	40 (78.4%)
Multiple	11 (21.6%)
Size	48.2 ± 45 mm
CT findings	
Ring enhancement	39 (73.6%)
No enhancement	6 (11.3%)
Heterogeneous or intralesional enhancement	5 (9.4%)
Peripheral nodular enhancement	3 (5.7%)
MRI (T1/T2)	
Low/high	40 (93.2%)
High/high	2 (4.5%)
Low/low	1 (2.3%)
Diagnostic confirmation	
Surgery	37 (64.9%)
Biopsy	13 (22.8%)
Autopsy	5 (8.8%)
Radiology	2 (3.5%)

M:F male:female, *CT* computed tomography, *MRI* magnetic resonance imaging

possibility of biliary lesion. The neoplastic cells were positive for CD34 and negative for CK7 confirm the vascular nature of neoplasm.

There is no consensus, however, as to the state of involution of hemangiomas. Several theories have been proposed. Takahashi et al. reported the role of VEGF in promoting angiogenesis and endothelial proliferation in the proliferating phase [1]. On the contrary, SMA was expressed in the pericytes and functioned through inhibition of endothelial cell proliferation in the involuting and involuted phases. Makhlouf and Ishak found high immunopositivity for CD34 and SMA in sclerosing rather than sclerosed hemangioma and the role of mast cells in the induction of angiogenesis, regression, and fibrogenesis [14]. In addition, Choi et al. reported a case of sclerosing hemangioma with predominant pericapillary smooth muscle proliferation [15]. Therefore, we performed a panel of IHC to estimate the possible phase of hemangioma. The endothelial cells were negative for VEGF indicating the arrested phase of proliferation. SMA highlighted perivascular smooth muscle proliferation and c-Kit was positive in the degenerated mast cells. These findings were inconsistent with the sclerosing phase of hemangioma.

Conclusion

Despite HSH are benign tumors that remain stable or even regressed over time, resection is necessary for large size lesions. The awareness of the imaging characteristics of HSH can alter patient management. Preoperative tissue biopsy or intraoperative frozen section should be considered to avoid unnecessary extended hepatic resection. However, if tumor malignancy cannot be ruled out or if the biopsy is hemorrhagic, hepatic resection should remain the choice for diagnostic surgery at present.

Abbreviations

ADC: Apparent diffusion coefficient; AFP: Alpha foetoprotein; CD34: Cluster of differentiation 34; CK: Cytokeratin; CT: Computed tomography; DW: Diffusion-weighted; HBV: Hepatitis B virus; HCC: Hepatocellular carcinoma; HCV: Hepatitis C virus; HSH: Hepatic sclerosing hemangioma; IHBRD: Intrahepatic biliary radicles dilatation; IHC: Immunohistochemical studies; IHCC: Intrahepatic cholangiocarcinoma; MRI: Magnetic resonance imaging; MT: Masson trichrome; NAFLD: Non-alcoholic fatty liver disease; SMA: Smooth muscle actin; VEGF: Vascular endothelial growth factor

Acknowledgements

Not applicable.

Authors' contributions

All authors of this paper have participated in its drafting and approved the final version submitted. DS, ZF, and ES wrote the case report. DS and ZF contributed to the pathological diagnosis. ES offered assistance for radiological diagnosis. MM performed technical immunohistochemical work. AS acquired and interpreted the clinical data. DS revised and edited the final version. All authors read and approved the final manuscript.

Competing interests

The authors declare that they have no competing interests.

Author details

[1]Pathology Department, National Liver Institute, Menoufia University, Al Menoufia, Egypt. [2]Radiology Department, Faculty of Medicine, Benha University, Benha, Egypt. [3]Hepato-pancreatobiliary Surgery and Liver Transplantation, National Liver Institute, Menoufia University, Al Menoufia, Egypt.

References

1. Takahashi K, Mulliken JB, Kozakewich HP, Rogers RA, Folkman J, Ezekowitz RA (1994) Cellular markers that distinguish the phases of hemangioma during infancy and childhood. J Clin Invest 93(6):2357–2364
2. Taseva A, Tasev V, Bulanov D, Dimitrov K, Popov V, Zivkov E et al (2013) Diagnosis of liver hemangioma. Khirurgiia (Sofiia) (3):8–13
3. Sugo H, Sekine Y, Miyano S, Watanobe I, Machida M, Kojima K et al (2018) Hepatic sclerosing hemangioma with predominance of the sclerosed area mimicking a biliary cystadenocarcinoma. Case Reports Hepatol 2018:6
4. Miyata T, Beppu T, Kuramoto K, Nakagawa S, Imai K, Hashimoto D et al (2018) Hepatic sclerosed hemangioma with special attention to diffusion-weighted magnetic resonance imaging. Surg Case Rep 4(1):3
5. Song JS, Kim YN, Moon WS (2013) A sclerosing hemangioma of the liver. Clin Mol Hepatol 19(4):426–430

6. Shepherd NA, Lee G (1983) Solitary necrotic nodules of the liver simulating hepatic metastases. J Clin Pathol 36(10):1181–1183
7. Berry CL (1985) Solitary "necrotic nodule" of the liver: a probable pathogenesis. J Clin Pathol 38:1278–1280
8. Yugawa K, Yoshizumi T, Harada N, Motomura T, Harimoto N, Itoh S et al (2018) Multiple hepatic sclerosing hemangiomas: a case report and review of the literature. Surg Case Rep 4(1):60
9. Caseiro-Alves F, Brito J, Araujo AE, Belo-Soares P, Rodrigues H, Cipriano A et al (2007 Jun) Liver haemangioma: common and uncommon findings and how to improve the differential diagnosis. Eur Radiol 17(6):1544–1554
10. Papafragkakis H, Moehlen M, Garcia-Buitrago MT, Madrazo B, Island E, Martin P (2011) A case of a ruptured sclerosing liver hemangioma. Int J Hepatol 2011:942360
11. Yang DM, Kim HS, Cho SW (2002) Pictorial review: various causes of hepatic capsular retraction: CT and MR findings. Br J Radiol 75(900):994–1002
12. Shin YM (2011) Sclerosing hemangioma in the liver. Korean J Hepatol 17(3): 242–246
13. Nunes LMAO, CDd M-A, Yamauchi FI, Baroni RH (2018) Atypical hepatic hemangioma: imaging features of hyalinized hemangioma. Einstein (Sao Paulo, Brazil) 16(2):eAI4256–eAI4eAI
14. Makhlouf HR, Ishak KG (2002) Sclerosed hemangioma and sclerosing cavernous hemangioma of the liver: a comparative clinicopathologic and immunohistochemical study with emphasis on the role of mast cells in their histogenesis. Liver 22(1):70–78
15. Choi YJ, Kim KW, Cha EY, Song JS, Yu E, Lee MG (2008) Case report. Sclerosing liver haemangioma with pericapillary smooth muscle proliferation: atypical CT and MR findings with pathological correlation. Br J Radiol 81(966):e162–e165

3

Antiproliferative effects on tumor cells of the synthesized gold nanoparticles against Hep2 liver cancer cell line

Kamala Priya M R and Priya R. Iyer*

Abstract

Background: Currently, nanomaterials (NMs) research and development is at a fastest pace due to the enhanced implication in different areas of applications. The synthesis of such NMs through biosynthesis methods is gaining much importance because of low cost involved and environment-friendly approach. In this present study, the nanoparticles (NPs) are synthesized using a medicinal plant, with anticancer properties so as to incorporate the therapeutic activity within the NPs, such that the NPs will have the attributes of NMs alongside the phytoactivity.

Results: The synthesis of gold nanoparticles (AuNPs) using Graviola, the fruit of *Annona muricata* (Ramaphal fruit) commonly referred as Mullu seetha fruit (Tamil), was successfully carried out. The initial confirmations of the NPs were using UV-vis spectra, which showed the characteristic peak for the NPs. HRSEM analysis gave an insight on the size and morphology of the NPs. The zeta potential was measured to check the stability of the NPs. The cytotoxicity was carried out in VERO cell line and anticancer study in Hep2 liver cancer cell line. The surface plasmon resonance (SPR) band showed the characteristic peak at 536 nm for the AuNPs. In SEM micrographs, the size was ranging between 20 and 30 nm, on an average of 15 nm with spherical morphology. On the various tested concentrations in VERO cell line, the nanoparticles were non-toxic to the cells. The anticancer study gave an IC50 value at 10.94 μg/ml.

Conclusions: The NPs showed anticancer activity in treated Hep2 liver cancer cell line and as well as commendable non-toxic effect on normal VERO cell line. The results pose a positive impact to expand further studies in the development of potential drug molecules to tackle the disease of interest.

Keywords: Nanoparticles, HRSEM, Zeta potential, Cytotoxicity, Anticancer, Hep2 liver cancer cell line

Background

Cancer—a major global public health issue

Alarmingly 8.8million people are dying each year of cancer, accounting to one out of six deaths and more than the number of deaths from HIV/AIDS, malaria, and tuberculosis combined. Particularly, in low-income and middle-income countries (LMICs), the disease management remains strenuous and the burden is greatest, where almost 75% of cancer deaths occur and the number of cancer cases is increasing steadily. It is estimated that cancer incidence will double by the year 2035 [1].

On an estimate, around 50% to 60% of patients will require radiotherapy at some time during their treatment; the International Atomic Energy Agency (IAEA) reported that in developing countries due to a shortage of 5000 machines, nearly 70% of cancer patients could not benefit from curative or palliative radiotherapy (International Atomic Energy Agency 2016). The IAEA are currently focusing to introduce radiotherapy to many of these countries. Moreover, it could be seen that investing in radiotherapy will save lives as well as have positive impact over economic benefits [2].

Liver cancer—global context

Liver cancer is the seventh most frequently occurring cancer in the world and the fourth most common cause of cancer mortality [3]. Its incidence rates have been

* Correspondence: brajuraj@yahoo.com
Post Graduate and Research Department of Biotechnology, Women's Christian College, College Road, Chennai 600006, India

gradually rising in many countries. The highest incidence rates of liver cancer in the world happen to be in Asia and Africa. A majority of cause lies within the chronic infections with hepatitis B virus (HBV) and hepatitis C virus (HCV) for almost three-quarters (73.4%) of hepatic cellular carcinoma in the world [4].

Barriers in current cancer therapy

Current cancer therapy involves three major approaches such as surgical oncology, chemotherapy, and radiotherapy [5]. The major obstacles in the current anticancer agents are the development of drug resistance [6]. Multidrug resistance (MDR) is the simultaneous resistance to a number of structurally and functionally unrelated chemotherapeutic drugs. During cancer treatment, many cancers initially respond well to chemotherapy but subsequently lead to acquired resistance such that more than 90% of patients with metastatic cancer either fail to respond or relapse from chemotherapeutics. To address all these issues, various efforts have been invested to elucidate both on inherent and acquired MDR mechanisms [7].

Inorganic compounds in cancer therapy

Selenite is one of the most studied inorganic compounds because of its outstanding chemopreventive and anticancer features. It effectively inhibits cell proliferation of various types of cancer cells. Of different human cancer cell lines tested, lung cancer cells appeared to be more sensitive to selenite. A study reported that selenite cytotoxicity was correlated with Se uptake of three lung cancer cell lines (H157, H611, and U2020) and high concentrations (> 1 mM) of selenate were non-toxic for these cell lines. Se plays a role as natural killer (NK) in cell-based anticancer immunotherapy where it increases the susceptibility of cancer cells to CD94/NK group, and has potential clinical applications in lung cancer patients. The combined effect of selenite and thioredoxin reductase inhibitors was detected in human ovarian and lung cancer cell lines. These results indicated the capacities of Se compounds to enhance the activity and reduce the toxicity of anticancer drugs. Additionally, these compounds appear to be more effective in inhibiting the growth of anticancer drug-resistant cancer cells compared with drug-sensitive cancer cells by means of deactivating various resistance mechanisms adapted by the cancer cells. Chemotherapeutic drug-resistant lung cancer cells were more sensitive to selenite compared to drug-sensitive cancer cells [8].

Microorganisms in cancer treatment

Microbes offer a feasible means of inducing anti-tumor immunity. Oncolytic viruses were among the first successfully used microbes in cancer therapy. An intratumoral injection of herpes virus, T-VEC received approval from the US Food and Drug Administration for metastatic melanoma in 2015. The authors used *Escherichia coli*, which are non-pathogenic, grow extracellularly, and persist for nearly 6 days after intratumoral injection. After the delivery of bacteria into the tumors, several rounds of bacterial lysis continues, a constant, high local concentration of CD47nb. It showed robust tumor-antigen-specific CD8 T cell responses that targeted non-injected tumors with established immunologic memory. These results strongly suggested the induction of adaptive immunity as the major therapeutic mechanism by which CD47 blockade operates in immune competent animals. Successful induction of T cell responses requires the presence of antigen as well as adjuvant to be present at the same time. The quorum-sensing bacteria achieve it through three major strategies. Initially, bacteria provide an abundance of adjuvant and persist at high levels for about a week in tumors. Followed by local delivery and quorum lysis prevent sepsis and leakage of therapeutics cargo into circulation, decreasing systemic exposure of the drug and generation of anti-drug antibodies. And finally, bacteria have a remarkable ability for genetic cargo and can be explored further with more therapeutics in a strand [9].

Cancer nanotechnology

Nanoparticles (NPs) targeted for cancer therapies basically comprise of nanocarrier and the active drug, few NPs formulations of the drug by itself also exist. The nanodrug systems are advantageous with higher metabolic stability, enhanced membrane permeability, improved bioavailability, and prolonged activity. Nano transporters allow specialized targeted drug delivery of the anti-cancer agents to the tissue as well as at the cellular level. The key factors that affect the mucosal or transdermal absorption are size, surface charge, and hydrophobicity. The size of the particles plays a crucial role; smaller NPs are inducing higher transcellular uptake than the larger particles. But NPs larger than 300 nm could not be absorbed by intestinal cells. And only smaller NPs less than 500 nm can penetrate the bloodstream [10].

Nanotechnology in biomedicine

There are an increasing numbers of nanoparticle-based treatments being approved for clinical use which involves mostly spherical liposomes. However, scientists are constantly working on a wider range of NPs designs with different core materials bearing magnetic, optical, and biochemical properties and NPs of varying size, shape, hardness, and surface properties. Adding on to their therapeutic applications, NPs as well enable effective capabilities in imaging [11].

Microbial-mediated synthesis of nanomaterials

The microbial-mediated synthesis of nanomaterials (NMs) has been considered due to the following advantages like synthetized NMs have definitive chemical composition, size, and morphology; biosynthesis is carried out under at mild physicochemical conditions; ease of handling and cultivation of microbial cells; and possibility of tunable NMs with required characteristics by varying key parameters of cell culture set up. One of the greatest challenges faced in microbial nano biosynthesis is the control of dispersity of nanostructure materials, which primarily influence electronic and optical properties. When going for large-scale productions, costs of culture media for microbial growth affects to a greater extent. For instance, currently, bacterial nanocellulose applications are much limited to a few biomedical devices, mainly due to the costs of culture medium [12].

Conventional chemical method of synthesis

The synthesis of gold nanoparticles (AuNPs) was first reported in 1940 upon reacting gold chloride (HAuCl4) and trisodium citrate (Na3C6H5O7 or NaCt) which resulted in the formation of colloidal gold. Further on, the detailed work carried out by Turkevich and his coworkers has become one of the milestones of AuNPs synthesis. From then onwards, the method has been modified and improvised in order to meet the requirements of diverse area such as development of chemical sensors for water quality analysis using surface enhanced Raman spectroscopy (SERS), surface-induced catalytic activities, and drug delivery in biological systems and nano-toxicology studies. There are certain significant features of AuNPs that make them more attractive to employ in wide applications like surface plasmon resonance (SPR), a size- and shape-dependent property, and biocompatibility. Even though of all the distinctive properties of AuNPs, there is a major challenge residing over its usage, which is the control of the particle size and size distribution due to the fact of batch-to-batch variation affected by three factors, local temperature gradient, the efficiency of reagent mixing, and the resulting local concentration gradient [13].

Green synthesis of nanomaterials

Different physical and chemical methods such as solvothermal method, hydrothermal route, pulsed laser ablation technique, sonochemical process, and microwave irradiation has been exploited for the synthesis of NPs [14]. Conventional methods have limitations such as expensiveness, undesirable end products, and hazardous toxic chemicals, involving high temperature and pressure, etc. Whereas green synthesis is an environment-friendly, cost-effective method to synthesize nanostructural material to have tunable structures, morphologies, and particle size distributions. Green synthesis methods employ organisms like plant, bacteria, fungi, etc. for the synthesis of NMs, and it has gained much interest in the rising area of research due to their less toxic or nontoxic nature, eco-friendly nature, and low cost of production. Plant extract are produced from leaves, stems, flower, and seeds of various plants. The extracts are rich in protein, amino acid, enzymes, vitamins, terpenoids, flavonoids, alkaloids, phenolic acids, etc., that act as capping and reducing agents that reduces metal ions during the bioreduction process to produce NPs or nanostructures in varied dimensions and morphologies [15].

Limitations in the application of nanomaterials

Nanotechnology has entered cancer therapy in the recent years. Upon then, many medical products have been approved for clinical use like albumin-bound-paclitaxel, liposomal doxorubicin, and liposomal irinotecan. At the moment, many anti-cancer nanodrugs are into various phases of clinical trials and preclinical research. But the major drawback is the increased cost of nanodrugs, compared with free drugs. Another limitation is the uptake of nanodrugs, which occurs through reticuloendothelial system (RES). Nanodrugs should avoid clearance through uptake by the (RES) which occurs primarily for particle size larger than 100 nm. On the other aspect, localization of nanodrugs in tumor-associated macrophages will definitely increase the concentration of the drug at the tumor sites [10].

AuNP's—as most preferred metallic nanoparticles

Significantly, AuNPs have become versatile candidates used for cancer detection and therapy due to their futuristic physicochemical properties. But still, the use of toxic chemicals in developing AuNPs is of great concern since it may create environmental issues. To combat with this, biological methods of fabricating AuNPs are the much preferred choice. Hence, synthesis of AuNPs using plants, seaweeds, and microbes are advantageous over physical and chemical methods. On this context, the phytocomponents present in the natural source contribute to added bio-compatibility and cytotoxicity by stabilizing the AuNPs. There have been numerous studies stating on the anticancer properties of AuNPs synthesized through biological approach. More studies about the comparative evaluation of AuNPs against cancer and normal cells are needed for further extended research [16].

Toxicity studies of metallic nanomaterials

Though there are several advantages of metallic nanoparticles, there is much concern regarding their safety on biological cells as reported in in-vitro/in-vivo toxicity studies. In higher metallic form/bulk form, gold is inert/

non-toxic, but at the nano dimensions based on the manner in which these NPs are developed using different synthetic procedures and the nature of capping/stabilizing agents may lead to toxicity. Though green synthesized NPs using of various plant extracts containing polysaccharides, biomass, phytochemicals, and synthetic molecules are less toxic, there is a major drawback at the polydispersity, yield, purity, and metabolite formation aspects. There are many inconclusive data in the literature discussing whether AuNPs are toxic or non-toxic. The toxicity of NPs is also influenced by the size, shape, and surface chemistry of NPs. Some NPs have demonstrated size-dependent toxicity, whereas others have shown surface chemistry-dependent toxicity. Therefore, predicting toxicity becomes difficult since similar sizes of NPs results in differential toxicity on the same cell line [17].

Anticancer effects of *Annona muricata's* Fruit—Graviola

Annona muricata is a tropical tree widely distributed in the regions of Africa, South America, and Southeast Asia. It belongs to the family Annonaceae. It is commonly referred as soursop, graviola, and guanabana. The fruit is edible in green heart-shaped and the tree comprises of large, glossy, dark green leaves. It has been reported in the literature that nearly 74 bioactive compounds of the plant exhibit a variety of anticancer effects in in vitro and in vivo animal model systems. *A. muricata*-derived preparations and formulations have been used for the treatment of different disease conditions, thereby proving its prominence in Ethnomedicine [18]. The bark, leaves, and roots of *Annona muricata* have been extensively applied globally in the disease management of various ailments, including inflammatory conditions, rheumatism, diabetes, hypertension, insomnia, cystitis, parasitic infections, and cancer [19].

Traditional medicines—treatment of liver disorders

Herbal and traditional medicines have been used to treat liver disorders for centuries. *A. muricata* is commonly used to treat various liver disorders, particularly jaundice. In a recent study, performed on phenyl hydrazine-induced jaundice in adult rats, treated with *A. muricata* aqueous extract at different doses, found a substantial reduction in elevated bilirubin. It has also been reported to protect against increased serum glutamic-oxaloacetic transaminase (SGOT), serum glutamic-pyruvic transaminase (SGPT), alkaline phosphatase (ALP), and liver and brain lipid peroxidation. In addition to the hepatoprotective properties, the aqueous extract was reported to protect against liver damage induced by CCl4 and acetaminophen. The glucosides of *A. muricata* mechanistically reduced the bilirubin levels by converting to glucuronic acid that conjugates with bilirubin for excretion. Apparently, the phytochemicals in the extract may act as regulators increasing the activity of enzymes and transporters, and thereby enhancing the overall activity involved in clearing bilirubin. Combining all these outcomes, the potential hepato-protective function *A. muricata* is clearly emphasized and its prominent role in liver function [19].

Hence, *A. muricata* was used for the synthesis of AuNPs in this study. Further, the synthesized nanoparticles were characterized and checked for the in vitro cytotoxicity in VERO cell line and anticancer activity in Hep2 liver cancer cell line.

Methods

Synthesis of the AuNPs

Preparation of gold chloride solution

Gold chloride was used in the synthesis of nanogold particles. Chloroauric solution was prepared by dissolving required volumes of HAuCl4 in 1000 ml of deionized double-distilled water. A stock solution of required molar concentration was prepared and from this the required working solution was used for the synthesis. The working solution was adjusted for the required pH and used as such without any further dilutions for the synthesis [20].

Preparation of the plant extract

The fruit of *Annona muricata*, Graviola (Soursop) was brought from the local fruit store in Purasaiwalkam, Chennai, India. The formal identification of the plant material used in the study was identified by Dr. G. Jeya Jothi, Taxonomist, Department of Plant Biology & Biotechnology, Loyola College, Chennai. I would like to confirm that no voucher specimen of this material has been deposited. About 5 g of the peel/pulp were taken and washed repeatedly to remove the soil and dirt over them. Then, 50 ml of double-distilled water was added to the finely cut leaves and taken in a conical flask. The flask was heated for 10–15 min on flame. Then, it was filtered and the extract was collected. The extract was stored at 4 °C and used for the further synthesis [21].

For the synthesis of AuNPs, the pH of the stock solution was checked and adjusted. To the required quantity of chloroauric acid solution, about 1 ml of plant extract was added. The plant extract served as the reducing and stabilizing agent for the synthesis. The pale yellow color of the chloroauric acid changed into a wine red, pink or purple color, confirming the formation of nanoparticle.

Characterization of nanoparticles using UV-vis spectra

The bioreduction of gold chloride in aqueous solution was monitored by periodic sampling of the aliquots of the suspension. One milliliter of the sample was diluted with 30 ml of double-distilled water and analyzed for the presence of nanoparticles. The UV-vis spectra of the AuNP's were recorded using a Systronic smart DBS 2303 UV-vis spectra operating in the wavelength of 400 to 700 nm.

HRSEM analysis

The NPs were diluted with Millipore water in the ratio of 1:20 such that the concentration of the NPs became much less, thus enabling better imaging of the NPs. About 10 µl of sample was placed on the aluminum foil and allowed to air dry. Then the scanning electron micrographs of the samples was carried out at SAIF (Sophisticated Analytical Instrumentation Facility), IIT Madras, Adyar [22].

Zeta potential

The stability of the NPs synthesized is elucidated on analysis of zeta potential. It is the measure of the charged species present at the NPs surface that prevents from aggregation and ensuring highly stable nanoformulations. The more the positive or the more the negative, the zeta measure possess the strongest stability.

Fourier-transform infrared spectroscopy analysis

The Fourier-transform infrared spectroscopy (FTIR) analysis method uses infrared light to scan the test samples and observe its chemical properties and other constituents. The synthesized NPs were analyzed for the presence of functional groups of plants that aided in the process of NPs formation. The study was performed using the FT-IR Spectrophotometer (Perkin Elmer) at Bharathidasan University, Trichy.

Phytochemical analysis of the green extracts of the plants tested

The plant extracts were tested for various phytochemicals such as terpenoids, flavonoids, saponins, tannins, phenols, Coumarins, Triterpenoids, and the results were recorded. These phytochemicals act as the reducing and stabilizing agents for the plant mediated synthesis of nanoparticles.

In vitro cytotoxicity of the AuNPs

Procedure

The VERO cell line was used to check cytotoxicity of the synthesized AuNPs. The cell line used was procured from Translational Research Platform for Veterinary Biologicals (TRPVB) TANUVAS, Chennai. About 1 × 10^4 cells (10, 000 total cells) were added into each well of 96-well plates and incubated overnight. To this, different concentration of AuNPs was added. The treated cells were incubated for 24 h at 37 °C in the CO_2 incubator. About 10 µl (5 mg/ml) of 3-(4,5-dimethylthiazol-2-yl)-2,5-diphenyltetrazolium bromide (MTT) was added to each well. The cells were incubated for about 3 hours for the formation of formazan crystals. About 100 µl of dimethyl sulfoxide (DMSO) solvent was added to dissolve the formazan crystals and incubated for about an hour. The absorbance was read at 540 nm with a reference filter of 620 nm. Percentage of cell viability was calculated. Formula for cell inhibition = (O.D of treated cells/O.D of control) × 100. Formula to check cell viability = (100 – cell inhibition)

Anticancer activity of the AuNPs

Procedure

The Hep2 liver cancer cell line was used to check antiproliferative activity of the synthesized nanoparticles. The cell line used was procured from Kings Institute, Guindy, Chennai. About 1 × 10^4 cells (10,000 total cells) were added into each well of 96-well plates and incubated overnight. To this, different concentration of AuNPs was added. The treated cells were incubated for 24 h at 37 °C in the CO_2 incubator [6]. About 10 µl (5 mg/ml) of MTT was added to each well. The cells were incubated for about 3 h for the formation of formazan crystals. About 100 µl of DMSO solvent was added to dissolve the formazan crystals and incubated for about an hour. The absorbance was read at 540 nm with a reference filter of 620 nm. Percentage of cell viability was calculated. Formula for cell inhibition = (O.D of treated cells/O.D of control) × 100. Formula to check cell viability = (100 – cell inhibition) [23].

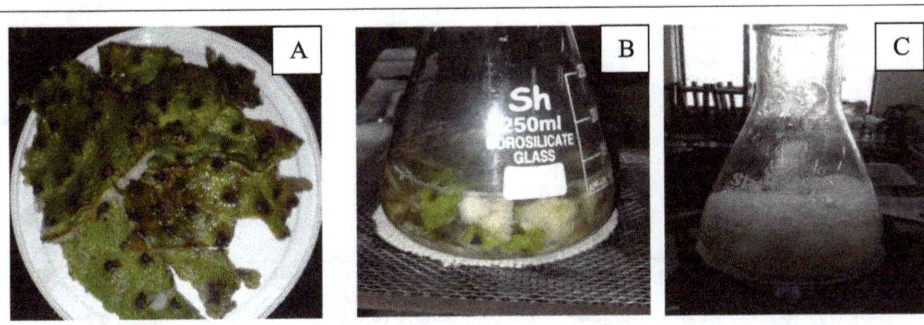

Fig 1 a–c Extracts of Graviola peel and pulp, preparation for the pulp extract

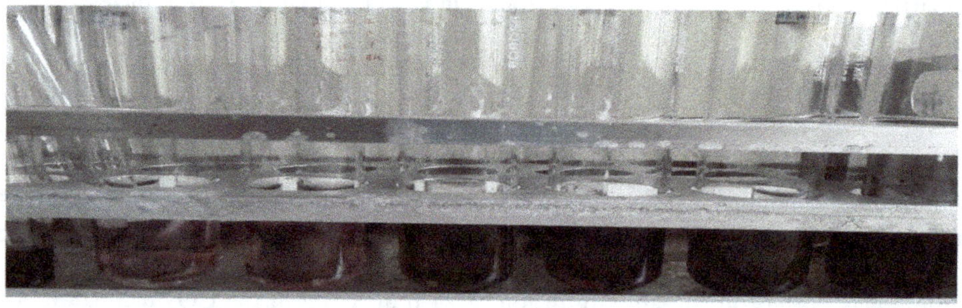

Fig. 2 The synthesized AuNPs using *A. muricata* peel and pulp extract

Results

Synthesis of AuNPs

The NPs were synthesized using the pulp and peel extract of the soursop fruit, *Annona muricata* on reduction with chloroauric acid. The synthesized NPs were pale pink to deep wine red in colour (Figs. 1 and 2).

Effect of pH on the synthesis

The pH has a prominent role in the synthesis of the NPs. A pH range of pH 6, pH 8, and pH 10 were tested. It was found that pH 8 to be the optimum pH for the synthesis of NPs. At other pH gradients, the reduction of chloroauric acid was not complete; a partial reduction was noted from the colour changes of the chloroauric solution [24].

UV Visible Spectrophotometry

The UV absorption peak is the respective wavelength at which the optical absorption spectra of metal nanoparticles are measured by the surface plasmon resonance. There exists a correlation between the wavelength and the particle size, wherein wavelength shifts to longer spectrum with increasing particle size. Based on the particle size, the position and shape of plasmon absorption of AuNPs highly varies. The initial confirmation of the NPs synthesis was through UV absorption spectrum, which was showing characteristic peaks for the synthesized AuNPs.

Similar results has been stated for nanoparticles synthesis by Jae Yong Song et al. 2009 (Fig. 3).

Zeta potential

The stability of the synthesized NPs were measured through zeta potential analysis. The zeta potential analysis the associated charges present at the surface of the NPs. This charge aids much more in the higher stability of the NMs. It helps the particles to stay monodispersed and prevents agglomerations. The zeta measures exist in polar ranges, it is either toward positivity or negativity. Both of these ranges assure high stability of the NPs. The zeta potential measurement also gives projection over the stability of the synthesized colloidal suspensions. In general, when the zeta potential value is about > 30 mV, there are less chances for agglomeration of the particles due to the electrostatic forces between the particles (Devika R. Bhumkar et al. 2007). The results observed were in concordance to similar reports by Devika R. Bhumkar et al. 2007 (Fig. 4).

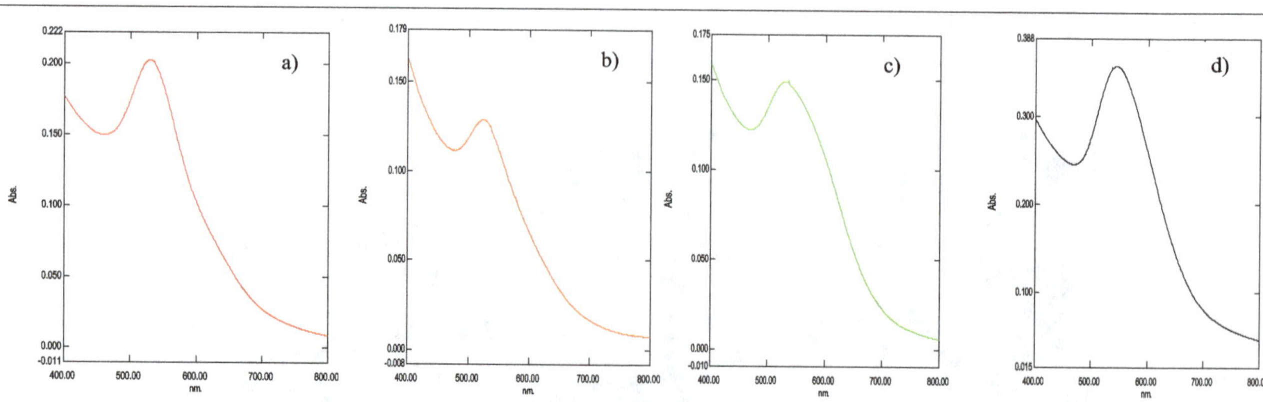

Fig. 3 a–d UV absorbance spectrum of AuNPs synthesized by *A. muricata* peel at 10^{-1} (λ_{max} – 529 nm), *A. muricata* pulp at 10^{-1} (λ_{max} – 525 nm), *A. muricata* peel at 10^{-3} (λ_{max} – 520 nm), *A. muricata* pulp at 10^{-3} (λ_{max} – 543 nm). The peak confirms the formation of AuNPs

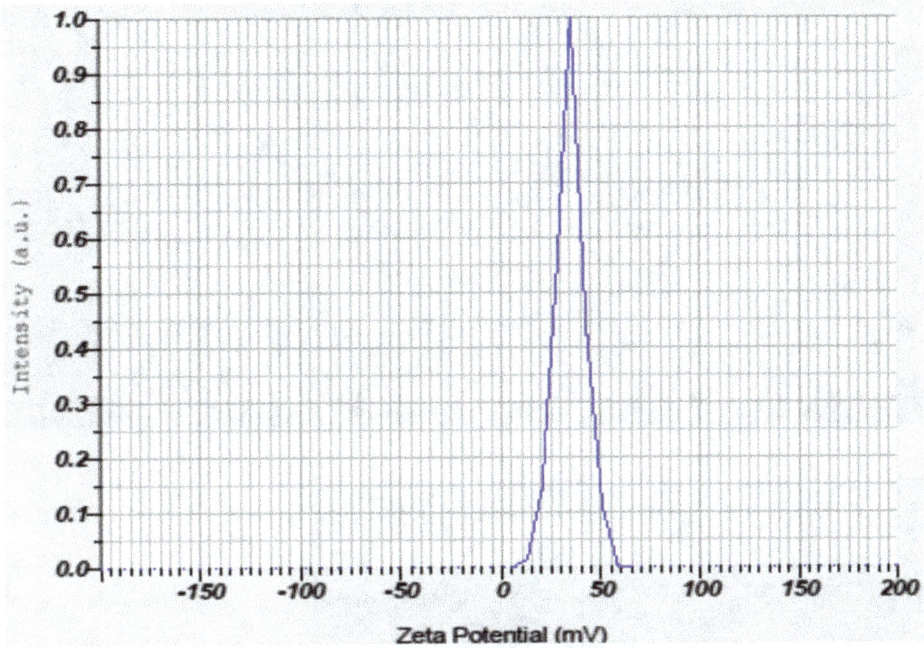

Fig. 4 Zeta potential analysis. Zeta potential (mean): − 30.9 mV. Zeta potential (mean): − 32.9 mV. Zeta potential (mean): − 34.9 mV

HRSEM analysis

The size of the NPs was 12 nm upwards, and an average about 20 nm; a commendable nano dimension achieved through plant-mediated synthesis. The NPs were spherical in morphology and evenly distributed. The significance on the size of the nanoparticles has been similarly stated by Jayanth and Vinod 2002 (Fig. 5).

FT-IR analysis

FT-IR analysis of A. muricata peel

Table 1 shows the FT-IR analysis of *A. muricata* peel.

Table 1 FT-IR analysis *A. muricata* peel

S. No.	Wave number (absorptions) (cm^{-1})	Functional groups
1.	1384.25	(-C-H) alkane
2.	1416.38	(C=C) aromatic
3.	1641.75	(C=C) Alkene

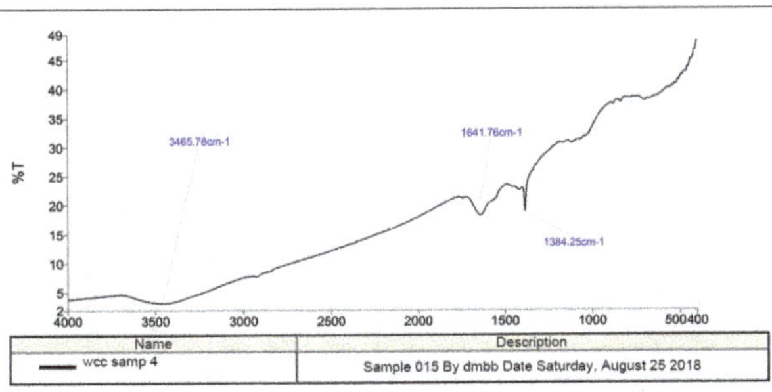

FT–IR analysis of A. muricata pulp

Table 2 shows the FT-IR analysis of *A. muricata* pulp.

The FT-IR spectra of organic compounds have two general areas, the functional group region (4000–1500 cm^{-1}) and the finger print region (1500–400 cm^{-1}). The peaks present in the functional group region correspond to the particular type of bonds present in the compound and hence can be used to identify the specific functional

Table 2 FT-IR analysis *A. muricata* pulp

S. No.	Wave number (absorptions) (cm^{-1})	Functional groups
1.	414.55	
2.	490.38	
3.	620.91	=(-C-H) alkane
4.	1113.78	(C-O) alcohol, (C-O) Ester
5.	1384.23	(-C-H) alkane
6.	1639.72	(C=C) Alkene
7.	3465.22	(N-H) Amine, (O-H) alcohol

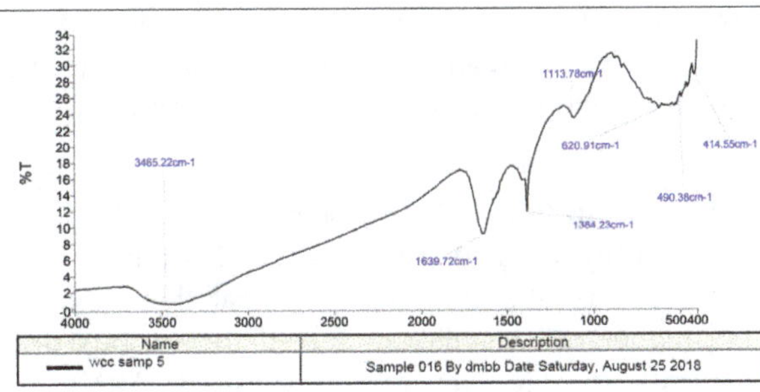

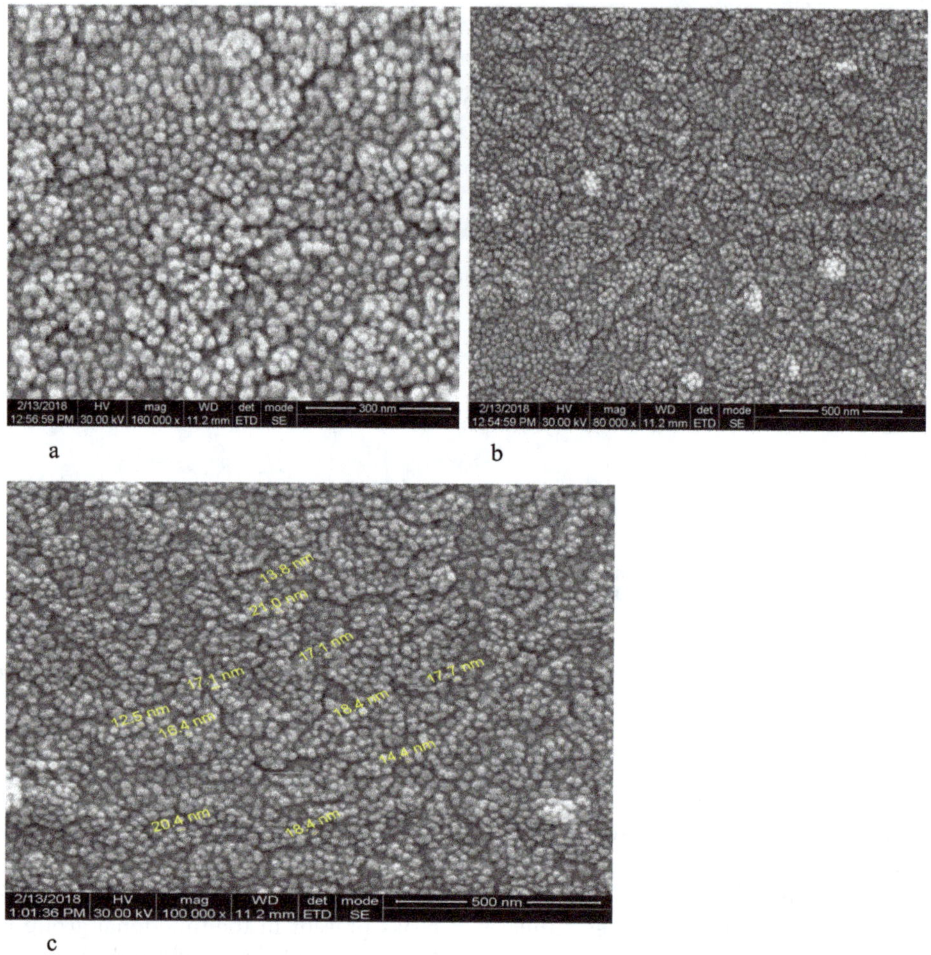

Fig. 5 a HRSEM images of the nanoparticles. **b** Nanoparticles showing spherical morphology. **c** Size of the nanoparticles measured

groups of the compound under study. The peaks present in the fingerprint region are a result of complex deformations of the molecule. In particular, they may be a characteristic of molecular symmetry or combination of bonds deforming simultaneously. Similar results have been reported by Jolly Mariam Johny et al. (2011).

Phytochemical analysis of the green extracts of the samples used

The phytochemistry of the plant extracts were carried out to check for the various secondary metabolites and constituents of the plant. The results showed the presence of many compounds as listed below (Table 3).

In vitro cytotoxicity in VERO cell line

The in vitro cytotoxicity assay was carried out in VERO cell line. The results obtained show that the AuNPs are having higher cell viability under all the various tested concentrations. Thereby the synthesized AuNPs are non-toxic over the treated VERO cell line.

The viability % of the AuNPs was illustrated through MTT assay in the VERO cell line, which showed that the AuNPs under study has good cell viability percentage at all the tested concentrations. Hence the synthesized AuNPs can be considered for further extended study (Fig. 6).

Table 3 The various phyto chemicals present in the plant extract

S. No.	Compounds	*A. muricata* peel	*A. muricata* pulp
1.	Coumarins	+	+
2.	Saponins	+	+
3.	Flavanoids	–	–
4.	Terpenoids	+	+
5.	Triterpenoids	–	–
6.	Carbohydrates	+	+
7.	Phenols	Yellow color	Yellow color
8.	Tannins	+	+
9.	Alkaloids	+	+

+ = Presence of the compound, – = absence of the compound
The number of signs indicates the intensity of results observed

In vitro anticancer activity in liver cancer Hep2 cell line

The results of the anticancer activity on the liver cancer Hep2 cell line showed that the Graviola mediated synthesized AuNPs, using pulp and peel, have demonstrated well antiproliferative activity against the cancer cell line. And proved to be efficient in most of the concentrations tested and the inhibition concentration 50 IC50 was at 17.98 µg/ml for NP1 and 13.08 µg/ml for NP 2 recorded out of the study. Based on the study, the AuNPs synthesized using Graviola peel extract has higher anticancer activity (Fig. 7).

Comparative anticancer activity between NP 1 & NP 2

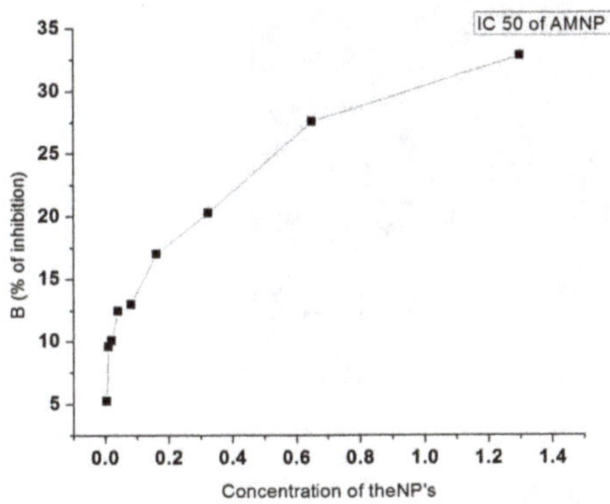

Inhibition Concentration 50 was at17.98 µg/ml for NP1 using pulp extract for synthesis.

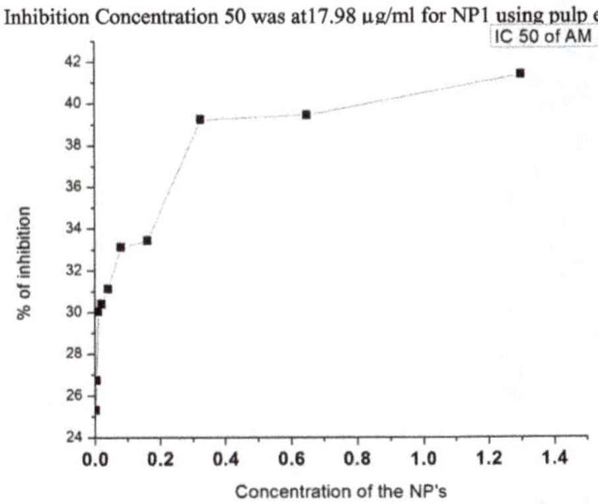

Inhibition Concentration 50 was at13.08 µg/ml for NP2 using pulp extract for synthesis.

Fluorescence assisted cell sorting—FACS analysis

Treated VERO cells

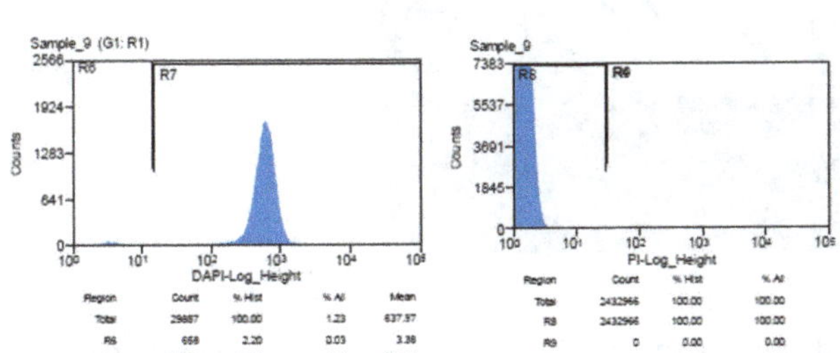

Treated Hep2 cells

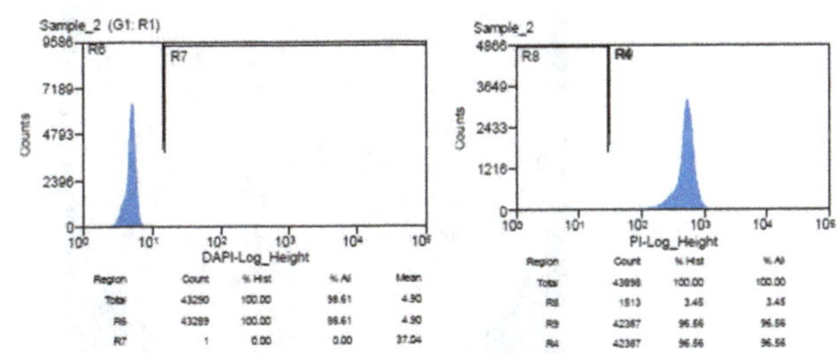

Fluorescence activated cell sorting (FACS) differentiates between the live and dead cells in the given population. The cells were labeled with PI (propidium iodide) and DAPI (4′,6-diamidino-2-phenylindole). DAPI was taken up by live cells, whereas PI stained the dead cells. In treated VERO cells, the percentage of live cells were highest and in treated Hep2 cells the PI log was seen in highest percentage. The results were much in concordance to the in vitro MTT assay. Similar analysis has been reported by Chih-Jen Lai, et al. 2019 [25].

Discussion

Ethnomedicine is emerging again from its dormancy. The traditional use of plants as therapeutic agents is an age old practice in many countries and cultures [26]. The results from the study imply a successful implication of an ethnomedically important plant for the treatment of cancer. The Graviola fruit is widely known for its anticancer activity as a crude extract. The present study has exploited the plant in the synthesis of nanoparticles and the anticancer activity of the synthesized nanoparticles is well demonstrated. Further, the bioactive compounds that are underlying this activity have to be elucidated. The extraction and purification of those bioactive compounds will help us to understand the mechanism of action against the disease. The anticancer studies can be extended targeting other types of cancer [27].

For a better oncotherapy and tumor targeting, nanotechnology-based drug delivery systems provides an exceptional opportunity. Among the various available nanotechnology-based strategies for tumor targeting, nanocrystals play a remarkable role since they are highly suitable for passive and active targeting with maximum possible drug content almost to 100%. In nanotechnology-based systems, there is a possibility to deliver together diagnostic probes along with the anticancer drugs. This combinational tumor theranostics approach results in the treatment of cancer, in a way simultaneously recognition, its evaluation, and transmission stages of the tumor. The multiple nanotechnology-based delivery systems utilized for tumor theranostics are polymeric nanoparticles, liposomes, micelles, polymersomes, etc. [28].

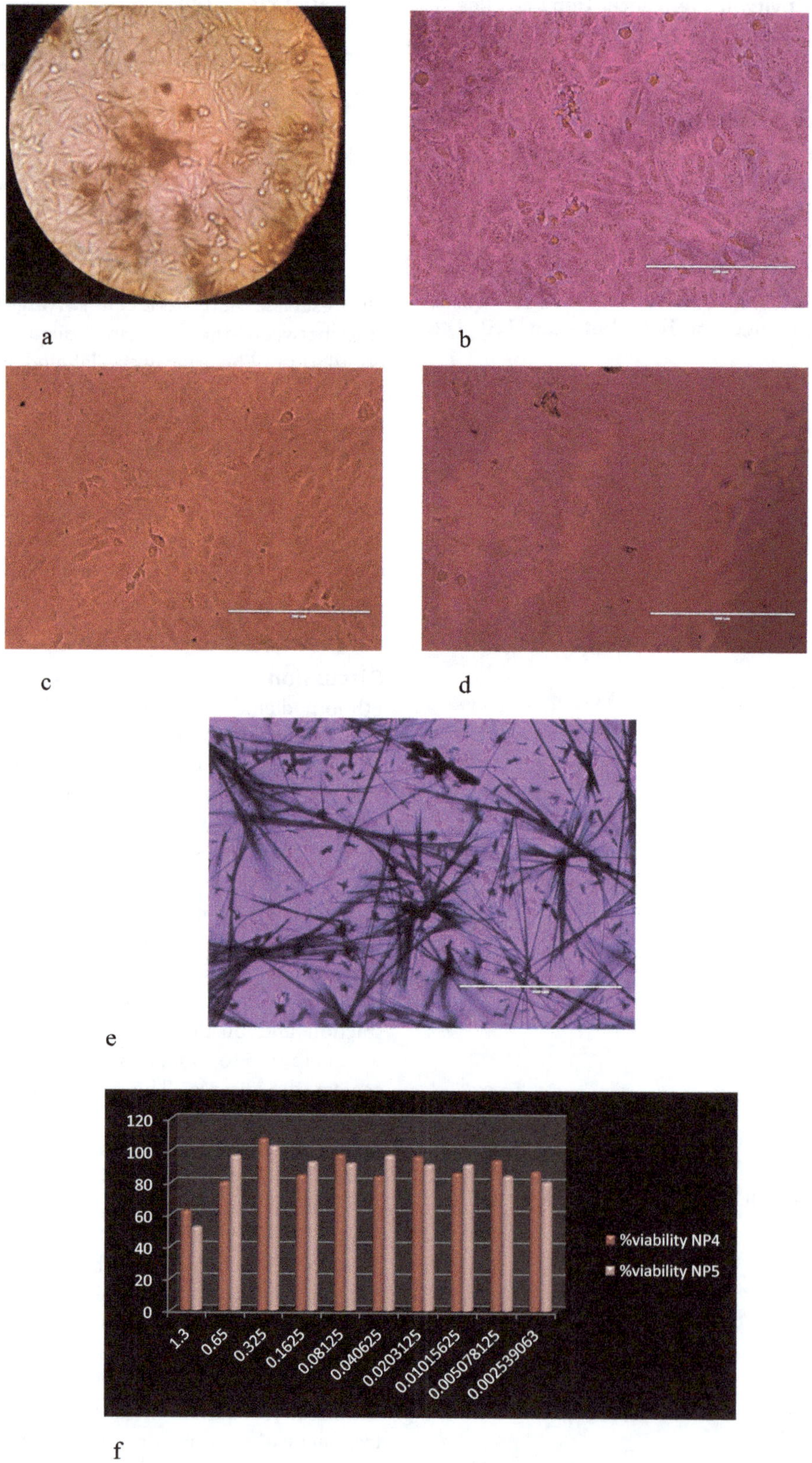

Fig. 6 **a** VERO cell line. **b** Control cell after 24 h. **c** After treated with AMNP1. **d** After treated with AMNP2. **e** The formazan crystals formed in treated VERO cells followed by MTT dye incubation. **f** Viability % in treated VERO cell line

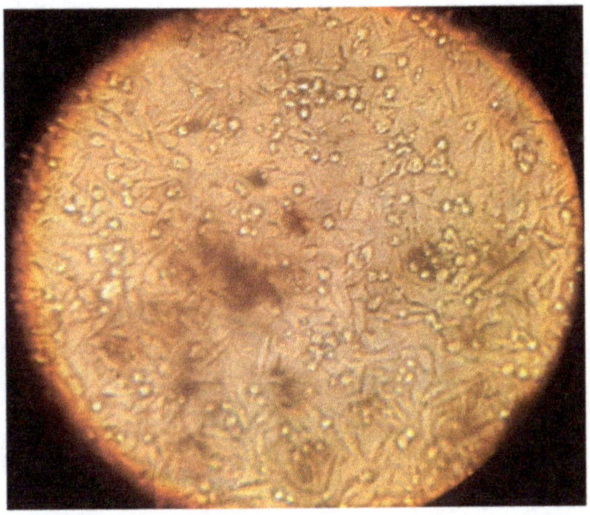

Fig. 7 a Hep2 liver cancer cell line

Presently, NPs have been extensively made use of topical drug delivery for wound healing. AuNPs have been much exploited for their potential antibacterial properties. Different types of nanocarriers have been used to enhance the permeation of drugs through skin as an alternative route to overcome the challenges of conventional oral and parenteral routes. Additionally to the use of lipid-based nanocarriers for dermal application of drugs, some polymeric nanocarriers showed an equally promising role in their places. The nanocapsules were used to deliver the antiandrogenic drug flutamide to the hair follicles thus providing a controlled and sustained drug release and thereby minimized penetration to the systemic circulation. Supportively, confocal microscopy imaging showed the follicular localization of the fluorescently labeled nanocapsules (NCs). To achieve long-term stability, NPs suspension can be converted to dry powder nanocomposites by spray-drying with inert carriers [4].

Conclusion

Currently, ethnomedicine is gaining its past glory and prominently being utilized at various treatments and therapies. On this context, the therapeutic properties pertaining to one of the medicinal plants, *Annona muricata*, was exploited in this study. The synthesis of AuNPs using pulp and peel extracts of the fruit of *A. muricata*, Soursop fruit was carried out successfully. The characterization of the synthesized nanoparticles was analyzed under UV-vis spectra, zeta potential, HRSEM, FTIR, and phytochemistry. The in vitro cytotoxicity showed that the synthesized gold NP's are non-toxic over VERO cell line and anticancer studies against Hep2 cell line proved that the NP's have good antiproliferative effect over the liver cancer cell line. Comparatively, the AuNPs mediated by peel extract have higher anticancer activity than AuNPs mediated by pulp extract. Finally, FACS analysis was performed to determine the live and dead cell populations in support of the in vitro results, which proved that the in vitro results were in concordance with the FACS analysis.

Abbreviations

AuNPs: Gold nanoparticles; DMSO: Dimethyl sulfoxide; FACS: Fluorescence assisted cell sorting; FTIR: Fourier-transform infrared spectroscopy analysis; HRSEM analysis: High-resolution scanning electron microscope; MNPs: Metallic nanoparticles; MTT: 3-(4,5-Dimethylthiazol-2-yl)-2,5-diphenyltetrazolium bromide; NMs: Nanomaterials; NPs: Nanoparticle

Acknowledgments

I would like to acknowledge Dr. Sathish Kota, Scientist, TRPVB, TANUVAS, Chennai and Dr. Harini Challa, Post-Doctoral Fellow, TRPVB, TANUVAS, Chennai for their courteous assistance all through the in vitro studies.

Authors' contributions

PI designed and directed the study and KP executed the entire research work from synthesis of NPs, its characterization, phytochemical analysis, in vitro studies, and was the major contributor in writing the manuscript. Both authors read and approved the final manuscript.

Competing interests

The authors declare that they have no competing interest.

References

1. Prager GW, Braga S, Bystricky B et al (2018) Global cancer control: responding to the growing burden, rising costs and inequalities in access. EMSO. 3:1–10
2. Olver I et al (2017) Cancer control—a global perspective. European Journal of Cancer Care 26(1):1–6
3. Jessica L. Petrick *et al.*, 2019, The changing epidemiology of primary liver cancer. Current Epidemiology Reports 6, 104–111
4. Elzoghby AO (2019) Pharmaceutical nanotechnology in Egypt: diverse applications and promising outcomes. Nanomedicine. 1-6
5. Nagajyothi PC et al (2017) Green synthesis: in-vitro anticancer activity of copper oxide nanoparticles against human cervical carcinoma cells. Arab J Chem 10:215–225
6. Zhai Lu *et al.*, 2017, Experimental study on the apoptosis of cervical cancer Hela cells induced by juglone through c-Jun N-terminal kinase/c-Jun pathway. Asian pacific journal of tropical medicine1-4
7. Arnst KE, Banerjee S, Chen H et al (2019) Current advances of tubulin inhibitors as dual acting small molecules for cancer therapy. Med Res Rev 1–29
8. Tan HW et al (2018) Selenium species: current status and potentials in cancer prevention and therapy. Int J Mol Sci 20(75):1–26
9. Dougan M, Dougan SK (2019) Programmable bacteria as cancer therapy. Nat Med 25:1030–1036
10. Kopeckovaa K et al (2019) Nanodrugs used in cancer therapy. Biomed Pap Med Fac Univ Palacky Olomouc Czech Repub 163(2):122–131
11. Grodzinski P et al (2019) Integrating nanotechnology into cancer care. ACS Nano 13:7370–7376
12. Grasso G et al (2019) Microbial nanotechnology: challenges and prospects for green biocatalytic synthesis of nanoscale materials for sensoristic and biomedical applications. Nanomaterials 2020(10):11
13. Dong J et al (2019) Synthesis of precision gold nanoparticles using Turkevich method. KONA Powder and Particle Journal 1-9
14. Govindaraju K et al (2019) Seaweed (Turbinaria ornata)-assisted green synthesis of magnesium hydroxide [Mg(OH)2] nanomaterials and their anti-mycobacterial activity. Mater Chem Phys 239:1–4
15. Surya Pratap Goutam *et al.*, 2019, Green synthesis of nanoparticles and their applications in water and wastewater treatment. Bioremediation of Industrial Waste for Environmental Safety, 349–379.
16. Jeyarani S et al (2019) Biomimetic gold nanoparticles for its cytotoxicity and biocompatibilityevidenced by fluorescence-based assays in cancer (MDA-MB-231) and non-cancerous (HEK-293) cells. J Photochem Photobiol B Biol 202:1–6

17. Akash Kumar *et al.*, 2019, A novel approach towards synthesis and characterization of non-cytotoxic gold nanoparticles using taurine as capping agent. Nanomaterials 2020, 10, 45, 1-19
18. Rady I et al (2018) Anticancer properties of Graviola (*Annona muricata*): a comprehensive mechanistic review, oxidative medicine and cellular longevity. 2018:1–39
19. Asif Khurshid Qazi *et al.*, 2018, Emerging Therapeutic Potential of Graviola and its Constituents in Cancers, https://academic.oup.com/carcin/advance-article abstract/doi/10.1093/carcin/bgy024/4859483
20. Kamala Priya MR, Iyer PR (2014) Extracellular rapid biosynthesis of AuNP's using various green extracts of plants. International journal of molecular biology & biochemistry 2:33–40
21. Kamala Priya MR, Iyer PR (2019) Anti-cancer study in hela cell line of phytosynthesized gold nanocompounds using *Andrographis paniculata* (nilavembu)—characterisation, optimization, phytochemical analysis & anti microbial study. Indian Journal of Applied Research 9:24–27
22. Kamala Priya MR, Iyer PR (2015) Comparitive study on the characterisation of AuNP's synthesized using various plant extracts. International Journal of Phytotherapy 5:17–21
23. M R Kamala Priya & Priya R. Iyer. 2014, Anticancer studies of the synthesized AuNP's against MCF 7 breast cancer cell line. Applied Nanoscience 443-448
24. Kamala Priya MR, Iyer PR (2014) Studies on the various parameters underlying the Synthesis of nanoparticles and the *in-vitro* stability of nanoparticles. Frontiers in Biotechnology 1-4
25. Lai C-J et al (2019) CD44 Promotes migration and invasion of docetaxel-resistant prostate cancer cells likely via induction of hippo-yap signaling. Cells 8(295):1–13
26. Li J et al (2008) queous extract of Solanum nigrum inhibit growth of cervical carcinoma (U14) via modulating immune response of tumor bearing mice and inducing apoptosis of tumor cells. Fitoterapia 79:548–556
27. Kamala Priya MR, Iyer PR (2015) Applications of the green synthesized AuNP's-antimicrobial activity, water purification system and drug delivery system. Symbiosis 1-4
28. Joseph E, Singhvi G et al (2019) Multifunctional nanocrystals for cancer therapy: a potential nanocarrier. Nanomaterials for Drug Delivery and Therapy 91–116

4

A novel serum index for accurate diagnosis of spontaneous bacterial peritonitis in cirrhotic patients without other infections

Hany M. Elsadek[1*], Soha A. Elhawari[2] and Ahmed Mokhtar[3]

Abstract

Background: The accurate non-invasive diagnosis of spontaneous bacterial peritonitis (SBP) in patients with decompensated liver cirrhosis has not been achieved yet. The aim of the study was to obtain an unmistakable diagnosis of SBP using a new simple serum bioscore, made by combined measurement of procalcitonin (PCT), erythrocyte sedimentation rate (ESR), and C-reactive protein (CRP), which we called the PEC index. This cross-sectional analytic study comprised 178 cirrhotic patients with ascites (60 patients with SBP and 118 patients with sterile ascites), after excluding non-SBP infection, during the period from March 2019 until September 2019. In all participants, serum levels of PCT, ESR, and CRP were measured, and PEC index was calculated [PEC index = PCT × (ESR + CRP)].

Results: Patients with SBP (n = 60) had significantly higher serum PEC index than those with sterile ascites (n = 118) (41.0/31.2–93.0 vs. 9.9/5.9–15.0, P < 0.001). PEC index distinguished culture positive cases significantly (P < 0.001). Using receiver operating characteristic (ROC) statistics, the sensitivity and specificity of PCT, at a cutoff value of 0.590 ng/mL, for SBP diagnosis, were 81.67% and 93.33%, respectively (area under the curve [AUC] = 0.879; 95% confidence interval [CI] 0.809–0.948). The sensitivity and specificity of ESR, at a cutoff value of 27.0 mm/hour, were 73.33% and 61.67%, respectively (AUC = 0.679; 95% CI 0.581–0.776). The sensitivity and specificity of CRP, at a cutoff value of 21.0 mg/L, were 93.33% and 51.67%, respectively (AUC = 0.736; 95% CI 0.639–0.833). While, the sensitivity and specificity of PEC index, at a cutoff value of 20, were highest (98.33% and 96.67%, respectively, AUC = 0.977; 95% CI 0.940–0.996).

Conclusion: Serum PEC index makes an accurate noninvasive diagnosis of SBP, after excluding other infections.

Keywords: Cirrhosis, Spontaneous bacterial peritonitis, Procalcitonin, PEC index

Background

Spontaneous bacterial peritonitis (SBP) is the commonest life-threatening infection encountered in cirrhotic patients with ascites. It accounts for more than half of all infections [1–3].The outpatient prevalence of SBP is 1.5–3.5% and exceeds 10% in hospitalized patients [4, 5].

The immune dysfunction in decompensated cirrhotic patients (DCPs) along with vulnerability of gut mucosa leading to translocation of bacteria and bacterial endotoxins from bowel lumen into ascitic fluid (AF), underlie the pathogenesis of SBP [1, 6–8].

* Correspondence: hanyelsadek75@yahoo.com
[1]Gastroenterology & Hepatology Unit, Internal Medicine Department, Faculty of Medicine, Zagazig University, Zagazig, Egypt

SBP precipitates several other complications of cirrhosis, e.g., impairment of hepatic status, hepatic encephalopathy, worsening of coagulopathy, variceal bleeding, renal failure, and even death [9]. In former decades, SBP was associated with > 90% mortality that has been reduced nowadays to ~ 20% with the development of prompt diagnosis and appropriate therapy [9, 10].

Typically, SBP presents with abdominal pain and tenderness associated with fever. However, it may present with other local symptoms and signs of peritonitis as vomiting, and ileus; other manifestations of systemic inflammation as hypothermia, chills, tachycardia, tachypnea, and shock; worsening of liver or kidney functions; or hepatic encephalopathy [11]. SBP may also be asymptomatic in 10% of cases [4].

Though, a positive AF culture for a pathogen is the gold standard for SBP diagnosis, about 60% of cases with clinical manifestations indicative of SBP and increased AF polymorphonuclear leukocytic (PMNL) count have negative cultures. Consequently, an AF PMNL count ≥ 250/μL is considered for SBP diagnosis, regardless of culture results [12–15]. In considerable number of cases, the absence of typical clinical characteristics of SBP makes its identification difficult [16].Therefore, an early non-invasive diagnosis of SBP in DCPs is sometimes recommended, especially in cases with irrelevant clinical manifestations, those newly admitted to hospital, or those with unexplained shock or deterioration of their liver functions [2, 3, 16].

Several non-invasive methods were tried in many studies for SBP diagnosis, as alternatives to diagnostic paracentesis, with variable accuracies, e.g., clinical scores [17], fecal calprotectin [18], and numerous serum inflammatory cytokines and chemokines such as monocyte chemotactic protein-1, interleukin-10 [19], human neutrophil peptide [20], platelet indices [21], macrophage inflammatory protein-1 beta [22], interferon-γ-induced protein-10, tumor necrosis factor-α, and interleukin-6 [23]. However, none of these methods was accurate enough to replace diagnostic paracentesis.

Procalcitonin (PCT) is a 116-amino acid polypeptide precursor of calcitonin with a molecular weight of 13 KDa produced by extra-thyroidal cells (e.g., monocytes) [24]. It has been proposed in highly cited studies as a potentially valuable serum biomarker to diagnose bacterial infections in general [24–26] and SBP in particular [27–30]. Normally, serum PCT level is undetectable (< 0.01 ng/mL), and it rapidly increases in case of infection [26].

Although the reported average estimate of sensitivity and specificity of serum PCT for SBP diagnosis in different clinical trials were relatively high (83% and 92%, respectively) [27], this performance was insufficient to make an acceptable accurate diagnosis. In order to achieve a more reliable diagnostic accuracy of PCT, we have tried a combined measurement of serum PCT with serum erythrocyte sedimentation rate (ESR) and C-reactive protein (CRP) to formulate a novel serum index for SBP diagnosis that we called, the PEC index.

Methods

Study design and sitting

This cross-sectional analytic study was carried out on 178 consecutive hospitalized cirrhotic patients with ascites admitted to internal medicine and tropical medicine departments, in collaboration with the Clinical Pathology Department, Faculty of Medicine, Zagazig University Hospital, Egypt, from March 2019 until September 2019.

Participants

Out of 257 consecutive hospital admissions of potentially eligible cirrhotic patients with ascites, 62 patients who had non-SBP infections were excluded and 7 patients died before the sampling procedures. Eligibility for the study was confirmed in 188 patients; of them, only 178 patients accepted to participate in the study.

Inclusion criteria

1. Adult patients ≥ 18 years
2. All consecutive hospitalized DCPs with moderate to severe ascites (that was detected clinically and confirmed with abdominal ultrasonography) who were admitted for different purposes like clinically suspected SBP, variceal bleeding, and hepatic encephalopathy. Participants were classified into an SBP group (either symptomatic or asymptomatic) (n = 60) and a sterile ascites group (n = 118).

The diagnosis of SBP was confirmed by an AFPMNL count ≥ 250/mm^3 with or without a positive ascitic fluid culture for pathogenic bacteria. Absence of both criteria meant the ascites was sterile [14, 15].

Exclusion criteria

1. Patients with a diagnosed infection other than AF infection, e.g., upper and lower respiratory tract infection, urinary tract infection, and otitis media
2. Patients with HCC or associated pancreatic disease, as these conditions could affect the components of PEC index.
3. Patients who received antibiotics 10 days prior to hospital admission.
4. Patients with AF culture positivity and AF PMNL count < 250/mm^3 (bacterascites)
5. Patients who refused to be enrolled in the study or refused to sign the consent.

Study tools

All included patients were subjected to thorough clinical assessment, abdominal ultrasound scanning, routine laboratory examination, e.g., complete blood picture, liver function and kidney function tests, coagulation profile and viral markers, and determination of serum levels of ESR (first hour), CRP (by Cobas 8000, Roch, Germany) and PCT, and peritoneal fluid examination.

Serum PCT measurement

This was done by the electrochemiluminescence immunoassay (ECLIA) on Cobas e 411 immunoassay analyzers, Roch, Germany, acting via the sandwich principle. The analyzer automatically calculates the analyte concentration of each sample in ng/ml with a measuring range of 0.02 to 100 ng/ml and the coefficient of variability of 8% [31].

Peritoneal fluid examination technique

Sterile bedside diagnostic paracentesis was done using a 23-G needle attached to a 20 cc syringe after applying local anesthesia. Then, aspirated ascitic fluid was collected into two tubes and analyzed within 2 h of aspiration. The first tube for culture and sensitivity and second tube with ethylene diamine tetraacetic acid were to be analyzed for biochemistry and leukocyte counts.

PEC index

This is a new serum bioscore, innovated in this study, which was calculated by the formula; PEC index = PCT × (ESR + CRP). This formula was chosen on a statistical base, after repeated trials and errors while trying several different formulae.

Statistical analysis

Statistical analysis was performed with SPSS software, version 22.0 (SPSS Inc., Chicago, IL, USA). The continuous variables were expressed as means ± standard deviation (SD) and the categorical variables as count numbers and proportions. The suitable test was used, e.g., Student's t test, Mann–Whitney U test, Pearson's chi-squared test, Fisher's exact test, and Pearson's correlation test. The result was considered significant if $P \leq 0.05$. In order to test the diagnostic accuracy of various markers as well as the novel PEC index for diagnosis of SBP, we used receiver operating characteristic (ROC) statistics and determined sensitivity, specificity, and area under the curve (AUC) for each.

Results

Comparison between SBP group (n = 60) and sterile ascites group (n = 118) regarding demographic, clinical, and laboratory characteristics revealed significantly higher serum PCT, ESR, and CRP, as well as significantly higher AF LDH and PMNL count in SBP group ($P < 0.001$, for all parameters). Also, PEC index was significantly higher in SBP group than in sterile ascites group (41.0/31.2–93.0 vs. 9.9/5.9–15.0, $P < 0.001$) (Table 1).

AF bacterial culture positivity was found in 41.67% (25/60) of SBP group, but not in sterile ascites group at all (0/60) (Table 1). The commonest pathogens encountered were Escherichia coli in 68.0% (17/25) and Klebsiella in 16.0% (4/25) of culture positive cases. Positivity of AF culture among patients with SBP was significantly associated with higher levels of serum PCT, PEC index, AF LDH, and AF PMNL count and with lower AF glucose level ($P < 0.001$, for all) (Table 2).

ROC statistics were used to assess diagnostic accuracy of tested serum markers in SBP diagnosis (Figs. 1 and 2). The sensitivity and specificity of PCT, at a cutoff value of 0.590 ng/mL, were 81.67% and 93.33% (AUC = 0.879; 95% confidence interval [CI] 0.809–0.948). The sensitivity and specificity of ESR, at a cutoff value of 27.0 mm/h, were 73.33% and 61.67% (AUC = 0.679; 95% CI 0.581–0.776). The sensitivity and specificity of CRP, at a cutoff value of 21.0 mg/L, were 93.33% and 51.67% (AUC = 0.736; 95% CI 0.639–0.833) (Fig. 1 and Table 3). Serum PEC index, at a cutoff value of 20, had much higher sensitivity and specificity for SBP diagnosis (98.33% and 96.67%, respectively, AUC = 0.977; 95% CI 0.940–0.996), with an overall diagnostic accuracy of 97.50% (Fig. 2 and Table 3).

Figures 3 and 4 and Table 3 show the diagnostic performances of PEC index and its components in discrimination between cases with culture-negative SBP and those with sterile ascites. PCT, at a cutoff value of 0.305 ng/mL, was associated with a better diagnostic accuracy (AUC = 0.825; 95% CI 0.742–0.907) than that of ESR, at a cutoff value of 27 mm/h (AUC = 0.649; 95% CI 0.521–0.776) and that of CRP at a cutoff value of 23.5 mg/L (AUC = 0.704; 95% CI 0.613–0.794) (Fig. 3). PEC index, at a cutoff value of 20, was associated with the best diagnostic performance (AUC = 0.970; 95% CI 0.934–1.0) (Fig. 4).

Discussion

The search for a non-invasive and readily available biomarker for unmistakable diagnosis of SBP in cirrhotic patients with ascites, is still under clinical trials [22, 23, 29, 30, 32, 33]. The current work, to the best of our knowledge, is the first to characterize the use of indexed combined measurement of serum PCT, ESR, and CRP for this purpose, after exclusion of non-SBP bacterial infections.

In this study, all SBP patients (n = 60) had AF inflammatory response due to bacterial infection as was identified by AF PMNL count ≥ 250/HPF. Other biochemical findings in AF analysis confirmed the presence of infection like high LDH and low glucose. These findings were in accordance with that of Badawy et al. [34] and EL-Motasem et al. [35].

In addition, serum levels of acute phase reactants; ESR, CRP, and PCT in the SBP group of our patients (31/23–36 mm/h, 27/24–29 mg/L, and 0.691/0.604–1.690 ng/mL, respectively) were significantly higher than in sterile ascites group (25/19–30 mm/h, 20/11–25 mg/L, and 0.259/0.159–0.350 ng/mL, respectively) ($P < 0.001$, for all). Likewise, Viallon et al. [36], Such et al. [37], Papp et al. [38], and Wu et al. [39] described elevations of inflammatory mediators in the setting of SBP. This could be explained by activation of cytokine synthesis and innate immunity in response to circulating bacterial endotoxins [40].

Table 1 Demographic, clinical, and laboratory data of the studied groups

	Sterile ascites n = 118	SBP n = 60	P
Age (mean ± SD, years)	57.3 ± 7.3	57.6 ± 6.8	0.824
Male sex	55 (46.6%)	38 (63.3%)	0.073
Hypertension	12 (10.2%)	9 (15.0%)	0.345
Diabetes mellitus	18 (15.3%)	11 (18.3%)	0.599
Cause of liver disease			0.727**
- HCV infection	94 (79.7%)	51 (85.5%)	
- HBV infection	20 (16.9%)	8 (13.3%)	
- Other causes	4 (3.4%)	1 (1.7%)	
Serum albumin (mean ± SD, g/dL)	2.53 ± 0.18	2.49 ± 0.21	0.178
Serum Total bilirubin (median/IQR, mg/dL)	2.11/0.91–3.29	2.00/1.50–3.42	0.167*
INR (mean ± SD)	1.47 ± 0.20	1.53 ± 0.28	0.095
ALT (median/IQR, IU/L)	27/18–38	34/15–44	0.387*
AST (median/IQR, IU/L)	48/36–60	47/29–74	0.892*
Serum creatinine (median/IQR, mg/dL)	1.00/1.00–1.00	1.00/1.00–1.75	0.158*
Serum LDH (mean ± SD, IU/L)	214 ± 54	226 ± 51	0.126
Blood TLC (median/IQR, × 10^3/mm^3)	6.10/4.00–8.00	7.00/4.43–8.90	0.158*
Hemoglobin (mean ± SD, g/dL)	10.07 ± 1.49	10.06 ± 1.33	0.952
Platelets count (median/IQR, × 10^3/mm^3)	90/66–144	82/66–144	0.550*
ESR (median/IQR, mm/hour)	25/19–30	31/23–36	< 0.001*
CRP (median/IQR, mg/L)	20/11–25	27/24–29	< 0.001*
PCT (median/IQR, ng/mL)	0.259/0.159–0.350	0.691/0.604–1.690	< 0.001*
PEC index [PCT × (ESR + CRP)] (median/IQR)	9.89/5.93–15.00	41.04/31.18–92.99	< 0.001*
Ascitic fluid albumin (mean ± SD, g/dL)	0.837 ± 0.148	0.875 ± 0.128	0.094
Ascitic fluid glucose (mean ± SD, g/dL)	112 ± 17	99 ± 12	< 0.001
Ascitic fluid LDH (mean ± SD, IU/L)	109 ± 18	157 ± 42	< 0.001
Ascitic fluid PMNL (median/IQR, cell/mm^3)	200/170–207	3334/274–641	< 0.001*
Ascitic fluid PMNL ≥ 250/mm^3	0 (0.0%)	60 (100.0%)	< 0.001
Positive ascitic fluid bacterial culture	0 (0.0%)	25 (41.7%)	< 0.001

SD standard deviation, *IQR* interquartile range, *HCV* hepatitis C virus, *HBV* hepatitis B virus, *INR* international normalized ratio, *ALT* alanine aminotransferase, *AST* aspartate aminotransferase, *IU* international unit, *LDH* lactate dehydrogenase, *TLC* total leukocytic count, *ESR* erythrocyte sedimentation rate, *CRP* C-reactive protein, *PCT* procalcitonin, *PMNL* polymorphonuclear leukocytes
*Mann–Whitney *U* test, ** Fisher's exact test

As a pro-inflammatory cytokine, PCT is elevated in acute bacterial infections and reaches the highest serum level in severe infections and sepsis as it is enhanced by systemic inflammatory response. It is not elevated by viral infection or autoimmune inflammation [24–26]. Serum PCT measurement has an established role in differentiation between bacterial infections and other inflammatory conditions [25, 41]; however, its use as a diagnostic biomarker for SBP has been reported frequently in the last decade, with conflicting results [22, 27–30, 38, 39].

In this work, with the exception that CRP was more sensitive than PCT for SBP diagnosis (93.33% versus 81.67%, respectively), the sensitivity and specificity of serum PCT at a cutoff value of 0.590 ng/mL for SBP diagnosis (81.67% and 93.33%, respectively, AUC: 0.879) were relatively higher than that of ESR at a cutoff value of 27.0 mm/h (73.33% and 61.67%, respectively, AUC 0.679) and that of CRP at a cutoff value > 21.0 mg/L (93.33% and 51.67%, respectively; AUC 0.736). PCT appears to be superior in detecting septic conditions to other pro-inflammatory markers like ESR and CRP, because of its earlier increase upon infection and its better specificity [36, 38, 39, 41].

A previous meta-analysis by Yang et al. [27] including18 studies on 1827 DCPs, published between 2000 and 2014, investigated the diagnostic performance of PCT as a marker of SBP. They reported a relatively good diagnostic performance with a summary estimate of sensitivity and specificity of 83.0% and 92.0%, respectively,

Table 2 Comparison between culture-positive and culture-negative SBP patients, regarding serum and AF biomarkers

	Culture negative n = 35	Culture-positive n = 25	P
ALT (median/IQR, IU/L)	38/15–45	26/15–39	0.413*
AST (median/IQR, IU/L)	44/31–74	48/22–79	0.554*
Serum LDH (mean ± SD, IU/L)	225 ± 46	229 ± 58	0.750
Blood TLC (median/IQR, × 10^3/mm3)	7.0/4.8–9.0	7.0/4.3–8.6	0.553*
Platelets count (median/IQR, × 10^3/mm^3)	82/66–145	80/68–133	0.887*
ESR (median/IQR, mm/hour)	32/22-36	30/28–35	0.952*
CRP (median/IQR, mg/L)	26/24–28	27/25–30	0.253
PCT (median/IQR, ng/mL)	0.614/0.410–0.649	1.733/1.256–2.500	< 0.001*
PEC index [PCT × (ESR + CRP)] (median/IQR)	36.34/25.22–40.19	101.48/70.79–136.89	< 0.001*
Ascitic fluid albumin (mean ± SD, g/dL)	0.865 ± 0.13	0.889 ± 0.13	0.467
Ascitic fluid glucose (mean ± SD, g/dL)	104 ± 9	93 ± 13	< 0.001
Ascitic fluid LDH (mean ± SD, IU/L)	142 ± 28	177 ± 50	< 0.001
Ascitic fluid PMNL (median/IQR, cell/mm^3)	275/260–310	655/463–6700	< 0.001*

SD standard deviation, *IQR* interquartile range, *ALT* alanine aminotransferase, *AST* aspartate aminotransferase, *LDH* lactate dehydrogenase, *TLC* total leukocytic count, *ESR* erythrocyte sedimentation rate, *CRP* C-reactive protein, *PCT* procalcitonin, *PMNL* polymorphonuclear leukocytes
*Mann-Whitney *U* test

which came very close to our results. On the other hand, Lesińska et al. [22] reported that serum PCT could not distinguish patients with and without SBP. The small sample size (n = 32) of their study [22] could explain this contradictory result.

Positive results of AF bacterial cultures, in this study, were found only in 41.6% (25/60) of SBP patients. Nearly the same result was frequently reported before [12, 14, 15]. The predominance of gram-negative over gram-positive bacteria among culture positive cases, in our study, goes with other studies [1, 42]. In the current work, serum PCT, opposite to ESR and CRP, was significantly elevated in culture positive cases of SBP ($P < 0.001$). This comes in accordance with the study of Cekin et al. [43], but it does not come in agreement with the studies of EL-Gendy et al. [44] or Cai et al. [28] who reported the lack of sensitivity of serum PCT to differentiate the culture results in SBP patients.

In this research, the newly advocated PEC index [calculated as PCT × (ESR + CRP)] was significantly higher in SBP group than in sterile ascites group ($P < 0.001$),

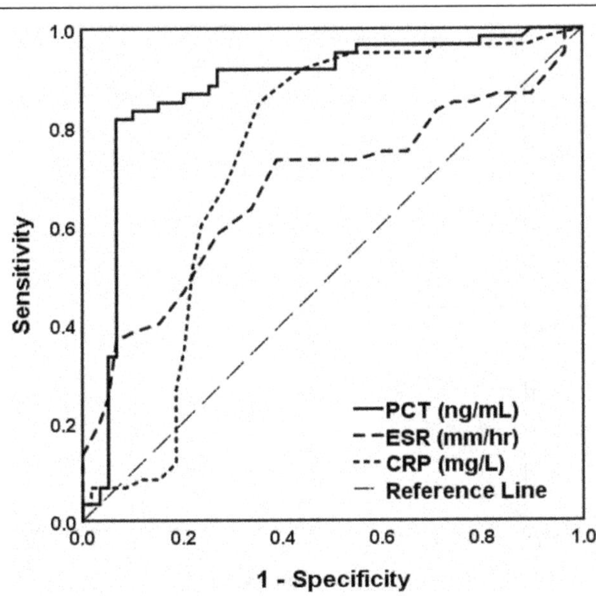

Fig. 1 Sensitivities and specificities of serum markers; ESR, CRP and PCT for SBP diagnosis

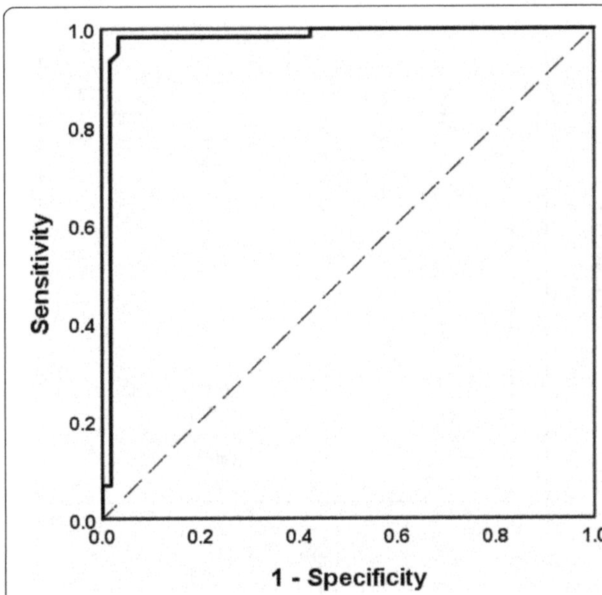

Fig. 2 Sensitivity and specificity of serum PEC index for SBP diagnosis

Table 3 Diagnostic accuracy of PEC index and its components for SBP diagnosis and for distinguishing culture-negative SBP from sterile ascites, using ROC statistics

Serum markers	SBP diagnosis					Discrimination between culture-negative SBP and sterile ascites				
	Cutoff value	Sensitivity	Specificity	AUC (95% CI)	*P*	Cutoff value	Sensitivity	Specificity	AUC (95% CI)	*P*
PCT ng/mL	> 0.590	81.67%	93.33%	0.879 0.809–0.948	*< 0.001*	> 0.305	85.70%	72.90%	0.825 0.742–0.907	*< 0.001*
ESR mm/hour	> 27.0	73.33%	61.67%	0.679 0.581–0.776	*< 0.001*	> 27.0	68.60%	61.00%	0.649 0.521–0.776	*0.008*
CRP mg/L	> 21.0	93.33%	51.67%	0.736 0.639–0.833	*< 0.001*	> 23.5	80.00%	64.40%	0.704 0.613–0.794	*< 0.001*
PEC index	> 20.0	98.33%	96.67%	0.977 0.940–0.996	*< 0.001*	> 20.0	97.10%	96.60%	0.970 0.934–1.0	*< 0.001*

ROC receiver operating characteristic, *PCT* procalcitonin, *ESR* erythrocyte sedimentation rate, *CRP* C-reactive protein, *AUC* area under the curve, *CI* confidence interval

and it was significantly more elevated in culture-positive than in culture-negative cases of SBP ($P < 0.001$).

In the present study, at a cutoff value of 20, the sensitivity and specificity of serum PEC index for SBP diagnosis (98.33% and 96.67%, respectively, AUC 0.977) were much higher than that of serum PCT, ESR, and CRP. Likewise, the sensitivity and specificity of serum PEC index, at a cutoff value of 20, to distinguish cases with culture-negative SBP from sterile ascites cases (97.1% and 96.6%, respectively, AUC 0.970), were much better than that of PEC components. The superiority of PEC index over any of its components, for diagnosis of SBP and even of its culture-negative subtype, could be explained simply by the mathematical compensatory effect of combining several markers with different degrees of sensitivity and specificity, helping escaping false positive and false negative results.

Furthermore, the above mentioned diagnostic accuracy of PEC index in SBP is better than that of other promising serum markers that were reported in the last few years [32, 33]. Although serum homocysteine had relatively high sensitivity and specificity for distinguishing SBP (95.1% and 89.3%, respectively; AUC 0.932) [32], it is less accurate than PEC index. A D-dimer cutoff value of 1500 ng/mL was determined optimal for ruling out SBP due to high sensitivity (96.8%); however, this marker was not useful for confirming SBP due to low specificity (40.6%) [33].

Similar to our study design, Wang et al. [45] have conducted a recently published study on 259 consecutive cirrhotic patients with ascites admitted to a Chinese

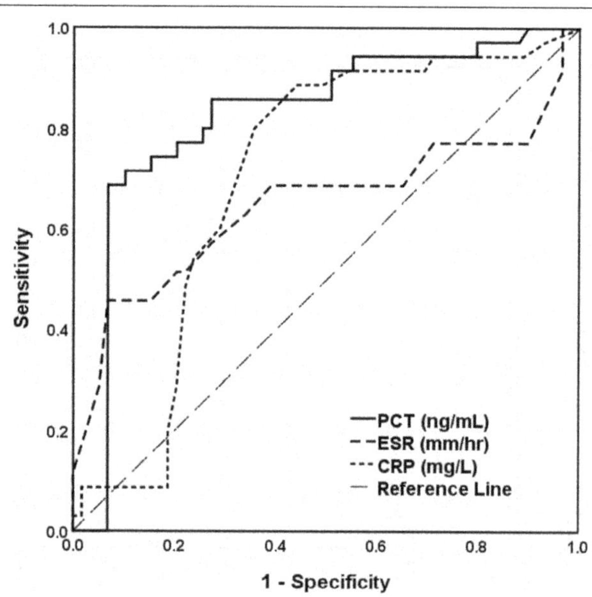

Fig. 3 Sensitivities and specificities of serum markers; ESR, CRP and PCT for discriminating culture-negative SBP from sterile ascites

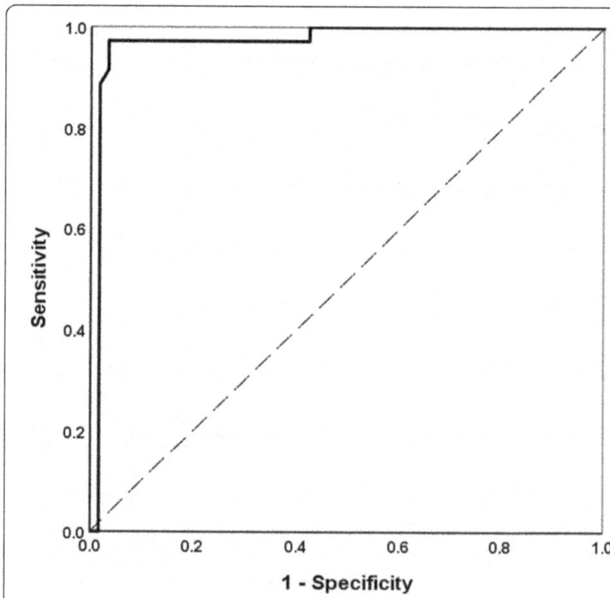

Fig. 4 Sensitivity and specificity of serum PEC index for discriminating culture-negative SBP from sterile ascites

military hospital to investigate the efficacy in SBP diagnosis of combined measurement of PCT, mean fluorescence intensity of mature neutrophils (sNFI) and difference in hemoglobin concentration between newly formed and mature red blood cells (dCHC). Of these, 51/259 (19.7%) had culture-positive SBP, 58/259 (22.4%) had culture-negative SBP, and 150/259 (57.9%) had sterile ascites. The total bioscore of those three markers used by Wang et al. [45], at a cutoff value of ≥3.40, had a sensitivity of 92.6%, a specificity of 95.3% and an AUC of 0.937 (95% CI 0.901–0.994, $P < 0.001$), which are less than that of PEC index innovated in our study.

Some limitations to our study are to be mentioned. First is the relatively small sample size. Second, we did not test for serum markers other than PEC index components to help making head to head comparison. Finally, it would have been more appropriate if we added one more group of DCPs with infections other than SBP to assess specificity of PEC index for SBP.

Conclusion

The novel serum PEC index seems sufficient to make a fairly accurate non-invasive diagnosis of SBP in cirrhotic patients with ascites, provided that non-SBP bacterial infections are excluded.

Recommendations

To validate the clinical use of serum PEC index for SBP diagnosis, further larger trials are needed that should involve assessment of PEC index in non-SBP infections and its comparison with other serum biomarkers.

Abbreviations

AF: Ascitic fluid; AUC: Area under the curve; CRP: C-reactive protein; DCPs: Decompensated cirrhotic patients; ESR: Erythrocyte sedimentation rate; PCT: Procalcitonin; PEC index: Index of combined measurement of PCT, ESR and PCT; PMNL: Polymorphonuclear leukocytes; ROC: Receiver operating characteristic; SBP: Spontaneous bacterial peritonitis

Acknowledgments

Great thanks to all patients who accepted enrollment in the study as well as to all nursing staff and technicians who helped accomplishing this work.

Authors contributions

HE had selected the idea and design of the work, had contributed in the data collection and interpretation, shared in drafting the work, and had made the final revision of data. SE had contributed in the data collection and interpretation and shared in drafting the work. AM had helped in the data collection and analysis and had performed the laboratory work. All authors have read and approved the final manuscript.

Competing interests

The authors declare that they have no competing interests.

Author details

Gastroenterology & Hepatology Unit, Internal Medicine Department, Faculty of Medicine, Zagazig University, Zagazig, Egypt. [2]Tropical Medicine Department, Faculty of Medicine, Zagazig University, Zagazig, Egypt. [3]Clinical Pathology Department, Faculty of Medicine, Zagazig University, Zagazig, Egypt.

References

1. Wiest R, Krag A, Gerbes A (2012) Spontaneous bacterial peritonitis: recent guidelines and beyond. Gut 61:297–310
2. Acharya SK (2013) Difficult to treat spontaneous bacterial peritonitis. Trop Gastroenterol 34:7–13
3. Jalan R, Fernandez J, Wiest R, Schnabl B, Moreau R, Angeli P et al (2014) Bacterial infections in cirrhosis: a position statement based on the EASL Special Conference 2013. J Hepatol 60:1310–1324
4. Evans LT, Kim WR, Poterucha JJ, Kamath PS (2003) Spontaneous bacterial peritonitis in asymptomatic outpatients with cirrhotic ascites. Hepatology 37:897–901
5. Nousbaum JB, Cadranel JF, Nahon P, Nguyen Khac E, Moreau R, Thévenot T et al (2007) Diagnostic accuracy of the Multistix 8 SG reagent strip in diagnosis of spontaneous bacterial peritonitis. Hepatology 45:1275–1281
6. Kalaitzakis E, Johansson J (2006) Intestinal permeability in cirrhotic patients with and without ascites. Scand J Gastroenterol 41:326–330
7. Gines P, Fernandez J, Durand F, Saliba F (2012) Management of critically-ill cirrhotic patients. J Hepatol 56(Suppl 1):S13–S24
8. Wiest R, Lawson M, Geuking M (2014) Pathological bacterial translocation in liver cirrhosis. J Hepatol 60:197–209
9. Tandon P, Garcia-Tsao G (2008) Bacterial infections, sepsis, and multiorgan failure in cirrhosis. Semin Liver Dis 28:26–42
10. Garcia-Tsao G (2001) Current management of the complications of cirrhosis and portal hypertension: variceal hemorrhage, ascites, and spontaneous bacterial peritonitis. Gastroenterology 120:726–748
11. Piddock LJ, Planas R, Bernard B, Inadomi JM (2000) Diagnosis, treatment and prophylaxis of spontaneous bacterial peritonitis: a consensus document. International ascites club. J Hepatol 32(1):142–153
12. Fernandez J, Navasa M (2002) Bacterial infections in cirrhosis: epidemiological changes with invasive procedures and norfloxacin prophylaxis. Hepatology 35:140–148
13. Wong CL, Holroyd-Leduc J (2008) Does this patient have bacterial peritonitis or portal hypertension? How do I perform a paracentesis and analyze the results? JAMA 299:1166–1178
14. European Association for the Study of the Liver (2010) EASL clinical practice guidelines on the management of ascites, spontaneous bacterial peritonitis, and hepatorenal syndrome in cirrhosis. J Hepatol 53:397–417
15. Runyon BA, AASLD (2013) Introduction to the revised American Association for the Study of Liver Diseases Practice Guideline management of adult patients with ascites due to cirrhosis 2012. Hepatology 57:1651–1653
16. Attar BM, George M (2014) Disease dependent qualitative and quantitative differences in the inflammatory response to ascites occurring in cirrhotics. World J Hepatol 6:85–91
17. Wehmeyer MH, Krohm S, Kastein F, Lohse AW, Lüth S (2014) Prediction of spontaneous bacterial peritonitis in cirrhotic ascites by a simple scoring system. Scand J Gastroenterol 49:595–603
18. Gundling F, Schmidtler F, Hapfelmeier A, Schulte B, Schmidt T, Pehl C et al (2011) Fecal calprotectin is a useful screening parameter for hepatic encephalopathy and spontaneous bacterial peritonitis in cirrhosis. Liver Int 31:1406–1415
19. Kim JK, Chon CY, Kim JH, Kim YJ, Cho JH, Bang SM et al (2007) Changes in serum and ascitic monocyte chemotactic protein-1 (MCP-1) and IL-10 levels in cirrhotic patients with spontaneous bacterial peritonitis. J Interf Cytokine Res 27:227–230
20. Gong Y, Cui S, Li L, Wang M, Guo N (2013) Diagnostic value of human neutrophil peptide in spontaneous bacterial peritonitis. Chin J Hepatol 21: 944–948 [abstract]
21. Abdel-Razik A, Eldars W, Rizk E (2014) Platelet indices and inflammatory markers as diagnostic predictors for ascitic fluid infection. Eur J Gastroenterol Hepatol 26:1342–1347
22. Lesińska M, Hartleb M, Gutkowski K, Nowakowska-Duława E (2014) Procalcitonin and macrophage inflammatory protein-1 beta (MIP-1β) in serum and peritoneal fluid of patients with decompensated cirrhosis and spontaneous bacterial peritonitis. Adv Med Sci 59:52–56
23. Abdel-Razik A, Mousa N, Elbaz S, Eissa M, Elhelaly R, Eldars W (2015) Diagnostic utility of interferon gamma-induced protein 10 kDa in spontaneous bacterial peritonitis: single-center study. Eur J Gastroenterol Hepatol 27:1087–1093
24. Uzzan B, Cohen R, Nicolas P, Cucherat M, Perret GY (2006) Procalcitonin as a diagnostic test for sepsis in critically ill adults and after surgery or trauma: a systematic review and meta-analysis. Crit Care Med 34(7):1996–2003

25. O'Grady NP, Barie PS, Bartlett JG, Bleck T, Carroll K, Kalil AC et al (2008) Guidelines for evaluation of new fever in critically ill adult patients: 2008 update from the American College of Critical Care Medicine and the Infectious Diseases Society of America. Crit Care Med 36(4):1330–1349
26. Wacker C, Prkno A, Brunkhorst FM, Schlattmann P (2013) Procalcitonin as a diagnostic marker for sepsis: a systematic review and meta-analysis. Lancet Infect Dis 13(5):426–435
27. Yang SK, Xiao L, Zhang H, Xu XX, Song PA, Liu FY, Sun L (2014) Significance of serum procalcitonin as biomarker for detection of bacterial peritonitis: a systematic review and meta-analysis. BMC Infect Dis 14:452
28. Cai ZH, Fan CL, Zheng JF, Zhang X, Zhao WM, Li B et al (2015) Measurement of serum procalcitonin levels for the early diagnosis of spontaneous bacterial peritonitis in patients with decompensated liver cirrhosis. BMC Infect Dis 15:55
29. Yang Y, Li L, Qu C, Zeng B, Liang S, Luo Z, Wang X, Zhong C (2015) Diagnostic accuracy of serum procalcitonin for spontaneous bacterial peritonitis due to end-stage liver disease: a meta-analysis. Medicine (Baltimore) 94(49):e2077
30. Abdel-Razik A, Mousa N, Elhammady D, Elhelaly R, Elzehery R, Elbaz S et al (2016) Ascitic fluid calprotectin and serum procalcitonin as accurate diagnostic markers for spontaneous bacterial peritonitis. Gut Liver 10(4):624–631
31. Kim SU, Kim DY, Lee CK, Park JY, Kim SH, Kim HM et al (2010) Ascitic fluid infection in patients with hepatitis B virus-related liver cirrhosis: culture-negative neutrocytic ascites versus spontaneous bacterial peritonitis. J Gastroenterol Hepatol 25(1):122–128
32. Abdel-Razik A, Eldars W, Elhelaly R, Eldeeb AA, Abdelsalam M, El-Wakeel N, Aboulmagd A (2018) Homocysteine a new diagnostic marker in spontaneous bacterial peritonitis. Eur J Gastroenterol Hepatol 30(7):779–785
33. Mikuła T, Sapuła M, Jabłońska J, Kozłowska J, Stańczak W, Krankowska D, Wiercińska-Drapało A (2018) Significance of heparin-binding protein and D-dimers in the early diagnosis of spontaneous bacterial peritonitis. Mediat Inflamm 2018:2018
34. Badawy AA, Zaher TI, Sharaf SM, Emara MH, Shaheen NE, Aly TF (2013) Effect of alternative antibiotics in treatment of cefotaxime resistant spontaneous bacterial peritonitis. World J Gastroenterol 19(8):1271
35. El Motasem EM, Heikal AA, El Haddad HE, Hamdy A, Samie RM, El Din HS (2015) Value of different diagnostic markers in spontaneous bacterial peritonitis in HCV Egyptian cirrhotic patients. Open J Gastroenterol 5(09):119
36. Viallon A, Zeni F, Pouzet V, Lambert C, Quenet S, Aubert G et al (2000) Serum and ascitic procalcitonin levels in cirrhotic patients with spontaneous bacterial peritonitis: diagnostic value and relationship to pro-inflammatory cytokines. Intensive Care Med 26(8):1082–1088
37. Such J, Hillebrand DJ, Guarner C, Berk L, Zapater P, Westengard J et al (2001) Tumor necrosis factor-α, interleukin-6, and nitric oxide in sterile ascitic fluid and serum from patients with cirrhosis who subsequently develop ascitic fluid infection. Digest Dis Sci 46(11):2360–2366
38. Papp M, Vitalis Z, Altorjay I, Tornai I, Udvardy M, Harsfalvi J et al (2012) Acute phase proteins in the diagnosis and prediction of cirrhosis associated bacterial infections. Liver Int 32(4):603–611
39. Wu H, Chen L, Sun Y, Meng C, Hou W (2016) The role of serum procalcitonin and C-reactive protein levels in predicting spontaneous bacterial peritonitis in patients with advanced liver cirrhosis. Pak J Med Sci 32(6):1484–1488
40. Deschénes M, Villeneuve JP (1999) Risk factors for the development of bacterial infections in hospitalized patients with cirrhosis. Am J Gastroenterol 94:2193–2197
41. Luzzani A, Polati E, Dorizzi R, Rungatscher A, Pavan R, Merlini A (2003) Comparison of procalcitonin and C-reactive protein as markers of sepsis. Crit Care Med 31(6):1737–1741
42. Lata J, Stiburek O, Kopacova M (2009) Spontaneous bacterial peritonitis: a severe complication of liver cirrhosis. World J Gastroenterol 15(44):5505
43. Cekin Y, Cekin AH, Duman A, Yilmaz U, Yesil B, Yolcular BO (2013) The role of serum procalcitonin levels in predicting ascitic fluid infection in hospitalized cirrhotic and non-cirrhotic patients. Int J Med Sci 10(10):1367–1374
44. El-Gendy NA, Tawfeek NA, Saleh RA, Radwan EE, Ahmad EE, Mohammed RA (2014) Diagnosis of spontaneous bacterial peritonitis. Egypt J Intern Med 26(2):53
45. Wang H, Li Y, Zhang F, Yang N, Xie N, Mao Y, Li B (2018) Combination of PCT, sNFI and dCHC for the diagnosis of ascites infection in cirrhotic patients. BMC Infect Dis 18(1):389

5

Comparison between NAFLD fibrosis score and retinoic acid serum level in NAFLD

Ahmed Samir Allam[1*], Mohamed Magdy Salama[1], Haytham Mohamed Nasser[2], Walaa Ahmed Yousry Kabiel[3] and Ehab H. Elsayed[4]

Abstract

Background: Non-alcoholic fatty liver disease (NAFLD) is described by the abnormal accumulation of fats in livers of individuals without significant alcohol intake. It includes a spectrum of diseases from simple steatosis to steatohepatitis (NASH) with fibrosis and cirrhosis. The prevalence of NAFLD is rising in association with increasing obesity worldwide. Retinoic acid (RA), a metabolite of vitamin A, mediates the functions of vitamin A required for growth and development. Also, RA has been shown to reduce adiposity not only in fat cells but also in the liver through increasing triglyceride hydrolysis and fat oxidation. This could put a future trial of preventing NASH and cirrhosis development by vitamin A supplementation. This work aimed to study the role of retinoic acid in NAFLD, whether it can differentiate simple steatosis from NASH and correlate the result with the NAFLD fibrosis score. It is a cross-sectional study done on 180 patients divided into three groups. Group 1 is composed of 80 patients with simple steatosis and normal ALT; group 2 is composed of 80 patients with NASH and high ALT in addition to group 3 with 20 healthy subjects served as a control group. All patients were proven to have fatty liver by ultrasonography. Serum RA was assayed by using enzyme-linked immunosorbent assay (ELISA) technique, and the NAFLD fibrosis score was calculated and compared with the retinoic acid level.

Result: Serum RA level was significantly decreased in the patient groups as compared to the controls; the lowest serum level was observed among the NASH group, followed by the steatosis group. NAFLD fibrosis score was calculated, and it was higher in the NASH group than in the steatosis group. Besides, there was a significant negative correlation between retinoic acid and NAFLD score among the patient groups.

Conclusion: Serum RA level was lower in patients with simple steatosis and NASH. RA had a high statistically significant difference in differentiation between the patient groups and the control group. The results were comparable to the NAFLD fibrosis score. Thus, retinoic acid could be used for diagnosis and accessing the degree of NAFLD.

Keywords: NAFLD, NASH, RA, ELISA, NAFLD fibrosis score

Background

Non-alcoholic fatty liver disease (NAFLD) is defined as the presence of hepatic steatosis in the absence of other causes of fat deposition in the liver. NAFLD includes simple steatosis, steatosis with various degrees of inflammation, and fibrosis, which is called non-alcoholic steatohepatitis (NASH). NAFLD is considered the most prevalent liver disease as a result of increased obesity incidence worldwide [1].

* Correspondence: ahm82allam@gmail.com
[1]Internal Medicine Department, Faculty of Medicine, Ain Shams University, Cairo 11211, Egypt

Simple steatosis is a benign disease; however, NASH is considered to be a potentially health-threatening inflammation that may progress to cirrhosis, liver cell failure, and Hepatocellular carcinoma (HCC) [2]. Recently, there has been an increase in the mortality rate and the number of liver transplantations as a result of NASH complications. Non-alcoholic steatohepatitis (NASH) is now the second indication for liver transplantation in the USA [3].

At present, the gold standard technique for NASH diagnosis is a liver biopsy; nonetheless, it is an invasive procedure with possible serious complications and limitations [4]. NAFLD diagnosis requires the presence of hepatic steatosis either by imaging or histology in the absence of significant alcohol consumption [5].

Scoring systems using clinical and/or laboratory parameters to identify patients with NASH from the larger pool of NAFLD patients have been evaluated [6]. The most commonly used is the NAFLD fibrosis scoring system, which uses six commonly measured parameters. These include age, hyperglycemia, body mass index (BMI), platelet count, albumin level, and AST/ALT ratio. By using a low cut-off score, the NPV for excluding advanced fibrosis was around 88%. When a high cut-off scores (0.676) was used, the PPV for predicting advanced fibrosis was almost 90% [7].

Many serum markers were proposed for diagnosis of the NAFLD, but all are still not yet approved [8]. Retinoic acid (RA), a metabolite of vitamin A (retinol), mediates the functions of vitamin A required for growth and development through binding with the retinoic acid receptor (RAR) and retinoic acid X receptor (RXR), which then regulates the target gene expression [9].

Vitamin A is linked to NAFLD as the liver is the primary storage site of vitamin A, and vitamin A has a role in the control of adipose tissue [10]. Vitamin A is stored in the quiescent hepatic stellate cells (qHSC), and these cells are responsible for fibrogenesis. When qHSC get activated to become profibrogenic HSC, the activated HSC lose their vitamin A content. The retinoic acid role was proposed to effectively reduce adiposity in the liver and enhance hepatic fat catabolism [11].

Aim of the work

The present work aimed to study the clinical relevance of retinoic acid in patients with NAFLD and to detect its ability to differentiate simple steatosis from NASH and correlate its results with NAFLD fibrosis score.

Methods

It is a cross-sectional study. Subjects in this study were recruited from the in-patient ward and the outpatient clinic of the Internal Medicine Department of Ain Shams University Hospitals from the period of October 2016 to January 2018. Informed written consent was obtained from each participant before enrolment in the study. Moreover, the study was approved by the Research Ethics Committee of Ain Shams University.

The included subjects were classified into group 1 which is composed of 80 patients with simple steatosis proved by ultrasound to have fatty liver, with normal ALT, and group 2 which is composed of 80 patients with non-alcoholic steatohepatitis (NASH) proved by ultrasound to have fatty liver, with high ALT. All other causes of hepatitis, fibrosis, and cirrhosis such as viral hepatitis B and C, alcoholic liver disease, drug-induced hepatitis, e.g., isoniazid and α-methyldopa, drug-induced fatty liver, e.g., corticosteroids and amiodarone, metabolic liver diseases including Wilson disease, α-1 antitrypsin and hemochromatosis, autoimmune hepatitis, primary biliary cirrhosis, and sclerosing cholangitis were excluded from the study. In addition to group 3, 20 age and sex-matched subjects, served as a healthy control group.

A full history was taken from all individuals included in this study with a thorough clinical examination with particular emphasis on anthropometric evaluation (measures of body weight and height) for calculation of body mass index. All participants in this study were subjected to routine laboratory hematology and chemistry assay including complete blood picture, liver function tests (albumin, INR, total and direct bilirubin, ALT, AST, and alkaline phosphatase), HCV Ab and HBsAg, kidney function tests (serum creatinine and blood urea), fasting blood sugar, HbA1C, lipid profile. Estimation of serum retinoic acid level throughout the enzyme-linked immunosorbent assay (ELISA) technique according to the manufacturer's instructions. Serum RA levels were measured using the commercial ELISA kit supplied by Life Science Company.

Abdominal ultrasonography was done for all subjects for diagnosis of non-alcoholic fatty liver and exclusion of other etiologies.

NAFLD fibrosis score was also calculated for all patients. It was calculated as per the following formula: $- 1.675 + 0.037 \times$ age (years) $+ 0.094 \times$ body mass index (BMI, kg/m^2) $+ 1.13 \times$ impaired fasting glucose/diabetes (yes = 1, no = 0) $+ 0.99 \times$ AST/ALT ratio $- 0.013 \times$ platelet ($\times$ 109/L) $- 0.66 \times$ albumin (g/dL). The result was interpreted as low NFS ($<- 1.445$), indeterminate NFS ($- 1.445$ to 0.676), and high NFS (> 0.676) [12].

Results

This study included 180 patients who were divided into three groups: group 1, 80 patients with simple steatosis and normal ALT; group 2, 80 patients with NASH with high ALT; and group 3, 20 healthy subjects.

Table 1 showed that there was no significant difference between the studied groups regarding sex, age, and BMI.

Table 2 showed that there were no significant differences between the studied groups regarding AST, albumin, HbA1c, total cholesterol, and triglycerides. Retinoic acid level had high statistically significant difference among the studied groups, as the lowest levels were in NASH group, and the highest levels were in the control group. NAFLD score was higher in the NASH group than in the steatosis group, with a high statistically significant difference between the control and the patient groups.

Figure 1 showed that the retinoic acid level lowest levels were in NASH group, and the highest levels were in the control group with a high statistically significant difference among the studied groups.

Table 1 Sex, age, and body mass index BMI among the studied groups

Variables	Measures	Group 1	Group 2	Group 3	P
Sex (n, %)	Male	52 (65.0%)	50 (62.5%)	14 (70.0%)	0.902[b]
	Female	28 (35.0%)	30 (37.5%)	6 (30.0%)	
Age (years)	Mean ± SD	53.5 ± 6.3	53.5 ± 5.2	52.5±6.3	0.880[a]
	Range	40.0–76.0	42.0–66.0	40.0–61.0	
BMI (kg/m^2)	Mean ± SD	30.9 ± 2.2	31.0 ± 2.2	29.0±1.2	0.82[a]
	Range	25.9–36.3	27.3–37.3	26.7–34.3	

Group 1 simple steatosis and normal ALT, *Group 2* NASH and high ALT, *Group 3* control group, *BMI* body mass index, *SD* standard deviation
[a]ANOVA test with post hoc Tukey test
[b]Chi square test

Figure 2 showed that the NAFLD score was higher in the NASH group than the steatosis group, with a high statistically significant difference in the differentiation between NASH Group and the steatosis group.

Table 3 showed that there were significant negative correlations between HbA1C, TC, retinoic acid, and NAFLD score among the patient groups.

Table 4 showed that retinoic acid level showed a high statistically significant difference among the studied groups. NAFLD score had a high statistically significant difference in the differentiation between the NASH group and the steatosis group.

Table 5 showed that in the differentiation between group 1 and group 3, retinoic acid value ≤ 120.0 had high diagnostic accuracy, while NAFLD score ≥− 3.25 had high sensitivity and PPV.

Table 6 showed that in differentiation between group 1 and group 2, retinoic acid value ≤ 87.0 had high sensitivity and negative predictive value, while NAFLD score ≥− 0.10 had a high specificity and positive predictive value.

Discussion

At present, non-alcoholic fatty liver disease (NAFLD) is assumed to be the most common chronic liver disease. Retinoic acid (RA) is primarily involved in the regulation of lipid metabolism and hepatic steatosis [13].

Although some studies showed that RA supplementation might be a promising therapeutic approach in fatty liver disease, the clinical relevance of RA in the pathogenesis of hepatic steatosis and NAFLD has not been carefully investigated. So, the present study was designed to study the role of retinoic acid in the development and progression of NAFLD from simple steatosis to NASH and to compare the results with the NAFLD fibrosis score. After approval of the institutional review board, this study was conducted at the Internal Medicine Department, Ain Shams University Hospitals. Informed consent was obtained from all subjects enrolled in the study.

Our study obtained samples from 80 patients in group 1 (52 males and 28 females), 80 patients in group 2 (50 males and 30 females), and 20 control patients (14 males and 6 females). There were no significant differences between the studied groups regarding age and sex. Also, Liu et al. (2015) [14] showed that were no significant differences in age or female to male ratio between subjects in control, NAFLD, and NASH groups. On the other hand, Chaves et al. (2008) [15] showed that the mean

Table 2 AST, albumin, HbA1C, total cholesterol, and triglycerides among the studied groups

Variables	Measures	Group 1	Group 2	Group 3	P
AST (IU/L)	Mean ± SD	27.1 ± 13.1	27.8 ± 16.2	26.2 ± 3.4	0.944
	Range	14.0–79.0	11.0–75.0	21.0–31.0	
Albumin (gm/dL)	Mean ± SD	3.7 ± 0.4	3.6 ± 0.4	4.2 ± 0.4	0.935
	Range	3.2–4.9	3.4–4.3	3.8–4.8	
HbA1C	Mean ± SD	5.9 ± 1.1	6.2 ± 1.8	4.9 ± 0.95	0.044
	Range	5.3–6.9	5.7–7.8	4.75–5.7	
Total cholesterol (mg/dl)	Mean ± SD	196 ± 36	176 ± 43	180 ± 42	0.079
	Range	180–213	216–263	160–190	
Triglycerides (mg/dl)	Mean ± SD	170 ± 32	186 ± 44	122 ± 28	0.064
	Range	140–210	153–237	110–150	
Retinoic Acid (ng/ml)	Mean ± SD	110.1 ± 39.9	54.7 ± 28.4	190.9 ± 37.2	< 0.001[a]
	Range	68–225	16–102	125–230	
NAFLD score	Mean ± SD	− 1.97 ± 1.63	0.68 ± 1.18	− 2.83 ± 0.57	< 0.001[a]
	Range	− 5.80 to − 1.12	− 2.27–6.12	− 3.66 to − 2.12	

Group 1 simple steatosis and normal ALT, *Group 2* NASH and high ALT, *Group 3* control group, *ALT* alanine aminotransferase, *AST* aspartate aminotransferase
ANOVA test with post hoc Tukey test
[a]Significant

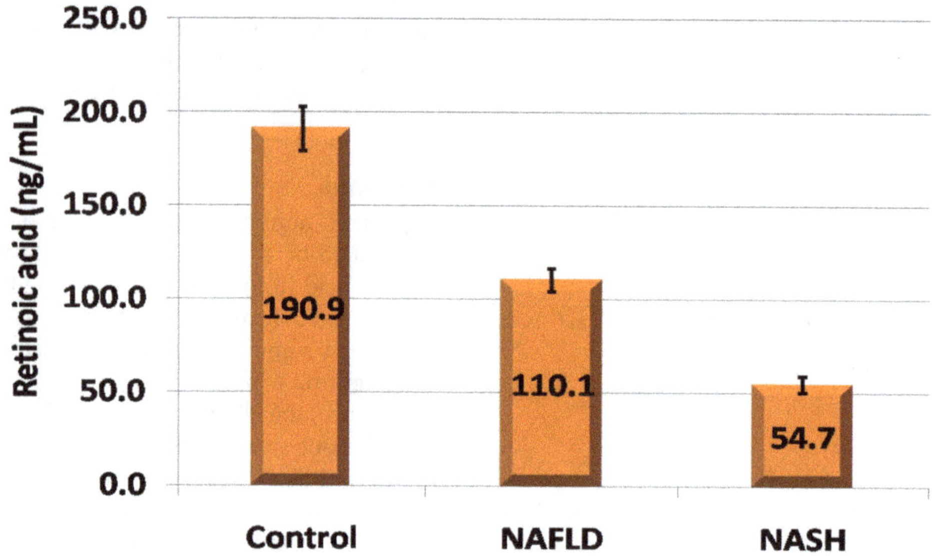

Fig. 1 Retinoic acid among the studied groups (normal level 9.3 ng/ml–300 ng/ml)

age was significantly higher within the NAFLD group with and without steatosis.

Also, there was no significant difference in BMI between the studied groups, and this in disagreement with the studies of Liu et al. (2015)(14) and Bottella et al. (2011) [16] who showed significant difference in BMI between studied groups with higher BMI in NAFLD than the control groups; however, in their study, they selected patient group to be obese from the start. The high prevalence of obesity could explain this in Egyptian people; that is why both patients and controls were obese from the start with no significant statistical difference between them.

The present study showed that FBG had the lowest levels among the control group, followed by the steatosis group and had the highest levels in the NASH group, with no significant differences between the studied groups. Liu et al. (2015) [14] stated that the concentration of fasting plasma glucose in subjects with NAFLD and NASH was significantly higher than that in control subjects.

Miyazaki et al. 2012 [17] showed that BMI, ALT, and LDH were significantly higher in NAFLD patients than in the control group. Nutritional parameters, including total cholesterol, triglyceride, and fasting plasma glucose levels, were higher in the NAFLD patients than in the control group, although these differences were not statistically significant.

HbA1C was significantly higher in the patient groups than the control group with no significant difference between the steatosis group and the NASH group, but TG and TC showed no significant difference between studied groups.

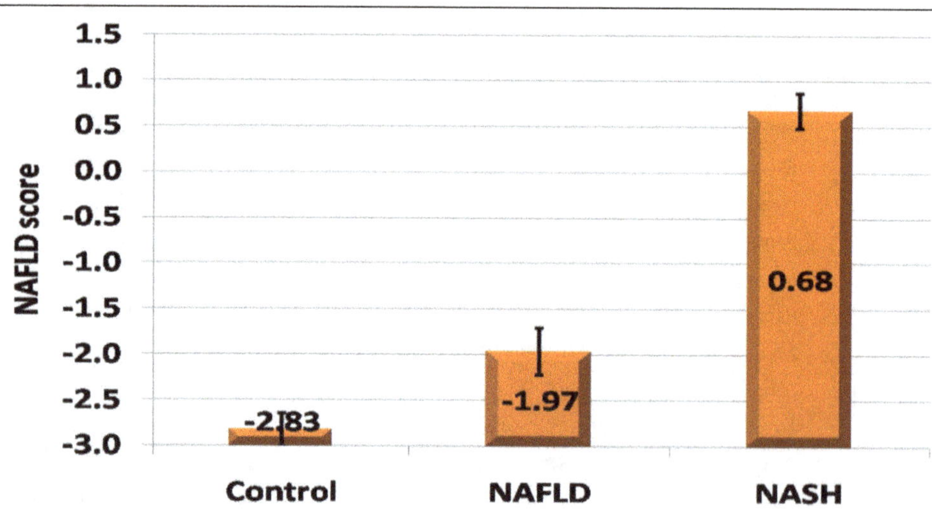

Fig. 2 NAFLD score among the studied groups

Table 3 Correlation between retinoic acid and other variables among the studied groups

Variables	Measures	Group 1	Group 2	Group 3
Age	*R*	− 0.023	− 0.135	− 0.084
	P	0.890	0.735	0.817
BMI	*R*	− 0.178	− 0.087	0.387
	P	0.271	0.598	0.270
FBG	*R*	− 0.213	− 0.171	0.203
	P	0.187	0.293	0.575
AST	*R*	− 0.072	− 0.005	0.028
	P	0.658	0.977	0.939
PLT	*R*	0.185	0.169	− 0.136
	P	0.874	0.298	0.708
Albumin	*R*	0.082	0.166	0.318
	P	0.613	0.306	0.371
NAFLD score	*R*	− 0.327	− 0.499	0.285
	P	0.039[a]	< 0.001[a]	0.424
HbA1C	*R*	− 0.427	− 0.627	− 0.072
	P	0.029[a]	0.019[a]	0.658
TC (mg/dl)	*R*	− 0.0.528	− 0.0.728	0.387
	P	0.0.015[a]	0.0.005[a]	0.270
T.G (mg)	*R*	− 0.359	− 0.659	− 0.087
	P	0.032[a]	0.244	0.598

Group 1 simple steatosis and normal ALT, *Group 2* NASH and high ALT, *Group 3* control group, *BMI* body mass index, *FBG* fasting blood glucose, *AST* aspartate aminotransferase, *PLT* platelets, *TC* total cholesterol, *TG* triglycerides Pearson correlation, [a]Significant

Our study showed that serum retinoic acid level was significantly different among the studied groups, was lowest in the NASH group, followed by the steatosis group and highest in the control group and this was in accordance with Mourad et al. 2018 [18] and Pettinelli et al. 2018 [19].

However, other studies displayed no significant differences between control and NAFLD adults as Cengiz et al. 2010 [20] or even higher serum retinol in patients with NAFLD compared with a control group in Alkhouri et al. 2009 [21]. Senno et al. 2010 [11] found a positive correlation between serum retinol values and concentrations of AST and ALT in NAFLD. Serum retinol was the only biochemical variable that could predict AST and ALT concentrations in these patients, pointing to retinol as a potential marker for liver damage.

Table 5 Diagnostic characteristics of retinoic acid and NAFLD score in differentiating group 1 from group 3

Characters	Value	95% CI
Retinoic acid ≤ 120.0		
Sensitivity	80.0%	64.4–90.9%
Specificity	76.3%	69.2–100.0%
Diagnostic accuracy (DA)	84.0%	70.9–92.8%
Positive predictive value (PPV)	74.2%	89.1–100.0%
Negative predictive value (NPV)	55.6%	30.8–78.5%
Positive likelihood ratio (LR+)	> 100.0	> 100.0–> 100.0
Negative likelihood ratio (LR–)	0.20	0.11–0.37
NAFLD score ≥− 3.25		
Sensitivity	85.0%	70.2–94.3%
Specificity	60.0%	26.2–87.8%
Diagnostic accuracy (DA)	80.0%	66.3–90.0%
Positive predictive value (PPV)	89.5%	75.2–97.1%
Negative predictive value (NPV)	50.0%	21.1–78.9%
Positive likelihood ratio (LR+)	2.13	0.98–4.59
Negative likelihood ratio (LR–)	0.25	0.10–0.61

CI confidence interval, *Group 1* simple steatosis and normal ALT, *Group 2* NASH and high ALT, *Group 3* control group

NAFLD score was higher in the NASH group than the steatosis group, with a high statistically significant difference in the differentiation between NASH group and the steatosis group.

The correlation analysis revealed a negative correlation between retinoic acid and NAFLD score among the steatosis group and the NASH group. The receiver operating characteristics (ROC) curve was used to define the best cutoff value of serum retinoic acid level. Retinoic acid had a significantly high statistical difference in the differentiation between the study groups similar to that of NAFLD fibrosis score.

Some limitations need to be discussed in the present study. First, more randomized controlled clinical trials in human subjects are required to confirm the fundamental role of low RA concentrations in NAFLD and to correlate the results with a liver biopsy; besides, the possible

Table 4 Diagnostic performance of retinoic acid and NAFLD score in differentiation between the studied groups

Group	Variable	AUC	SE	*P*	95% CI	Cut-off
Group 1 from group 3	Retinoic	0.920	0.038	< 0.001[a]	0.845–0.995	≤ 120.0
	Score	0.785	0.063	0.006[a]	0.662–0.908	≥− 3.25
Group 2 from group 1	Retinoic	0.912	0.030	< 0.001[a]	0.852–0.971	≤ 87.0
	Score	0.942	0.025	< 0.001[a]	0.893–0.991	≥− 0.10

AUC area under curve, *SE* standard error, *CI* confidence interval, *Group 1* simple steatosis and normal ALT, *Group 2* NASH and high ALT, *Group 3* control group
[a]Significant

Table 6 Diagnostic characteristics of retinoic acid and NAFLD score in differentiating group 1 from group 2

Characters	Value	95% CI
Retinoic acid ≤ 87.0		
Sensitivity	82.5%	67.2–92.7%
Specificity	77.5%	61.5–89.2%
Diagnostic accuracy (DA)	80.0%	69.6–88.1%
Positive predictive value (PPV)	78.6%	63.2–89.7%
Negative predictive value (NPV)	81.6%	65.7–92.3%
Positive likelihood ratio (LR+)	3.67	2.03–6.63
Negative likelihood ratio (LR–)	0.23	0.11–0.45
NAFLD score ≥– 0.10		
Sensitivity	80.0%	64.4–90.9%
Specificity	97.5%	86.8–99.9%
Diagnostic accuracy (DA)	88.8%	79.7–94.7%
Positive predictive value (PPV)	97.0%	84.2–99.9%
Negative predictive value (NPV)	83.0%	69.2–92.4%
Positive likelihood ratio (LR+)	32.00	4.59–223.01
Negative likelihood ratio (LR–)	0.21	0.11–0.38

CI confidence interval, *Group 1* simple steatosis and normal ALT, *Group 2* NASH and high ALT, *Group 3* control group

preventive or therapeutic advantage of RA needs to be evaluated to confirm its benefits and safety.

Furthermore, in diagnosing NAFLD in the studied groups, most of the previous studies used ultrasound only, which is limited by its inability to differentiate mild steatosis from fibrosis and to accurately quantify fatty infiltration; besides, it is an operator dependent. Others used a liver biopsy, which is an invasive method with possible serious complications. Nevertheless, in our study, we used, in addition to ultrasound, NAFLD fibrosis score, which is one of the accurate scores in diagnosing and differentiation simple steatosis from NASH and compared its results with RA serum levels.

Magnetic resonance elastography (MRE) is a non-invasive medical imaging technique that measures liver stiffness can also be used; however, the issue of the cost and the availability of the MRI needs to be discussed. This may open new insights on the use of serum retinoic acid in NAFLD as regards the cost per test, and being a single biomarker could be less costly than variable laboratory parameters already used right now or imaging techniques as MRE.

Conclusion

The present study showed that serum RA was lower in patients with simple steatosis and NASH with high statistical significant differences in differentiation between the patient groups and the control group. NAFLD fibrosis score had high sensitivity in differentiating the NAFLD groups from the control group and in differentiating the steatosis group from the NASH group. Additionally, there were significant negative correlations between retinoic acid and NAFLD score among steatosis and NASH groups. Serum RA concentration is lowest in the NASH group. Consequently, Retinoic Acid can be used as a single non-invasive tool for diagnosis and assessing the degree of NAFLD and possibly differentiating simple steatosis from NASH.

Abbreviations

ALT : Alanine aminotransferase; ANOVA: Analysis of variance; AST: Aspartate aminotransferase; AUC: Area under the curve; BMI: Body mass index; CBC: Complete blood count; CI: Confidence interval; DA: Diagnostic accuracy; ELISA: Enzyme-linked immunosorbent assay; FBG: Fasting blood glucose; Hb: Hemoglobin; HBV: Hepatitis B virus; HCC: Hepatocellular carcinoma; HCV: Hepatitis C virus; HSC: Hepatic stellate cells; INR: International normalized ratio; K: Potassium; LR+: Positive likelihood ratio; LR–: Negative likelihood ratio; MR: Magnetic resonance elastography; Na: Sodium; NAFLD: Non-alcoholic fatty liver disease; NASH: Non-alcoholic steatohepatitis.; NFS: NAFLD fibrosis score; NPV: Negative predictive value; PLT: Platelets; PPV: Positive predictive value; qHSC: quiescent hepatic stellate cells; RA: Retinoic acid; RAR: Retinoic acid receptor; ROC-curve: Receiver operating characteristic curve; RXR: Retinoic acid X receptor; SD: Standard deviation; TC: Total cholesterol; TG: Triglycerides

Acknowledgements
Not applicable

Authors' contributions

ASA and MMS conceived and planned the experiments. WAK contributed to sample preparation. HMN performed the ultrasound to the patients. EE contributed to final manuscript editing and revision. All authors provided critical feedback and helped shape the research, analysis and manuscript. All authors have read and approved the manuscript

Competing interests

The authors declare that they have no competing interest.

Author details
Internal Medicine Department, Faculty of Medicine, Ain Shams University, Cairo 11211, Egypt. [2]Radiology Department, Faculty of Medicine, Ain Shams University, Cairo, Egypt. [3]Clinical Pathology Department, Faculty of Medicine, Ain Shams University, Cairo 11211, Egypt. [4]Tropical Medicine Department, National Research Center, Cairo 11211, Egypt.

References

1. Hazlehurst JM, and Tomlinson JW (2013)Non-alcoholic fatty liver disease in common endocrine disorders 169:R27-37. doi: https//doi.org/10.1530/EJE-13-0296
2. Nascimbeni F, Pais R, Bellentani S et al (2013) From NAFLD in clinical practice to answers from guidelines. J Hepatol 59:859–871
3. Zhu JZ, Dai YN, Wang YM et al (2015) Prevalence of nonalcoholic fatty liver disease and economy. Dig Dis Sci 60:3194–3202
4. Bell LN, Theodorakis JL, Vuppalanchi R et al (2010) Serum proteomics and biomarker discovery across the spectrum of nonalcoholic fatty liver disease. Hepatology 51:111–120
5. Chalasani N, Younossi Z, Lavine JE et al (2012) The diagnosis and management of non-alcoholic fatty liver disease: practice guideline by the American Association for the Study of Liver Diseases, American College of Gastroenterology, and the Amer-ican Gastroenterological Association. Hepatology 55:2005–2023
6. Ratziu V, Giral P, Charlotte F et al (2000) Liver fibrosis in overweight patients. Gastroenterology 118:1117–1123
7. Angulo P, Hui JM, Marchesini G et al (2007) The NAFLD fibrosis score: a noninvasive system that identifies liver fibrosis in patients with NAFLD. Hepatology 45:846–854

8. Machado MV, Cortex-Pinto H (2013) Noninvasive diagnosis of non-alcoholic fatty liver disease: A critical appraisal. J Hepatol 58:1007–1019
9. Kam RK, Deng Y, Chen Y. et al. (2012) Retinoic acid synthesis and functions in early embyronic developement Cell Biosci 2: 11.
10. Mondul A, Mancina RM, Merlo A et al (2015) PNPLA3 I148M variant influences circulating retinol in adults with nonalcoholic fatty liver disease or obesity. J Nutr 145:1687–1691
11. Senoo H, Yoshikawa K, Morii M et al (2010) Hepatic stellate cell (vitamin A-stor-ing cell) and it's relative – past, present and future. Cell Biol Int 34: 1247–1272
12. Rinella M.(2015)Non-alcoholic fatty liver disease: a systematic review313: 2263-73. doi: https://doi.org/10.1001/jama.2015.5370.
13. Bonet ML, Ribot J, Palou A (2012) Lipid metabolism in mammalian tissues and its control by retinoic acid. Biochim Biophys Acta 1821:177–189
14. Liu Y, Chen H, Wang J et al (2015) Association of serum retinoic acid with hepatic steatosis and liver injury in non-alcoholic fatty liver disease. Am J Clin Nutr 102:130–137
15. Chaves G, Pereira SE, Saboya CJ et al (2008) Non-alcoholic Fatty Liver Disease and Its Relationship with the Nutritional Status of Vitamin A in Individuals with Class III Obesity. Obes Surg 18:378. https://doi.org/10.1007/s11695-007-9361-2
16. Botella-Carretero JI, Balsa JA, Vázquez C et al (2010) Retinol and alpha-tocopherol in morbid obesity and nonalcoholic fatty liver disease. Obes Surg 20:69–76
17. Miyazaki M, Kato M, Tanaka K et al (2012) Increased hepatic expression of dipeptidyl peptidase-4 in non-alcoholic fatty liver disease and its association with insulin resistance and glucose metabolism. Mol Med Rep 5:729–733
18. Mourad F, El Sayeda Z, Showmana H, Abo RM, Mohamed N (2018) The role of serum retinol in nonalcoholic fatty liver disease. Sci J Al-Azhar Med Fac Girls 2:115–122
19. Pettinelli P, Arendt BM, Teterina A, McGilvray I, Comelli EM, Fung SK, Fischer SE, Allard JP (2018) Altered hepatic genes related to retinol metabolism and plasma retinol in patients with non-alcoholic fatty liver disease. PLoS One. 13:e0205747
20. Cengiz C, Ardicoglu Y, Bulut S, Boyacioglu S (2010) Serum retinol-binding protein 4 in patients with nonalcoholic fatty liver disease: does it have a significant impact on pathogenesis? Eur J Gastroenterol Hepatol 22:813–819
21. Alkhouri N, Lopez R, Berk M, Feldstein A (2009) Serum retinol-binding protein 4 levels in patients with nonalcoholic fatty liver disease. J Clin Gastroenterol 43:985–989

6

Liver biopsy is still needed in liver transplantation recipients: a single center experience

Eman Abdelsameea[1*], Ayman Alsebaey[1], Nermine Ehsan[2], Ahmed Elrefaey[2], Khalid Aboelela[3], El-Sayed Ibrahim[1] and Maha Elsabaawy[1]

Abstract

Background: Liver transplantation is a final treatment for decompensated liver disease.

Aim: Description of post-liver transplant histopathology. We enrolled 89 patients divided into two groups according to if they underwent on demand liver biopsy (n = 34; 38.2%) or not (n = 55; 61.8%). Albumin-bilirubin (ALBI) score and model for end-stage liver disease (MELD) assessed the degree of liver dysfunction.

Results: Patient underwent liver biopsy (LB) was 44.65 ± 8.46 years old, mainly males (88.2%) with average MELD of 8.74 ± 4.71. Most patients were positive pre-transplant for HCV (91.2%) and 29.4% had hepatocellular carcinoma on top of hepatitis C. Patients underwent LB had worse liver dysfunction by ALBI score (− 2.62 ± 0.6 vs. − 2.96 ± 0.5; p = 0.014) but comparable MELD. The time till first biopsy was 19.88 ± 11.22 (4-44) months. It was not different statistically with various histopathology ($p > 0.05$). Histopathology of first biopsy was viral chronic hepatitis (50%), acute rejection (20.6%), steatohepatitis (11.8%), chronic rejection (5.9%), chronic hepatitis (5.9%), biliary obstruction (2.9%), and cytomegalovirus hepatitis (2.9%). Most patients were F1 (38.2%) and A1 (35.3%). The immunosuppressive drug regimen had no impact on the histopathology ($p > 0.05$). Patients with hepatitis C pre-transplant had in a descending manner the following histological diagnosis (p = 0.001): viral chronic hepatitis 16 (51.6%), acute rejection 7 (22.6%), steatohepatitis 4 (12.9%), chronic rejection 2 (6.5%), biliary obstruction 1 (3.2%), and CMV hepatitis 1(3.2%). Some patients required on demand second (n = 9) and third biopsied (n = 5) that were the same as the first biopsy or completely different.

Conclusion: Liver biopsy is a useful tool for diagnosis of liver transplantation complications.

Keywords: Liver, Biopsy, Liver transplantation, Rejection, Recurrent post-transplant

Background

Liver transplantation (LT) is a final treatment for end stage liver diseases. LT improves the quality of life and is a definitive therapy for metabolic liver diseases as Wilson's disease and hemochromatosis. Liver transplantation is associated with a lot of complications for example nonfunctioning graft, rejection, vascular complications, biliary complications, infections, and viral recurrence [1].

The diagnosis of the various events or complications can be done noninvasively with laboratory and radiological investigations as with vascular and biliary complications [2]. Nonetheless, some complications can be diagnosed only with the aid of liver biopsy as acute cellular rejection, recurrent autoimmune hepatitis, and steatohepatitis [3, 4].

Liver biopsy is invasive technique for obtaining samples from the liver tissue for histopathology. In fact, it is the golden standard for diagnosis of liver fibrosis and

* Correspondence: dreman555@yahoo.co.uk
[1]Department of Hepatology and Gastroenterology, National Liver Institute, Menoufia University, Shebeen El-Koom 32511, Egypt

inflammation [5]. Besides, it can detect other associated diseases as steatosis and sarcoidosis. It is useful also for follow up, assessing progression, or regression of the disease and efficacy of therapy. Although liver biopsy is a safe maneuver, yet it is associated with some disadvantages, some of them may be life dangerous as bleeding. The common complications range from pain, hematoma, organ injury, and fistulation. Another point that may affect the histopathology is the heterogeneous distribution of the disease within the liver, along with inter and intra-observer variation [6].

This study aimed to describe the diagnostic role of liver biopsy in the recipients of liver transplantation.

Methods

This is a retrospective study that was conducted at National Liver Institute Hospitals, Menoufia University after approval by the institutional review board. Data were taken from the medical records in the liver transplantation unit.

From 2003 to 2015, about 198 adult patients underwent living donor liver transplantation. Eighty-nine patients were included in the study as 99 patients died and 10 patients travelled abroad and their data was not available. The patients were divided into two groups according to if they underwent on demand liver biopsy (n = 34; 38.2%) or not (n = 55; 61.8%).

All the patients received intraoperative methylprednisolone as 10 mg/kg during the anhepatic phase and after operation they were shifted to the intensive care unit (ICU) [7]. In the ICU, the following lab tests were done every 12 h: liver functions, renal functions, complete blood counts, international normalized ratio (INR), uric acid, electrolytes, C-reactive protein, cholesterol, serum phosphate, serum lactate, fibrinogen, and fibrin degradation products. Doppler on the hepatic artery, portal vein, and hepatic veins was done every 4 h. Prophylactic antibiotics, antifungals, anticoagulants, and antiviral as acyclovir were given [1].

The patients were usually shifted to ward on the 8th day where anticoagulant therapies are shifted to antiplatelets as dipyridamole, and the investigations were done once daily. After discharge, the patients had a visit every week for 2 months then monthly till the end of the first year after which the visit was every 3 months.

In that era, the only available treatment for hepatitis C virus (HCV) infection was pegylated interferon/ribavirin with poor results. The direct acting antivirals for hepatitis C were not available. The treatment was deferred after 6-12 months and was given if the fibrosis stage was F3-4 Metavir by liver biopsy with features of recurrent viral hepatitis. Lamivudine and hepatitis B immunoglobulin were given for patients with hepatitis B.

The following immunosuppressive drugs were used: calcineurin inhibitors (tacrolimus, cyclosporine), steroids, mTOR inhibitors (sirolimus, everolimus), mycophenolate mofetil, or mycophenolic acid. Induction with basiliximab was used for patients with pre-transplant renal impairment or calcineurin inhibitors sparing.

The usual applied immunosuppressive therapy was the triple steroids, tacrolimus, and mycophenolate mofetil per os. Patients intolerant to mycophenolate mofetil were shifted to mycophenolic acid per os. Patients developed side effects with tacrolimus were shifted to oral cyclosporine. Patients with renal impairment shifted to sirolimus and in the last years to everolimus [8, 9].

On the time of biopsy, the following regimens were applied: 17.6% (cyclosporine and mycophenolate mofetil), 17.6% (sirolimus and mycophenolic acid), 17.6% (tacrolimus and mycophenolate mofetil), 14.7% (cyclosporine, sirolimus, and mycophenolate mofetil), 14.7% (tacrolimus monotherapy), 5.9% (sirolimus monotherapy), 2.9% (tacrolimus, everolimus, and mycophenolate mofetil), 2.9% (tacrolimus, sirolimus, and mycophenolate mofetil), 2.9% (everolimus and mycophenolate mofetil), and 2.9% (cyclosporine monotherapy).

Protocol biopsies were not adopted by our center. Only on demand biopsies were applied with the following conditions: sudden elevation or deterioration of the liver enzymes not responding to adjustment of the immunosuppressive drugs, confirmation of cytomegalovirus hepatitis, pre-pegylated interferon/ribavirin therapy, cholestasis of unclear diagnosis, unclear diagnosis of liver focal lesions, suspicion of recurrent disease, or steatohepatitis. It is to be noted that the vascular causes were excluded by Doppler ultrasonography and CT angiography. The biliary causes were excluded by preliminary ultrasonography confirmed by magnetic resonance cholangiopancreatography.

Sonar guided transcutaneous liver biopsy under complete aseptic technique was done [10]. The slides were read by 2 blinded pathologists to avoid interobserver variation. Fibrosis stage and the histological activity were assessed by Metavir score [10].

Calculations for assessing degree of liver dysfunction: Albumin-bilirubin (ALBI) score [11] = ($\log_{10}$ bilirubin μmol/L × 0.66) + (albumin g/L × −0.085).

Model for end-stage liver disease (MELD) [12] = 3:78 ln [serum total bilirubin (mg/dL)] + 11:2 ln [INR] + 9:57 ln [serum creatinine (mg/dL)] + 6:43.

Statistical analysis

Data were statistically analyzed using IBM® SPSS® Statistics® version 21 for Windows (IBM Corporation, North Castle Drive, Armonk, NY, USA). Data were expressed as mean ± standard deviation and number percentage for nominal data. All p values are 2 tailed, with values <

0.05 considered statistically significant. Comparisons between two groups were performed using the Student's *t* test for normally distributed data, and Mann-Whitney test for nonparametric data that lacks the normal distribution. CHI-squared test (χ^2) was done for nominal data comparison.

Results

In the current study as shown in Tables 1 and 2, most patients who underwent liver biopsy (n = 34) were 44.65 ± 8.46 years old and mainly males 30 (88.2%). The age ranged from 25 to 58 years old. They had average 8.74 ± 4.71 MELD score. The laboratory parameters were as follows: total bilirubin 1.96 ± 2.50 mg/dL, serum albumin 4.11 ± 0.62 g/dL, aspartate aminotransferase (AST) 111.79 ± 67.08 U/L, alanine aminotransferase (ALT) 125.59 ± 70.42 U/L, alkaline phosphatase (ALP) 541.45 ± 1185.65 U/L, gamma glutamyl transpeptidase (GGT) 486.3 ± 653.2 U/L, serum creatinine 0.98 ± 0.29 mg/dL, WBCs 6 ± 2.27 10^9/L, platelets 167.82 ± 83.32 10^9/L, and INR was 1.05 ± 0.22.

Wide fluctuations were found in the liver tests where with AST that ranged 30-270 U/L, ALT ranged 20-303 U/L, GGT 11-3408 U/L, and finally marked fluctuation with ALP 81-7120 U/L.

The indications of liver transplantation were diverse. From virological point, most patients who underwent liver biopsy were mainly HCV positive: 31(91.2%) and one case 1(2.9%) had dual hepatitis B virus (HBV) and HCV coinfection. Two patients were virus free. In fact patients who underwent liver biopsy had multiple indications as follows: HCV; 21(61.8%), hepatocellular carcinoma (HCC) on top of HCV; 10(29.4%), HCC on top of dual HBV and HCV coinfection; 1(2.9%), primary sclerosing cholangitis (PSC); 1(2.9%) and autoimmune hepatitis (AIH); 1(2.9%).

Patients were followed up for 51.53 ± 15.92 (10.0-93 months). The average time from transplant operation to the first biopsy was 19.88 ± 11.22 ranging from 4-44 months.

The histopathology revealed 7 diagnoses in a descending pattern as the following (Fig. 1): chronic viral hepatitis, 17 (50%); acute rejection, 7 (20.6%); steatohepatitis, 4 (11.8%); chronic rejection, 2 (5.9%), chronic hepatitis, 2 (5.9%); biliary obstruction, 1 (2.9%); and cytomegalovirus (CMV) infection, 1 (2.9%).

Chronic viral hepatitis was defined histologically by portal tract mononuclear inflammatory infiltrate with lymphoid aggregate formation, interface hepatitis, parenchymal necroinflammation, and steatosis as shown in Fig. 1a. Portal tract fibrosis varied in different cases, ranged from F0-F4 according to METAVAIR scoring system. Acute cellular rejection (ACR) revealed a wide range of histological presentations. A portal tract triad of histopathological findings in the form of mixed inflammatory cellular infiltrate, venular endothelietis, and bile duct injury was a typical diagnosis for ACR (Fig. 1b). Other histopathological changes were also noticed

Table 1 Characteristics of the liver transplant recipients that were biopsied

	M ± SD	Range
Age years	44.65 ± 8.46	25-58
Time till biopsy months	19.88 ± 11.22	4-44
Follow-up months	51.53 ± 15.92	10.0-93
Total bilirubin mg/dL	1.96 ± 2.50	0.3-9.9
Serum albumin g/dL	4.11 ± 0.62	2.7-5.1
AST U/L	111.79 ± 67.08	30-270
ALT U/L	125.59 ± 70.42	20-303
ALP U/L	541.45 ± 1185.65	81-7120
GGT U/L	486.3 ± 653.2	11-3408
Urea mg/dL	41.97 ± 16.98	20-105
Serum creatinine mg/dL	0.98 ± 0.29	0.5-1.7
Serum sodium mmol/L	138.44 ± 4.04	129-146
Serum potassium mmol/L	4.31 ± 0.46	3.8-5.7
Hemoglobin g/dL	12.71 ± 2.09	7.7-17.6
WBCs 10^9/L	6 ± 2.27	2.3-14.2
Platelets 10^9/L	167.82 ± 83.32	59-398
INR	1.05 ± 0.22	0.8-2.1
MELD	8.74 ± 4.71	3-28
Liver Fibrosis		
None	16 (47.1%)	
F1	13 (38.2%)	
F2	3 (8.8%)	
F3	2 (5.9%)	
Liver Activity		
None	16 (47.1%)	
A1	12 (35.3%)	
A2	5 (14.7%)	
A3	1 (2.9%)	
Histopathology		
Acute rejection	7 (20.6%)	
Viral chronic hepatitis	17 (50%)	
Steatohepatitis	4 (11.8%)	
Biliary obstruction	1 (2.9%)	
CMV infection	1 (2.9%)	
Chronic rejection	2 (5.9%)	
Chronic hepatitis	2 (5.9%)	

M ± SD mean ± standard deviation, *AST* aspartate aminotransferase, *ALT* alanine aminotransferase, *ALP* alkaline phosphatase, *GGT* gamma-glutamyl transferase, *WBC* white blood cell, *INR* international normalized ratio, *MELD* model for end-stage liver disease, *CMV* cytomegalovirus

Table 2 Comparison of liver transplant recipients who did and did not undergo liver biopsy

	Recipients (n = 89)			p
	Non-biopsied	Biopsied		
	n = 55 (61.8%)	n = 34 (38.2%)		
Age years	46.96 ± 8.74	44.65 ± 8.46		0.222
MELD	8.82 ± 2.86	8.74 ± 4.71		0.258#
ALBI score	− 2.96 ± 0.50	− 2.62 ± 0.60		0.014#
Follow-up months	38.40 ± 20.42	51.53 ± 15.92		0.001#
Sex				
Male	53 (96.4%)	30 (88.2%)	83 (93.3%)	0.197
Female	2 (3.6%)	4 (11.8%)	6 (6.7%)	
Indication of LT				
HCV	33 (60%)	21 (61.8%)	54 (60.7%)	0.192
HCV + HCC	18 (32.7%)	10 (29.4%)	28 (31.5%)	
HBV	4 (7.3%)	0	4 (4.5%)	
HCV + HBV + HCC	0	1 (2.9%)	1 (1.1%)	
PSC	0	1 (2.9%)	1 (1.1%)	
AIH	0	1 (2.9%)	1 (1.1%)	

MELD model for end-stage liver disease, *ALBI* albumin-bilirubin, *HCV* hepatitis C virus, *HBV* hepatitis B virus, *HCC* hepatocellular carcinoma, *PSC* primary biliary cholangitis, *AIH* autoimmune hepatitis
#Mann–Whitney *U* test

in cases of ACR such as interface hepatitis and perivenular parenchymal collapse. Steatohepatitis was diagnosed histologically by the presence of steatosis in hepatocytes, ballooning, and lobular inflammation with neutrophil rich (Fig. 1c). Liver biopsy diagnosed as chronic rejection revealed missing major bile ducts in portal tracts and arteriopathy. Chronic hepatitis other than viral etiology exhibited portal tract inflammation with spill over the interface and lobular inflammation in the form of apoptotic bodies, spotty, and confluent necrosis. Liver biopsy diagnosed as biliary obstruction revealed portal tract edema, mixed acute and chronic inflammatory cellular infiltrate, and ductular proliferation with intraluminal bile plugs as shown in Fig. 1d.

About 52.9% of patients had variable degrees of liver fibrosis mainly F1, 13 (38.2%),then F2, 3 (8.8%) and at last F3, 2 (5.9%). None of them had F4 fibrosis. As regards, the histological activity of most of the patients had A1, 12 (35.3%) then A2, 5 (14.7%) and few were A3, 1 (2.9%).

There was no statistically significant difference of the time till the first biopsy among the different diagnosis groups (p = 0.737). The time for each one was as follows: acute rejection, 15.14 ± 13.69 (04-44 months); viral chronic hepatitis, 20.76 ± 10.3 (06-44 months); steatohepatitis, 25.25 ± 14.17 (10-44 months); biliary obstruction, 11 (11-11 months); CMV infection, 15 (15-15 months); chronic rejection, 18.5 ± 14.85 (08-29 months); and chronic hepatitis, 26.5 ± 4.95 (23-30 months).

Patients that did (n = 34) and did not (n = 55) undergo liver biopsy were matched (p > 0.05) for age, sex, MELD score, indication of liver transplantation, and virology. The follow up period was statistically higher in the biopsied patients (51.53 ± 15.92 vs. 38.40 ± 20.42 months, p = 0.001). The liver dysfunction reflected by the ALBI score (Fig. 2) was statistically higher in the biopsied group (− 2.62 ± 0.6 vs. − 2.96 ± 0.5; p = 0.014).

Figure 3 shows the pattern of the histopathology in relation to the indication of liver transplantation. Patients with HCV had in a descending manner the following (p = 0.001): viral chronic hepatitis 16 (51.6%), acute rejection 7 (22.6%), steatohepatitis 4 (12.9%), chronic rejection 2 (6.5%), biliary obstruction 1 (3.2%), and CMV hepatitis 1 (3.2%). The patient with dual HBV and HCV had viral chronic hepatitis related to HCV. The two viral free patients had chronic hepatitis.

On sub analysis (p = 0.024) as in Table 2, patients with HCV had viral hepatitis (47.6%), patients with HCC on top of HCV had viral hepatitis (60%), patient with dual HBV and HCV had viral hepatitis, PSC and AIH had viral hepatitis. There was no statistically significant impact (p = 0.81) of the applied immunosuppressive drug regimen on the histopathology as shown in Table 3 and Fig. 4.

Some patients required a second and third biopsy. In the second biopsy (n = 9) the histopathology was acute rejection; 3 (33.3%), viral chronic hepatitis; 3 (33.3%), chronic rejection; 2 (22.2%) and chronic hepatitis; 1 (11.1%). In the third biopsy (n = 5) the histopathology

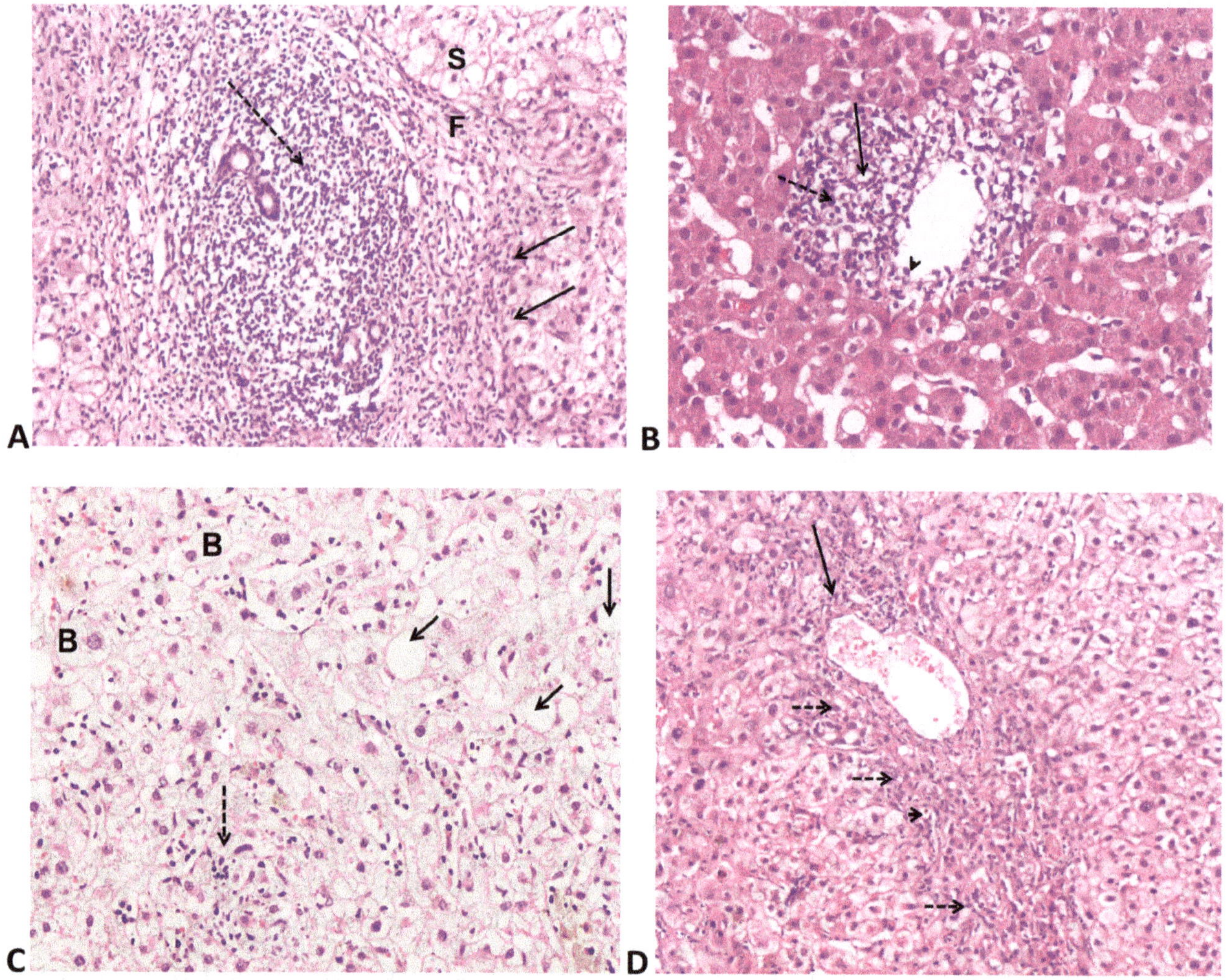

Fig. 1 Liver biopsy findings post liver transplantation: **a** Recurrent HCV infection showing portal tract mononuclear inflammatory infiltrate forming lymphoid aggregate (dashed arrow), interface hepatitis (arrow), fibrosis (F), and steatosis (S). **b** Acute cellular rejection demonstrating diagnostic portal tract triad of mixed cellular infiltrate (dashed arrow), bile duct injury (arrow), and venular endothelietis (arrow head). **c** Steatohepatitis exhibiting steatosis (arrows), ballooned hepatocytes (B), and neutrophilic rich infiltrate around hepatocytes (dashed arrow). **d** Biliary obstruction revealing mixed acute and chronic inflammatory cellular infiltrate (arrow), ductular proliferation (dashed arrow), and intraluminal bile plugs (arrow head)

was acute rejection, viral chronic hepatitis, biliary obstruction, CMV infection, and chronic rejection.

The findings of the second and the third biopsy may be the same as the first one or changing to another histopathology as in Table 4. One patient with acute rejection developed another attack and one proceeded to chronic rejection. Patients with viral hepatitis: some had the same diagnosis and some developed acute rejection, chronic rejection, biliary obstruction, and finally CMV hepatitis.

Discussion

Liver biopsy is the gold standard for diagnosis of many liver diseases and is a useful tool for follow-up. Despite the many advantages it has also drawbacks. It is an invasive maneuver that causes pain and liability for bleeding that may be life threatening. Organ perforation is one of the reported complications. Sometimes it may miss or underestimate the diagnosis as some diseases do not affect all parts of the liver evenly requiring both right and left lobe biopsy. Besides, there is inter-observer variation [13].

In the context of liver transplantation liver biopsy may be done early or late. The early indications are worsening or non-decreasing liver functions, re-rise of the liver functions after improvement and protocol biopsy. The late indications are rise of the liver enzymes from baseline, failed normalization after treated event, imaging abnormalities, and protocol biopsies [3].

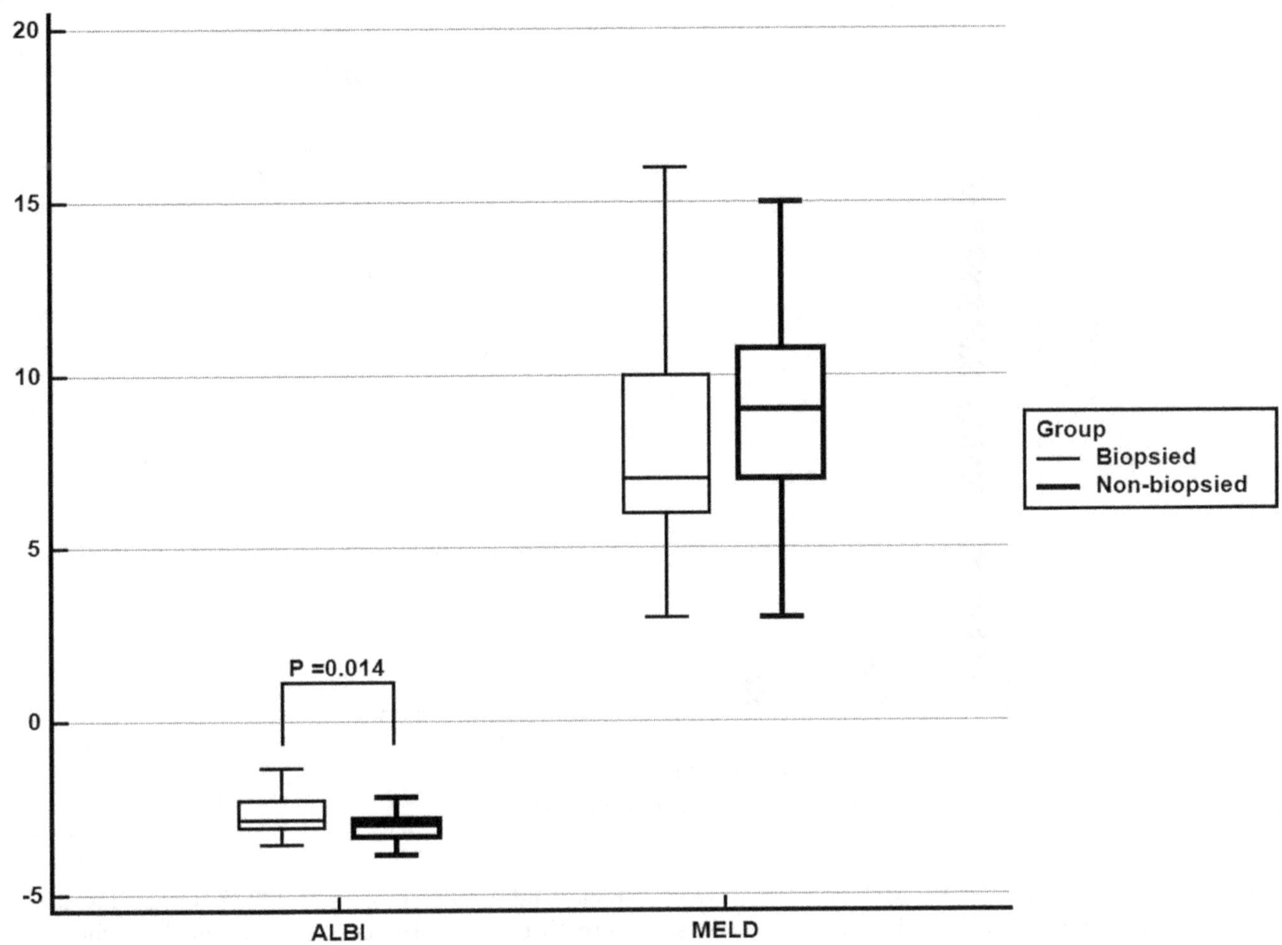

Fig. 2 Comparisons of the MELD and ALBI score in patients who did and did not undergo liver biopsy

The common histopathology depends on the time of the liver biopsy. Early, the diagnosis is usually small for size, acute cellular rejection, confirmation of vascular event, or severe recurrent of diseases as fibrosing cholestatic hepatitis. In the late one, it is common to find recurrent diseases as viral hepatitis, acute, or chronic rejection and sometimes recurrent malignancies [3, 4].

The need of liver biopsy till now is mandatory for diagnosis and assessment of some diseases as acute, chronic rejection, steatohepatitis, and de novo autoimmune hepatitis. Liver biopsy is needed for confirmation of uncertain laboratory or radiology diagnosis as with CMV or liver tumors. The enthusiasm of liver biopsy has faded away in many aspects and supplanted nowadays by noninvasive parameters as seen with recurrent viral hepatitis where laboratory and radiological parameters are sufficient to commence antiviral therapy.

On reviewing the studies on the utility of liver biopsy post-transplant; Yu et al. [14] analyzed 50 biopsies out of 27 patients (2002-2003). The time till biopsy ranged from 5 h to 330 days. The main histological diagnosis was acute rejection (48.2%), preservation-reperfusion injury (25.9%), chronic rejection (14.8%), hepatic artery thrombosis (11.1%), drug induced hepatitis (11.1%), CMV (3.7%), and recurrent hepatitis (3.7%).

An Iranian study [15] analyzed 382 post LT biopsies from 287 patients. The average age was 28 (1-64 years). The main indication of liver transplantation was HBV (20.2%) followed by AIH (17.7%). The time till biopsy varied from few hours till 261 days post-transplant. Acute cellular rejection was the most common finding (47%) followed by hepatic artery related ischemic changes. Some patients had normal liver histopathology (17.7%).

In another study, Kanodia et al. [16] studied 57 biopsies from 35 patients (January 2010 to July 2014). Some patients underwent repeated biopsies. The average age was 53 years and most of them were males. The mean bilirubin was 5.54 mg/dL, AST (197 U/L), ALT (298 U/L), and ALP (256 U/L). The most common indication for LT was alcoholic cirrhosis (25.71%), cryptogenic (17.14%), HBV related (17.14%), and Wilson's disease

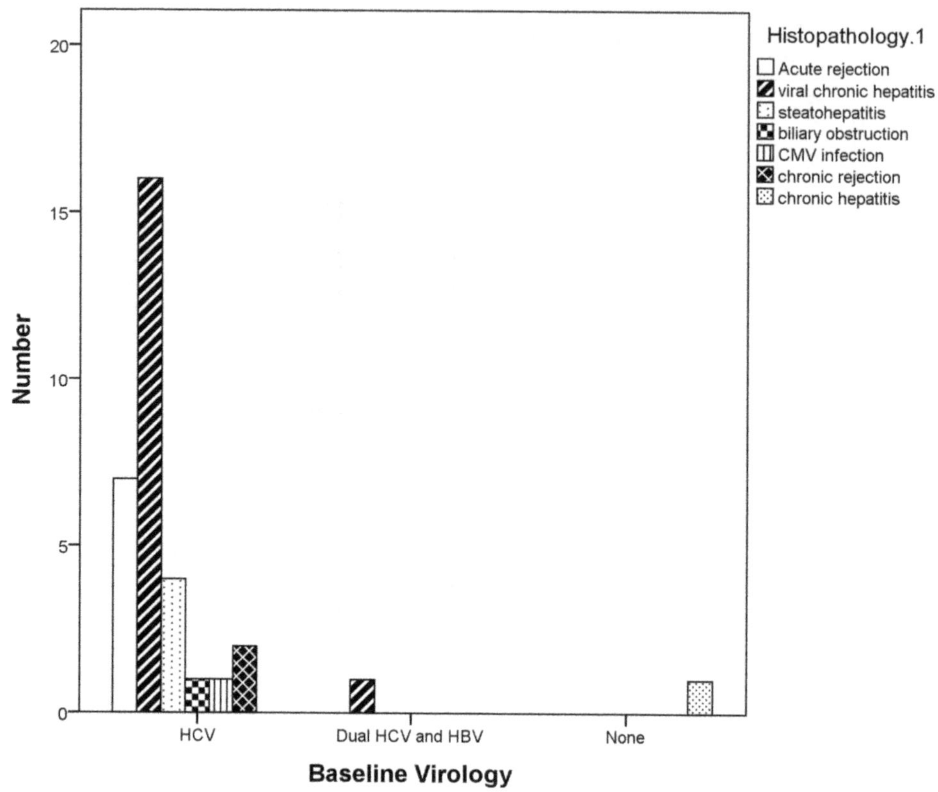

Fig. 3 Correlations between the indication of liver transplantation and the histopathology

(11.42%). Few cases with HCV, AIH, and PSC were present. The time till biopsy ranged from 1 to 980 days. The most common histological diagnosis was acute rejection (55.36%), preservation-reperfusion injury (17.86%), drug toxicity (14.29%), and recurrent HCV infection (5.36%).

Voigtlander et al. [17] reported 496 liver biopsies obtained from 312 liver transplant patients. The main indications of LT were mainly viral hepatitis (28%), PSC (19%), and acute liver cell failure (8%). The main indications for doing liver biopsy were suspected rejection (66%) and protocol biopsies (22%). Other indications were disease recurrence (7%) and unclear cholestasis (3%). The average time till liver biopsy was 27 months. The histological findings were acute cellular rejection (36%), chronic hepatitis (28%), obstructive cholangiopathy (7%), and fatty liver disease (6%).

In another report, Fonseca et al. [18] analyzed liver biopsies in Indian liver transplant center. He analyzed the explants, donor liver histopathology, and biopsies done after liver transplantation for pediatric and adult cases. About 58 biopsies were done for 42 patients (adult and

Table 3 Effect of the immunosuppressive drug regimen on the liver histopathological diagnosis

Histopathology.1	Immunosuppressive drug regimen				
	CNI based	mTOR based	Dual CNI and mTOR	Total	*p*
	n = 18	*n* = 9	*n* = 7	*n* = 34	
Acute rejection	3 (16.7%)	3 (33.3%)	1 (14.3%)	7 (20.6%)	0.81
Viral chronic hepatitis	10 (55.6%)	4 (44.4%)	3 (42.9%)	17 (50%)	
Steatohepatitis	2 (11.1%)	1 (11.1%)	1 (14.3%)	4 (11.8%)	
Biliary obstruction	1 (5.6%)	0 (0%)	0 (0%)	1 (2.9%)	
CMV infection	0 (0%)	1 (11.1%)	0 (0%)	1 (2.9%)	
Chronic rejection	1 (5.6%)	0 (0%)	1 (14.3%)	2 (5.9%)	
Chronic hepatitis	1 (5.6%)	0 (0%)	1 (14.3%)	2 (5.9%)	

CMV cytomegalovirus, *CNI* calcineurin inhibitors, *mTOR* mechanistic target of rapamycin

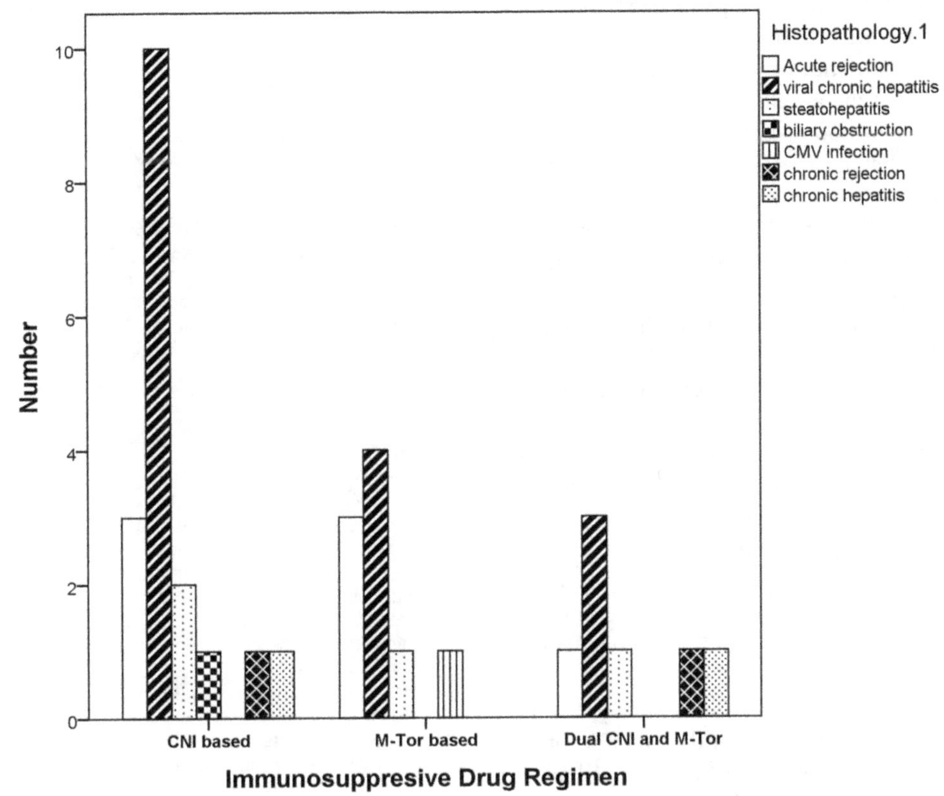

Fig. 4 Impact of the immunosuppressive drug regimen on the histopathology

pediatric). Some patients underwent repeated biopsies. In adults, the most common histopathology was acute cellular rejection.

In the current study, 89 patients were followed up where 38.2% underwent liver biopsy mainly for suspecting acute rejection or recurrent diseases especially viral ones. Some patients underwent single biopsy and some patients underwent repeated biopsies consistent with other studies [14–16, 18]. The average age was 44 years that is lower than Kanodia et al. [16], and higher than Geramizadeh et al. [15] as he enrolled pediatric cases.

Table 4 Sequential finding of the first, second, and third liver biopsy

	First biopsy	Second biopsy	Third biopsy
Case 1	Acute rejection	Chronic rejection	
Case 2	Acute rejection	Acute rejection	
Case 3	Biliary obstruction	Chronic rejection	
Case 4	Chronic hepatitis	Chronic hepatitis	Chronic hepatitis
Case 5	Chronic rejection	Viral chronic hepatitis	Acute rejection
Case 6	Viral chronic hepatitis	Viral chronic hepatitis	
Case 7	Viral chronic hepatitis	Viral chronic hepatitis	Chronic rejection
Case 8	Viral chronic hepatitis	Acute rejection	Biliary obstruction
Case 9	Viral chronic hepatitis	Acute rejection	CMV infection

Most patients were males in agreement with Kanodia et al. [16]. In comparison to biopsy free patients, most patients had more liver dysfunction that was assessed by the ALBI score

Most of the liver functions are elevated more than 2-3 folds and the wide fluctuations were with AST, ALT, GGT, and ALP. In our center, 91.2% of cases were positive for HCV. Regarding indications of liver transplantation, the first one was HCV related decompensated liver disease followed by HCC on top of HCV related liver disease. In the other studies, the indication was different according to the geographical distribution, so in the Iranian study HBV was the main one [15], whereas alcohol in the Indian study [16].

The average time till the 1st liver biopsy was 19.88 (10-93) months. Some centers did very early liver biopsy within hours postoperatively as with Geramizadeh et al. [15], Kanodia et al. [16], and some center earlier time as with Voigtlander et al. [17]. The different histopathological diagnosis was not affected by the time till biopsy.

The first histopathological diagnosis was recurrent viral hepatitis in 50% of cases followed by acute cellular rejection, steatohepatitis, and chronic rejection. In fact, the incidence of acute cellular rejection is low (20.6%) in our study compared to 48.2% [14], 36% [17], 47% [15], and 55.36% [16]. The most probable explanation that some studies applied protocol biopsies [18] and they began earlier postoperative biopsies [15–17]. Acute cellular rejection is very common in the early 3 months post-transplant. Maybe the application of induction therapy with basiliximab in some cases and the triple regimen has decreased the occurrence of acute rejection in our center.

Since three studies did early biopsies, so it was common to report preservation-reperfusion injury [14, 16] and hepatic artery thrombosis [14, 15].

The incidence of recurrent viral hepatitis especially HCV was high (50%) compared to 3.7% [14], 5.36% [16], and 28% [17]. The explanation that Egypt is one of the countries of high prevalence of chronic hepatitis C [19].

Regarding liver fibrosis and histological activity, most cases were free of F4 fibrosis where most of them were F1 (38.2%) and A1 (35.3%). This was due to regular follow-up and early management of the complications.

None of the patients who underwent biopsy were free of positive diagnostic findings in contrast to Geramizadeh et al. [15], who reported that 17.7% of the patients had normal histopathology.

On correlation of the indication of liver transplant and the found histopathology, it was found that 50% of the patients with pre-transplant chronic hepatitis C had recurrent viral hepatitis.

The varied immunosuppressive drug regimen did not affect that pattern of histopathology. Few patients needed on demand second (n = 9) and third biopsy (n = 5). Sometimes the diagnosis was the same as acute rejection and some proceeded to chronic rejection. Patients with viral hepatitis proceeded to other events as rejection in the other biopsies.

The limitations of the study were small number, single centered experienced, and absence of protocol biopsies.

Conclusion

Liver biopsy is still a useful diagnostic tool in liver transplant recipients.

Abbreviations

AIH: Autoimmune hepatitis; ALBI: Albumin-bilirubin; ALP: Alkaline phosphatase; ALT: Alanine aminotransferase; AST: Aspartate aminotransferase; CMV: Cytomegalovirus; CNI: Calcineurin inhibitors; GGT: Gamma-glutamyl transferase; HBV: Hepatitis B virus; HCC: Hhepatocellular carcinoma; HCV: Hepatitis C virus; INR: International normalized ratio; LT: Liver transplantation; MELD: Model for end-stage liver disease; mTOR: Mechanistic target of rapamycin; PSC: Primary biliary cholangitis; WBC: White blood cell

Acknowledgements

All authors are greatly indebted to members of all departments of National Liver Institute, Menoufia University, Egypt.

Authors' contributions

EA: initiated the project, designed and implemented the study for application, drafted and revised the paper, AA: analyzed the data, drafted and revised the paper, NE: histopathological examination and interpretation, AE: histopathological examination and interpretation, KA: analyzed the data, one of the surgical team, revised the paper. EI: analyzed the data, drafted and revised the paper. ME: analyzed the data, drafted and revised the paper. All authors have read and approved the manuscript.
A poster from this abstract was presented at the Asian Pacific Association for the Study of the Liver 2019.

Competing interests

The authors declare that they have no competing interests.

Author details

Department of Hepatology and Gastroenterology, National Liver Institute, Menoufia University, Shebeen El-Koom 32511, Egypt. [2]Department of Pathology, National Liver Institute, Menoufia University, Shebeen El-Koom, Egypt. [3]Department of Hepatobiliary Surgery, National Liver Institute, Menoufia University, Shebeen El-Koom, Egypt.

References

1. Gad EH, Alsebaey A, Lotfy M, Eltabbakh M, Sherif AA (2015) Complications and mortality after adult to adult living donor liver transplantation: a retrospective cohort study. Ann Med Surg (Lond) 4:162–171
2. Caiado AH, Blasbalg R, Marcelino AS, da Cunha PM, Chammas MC, da Costa LC et al (2007) Complications of liver transplantation: multimodality imaging approach. Radiographics 27:1401–1417
3. Adeyi O, Fischer SE, Guindi M (2010) Liver allograft pathology: approach to interpretation of needle biopsies with clinicopathological correlation. J Clin Pathol 63:47–74
4. Da J (2006) Liver biopsy interpretation for causes of late liver allograft dysfunction. Hepatology (Baltimore, Md) 44:489–501
5. Abdelsameea E, Alsebaey A, Abdel-Razek W, Ehsan N, Morad W, Salama M et al (2020) Elastography and serum markers of fibrosis versus liver biopsy in 1270 Egyptian patients with hepatitis C. Eur J Gastroenterol Hepatol
6. C. RD, H. CS, D. GZ, C. NR, D. SA. Liver biopsy. Hepatology (Baltimore, Md) 2009;49:1017-1044.
7. Hiraoka A, Kumada T, Kudo M, Hirooka M, Tsuji K, Itobayashi E et al (2017) Albumin-Bilirubin (ALBI) grade as part of the evidence-based clinical practice guideline for HCC of the Japan Society of Hepatology: a comparison with the liver damage and child-pugh classifications. Liver Cancer 6:204–215
8. De Simone P, Fagiuoli S, Cescon M, De Carlis L, Tisone G, Volpes R et al (2017) Use of everolimus in liver transplantation: recommendations from a working group. Transplantation 101:239–251
9. Cholongitas E, Goulis I, Theocharidou E, Antoniadis N, Fouzas I, Giakoustidis D et al (2014) Everolimus-based immunosuppression in liver transplant recipients: a single-centre experience. Hepatol Int 8:137–145
10. Intraobserver and interobserver variations in liver biopsy interpretation in patients with chronic hepatitis C. The French METAVIR Cooperative Study Group. Hepatology (Baltimore, Md) 1994;20:15-20.
11. Johnson PJ, Berhane S, Kagebayashi C, Satomura S, Teng M, Reeves HL et al (2015) Assessment of liver function in patients with hepatocellular carcinoma: a new evidence-based approach—the ALBI grade. J Clin Oncol 33:550–558
12. P. WJ, M. HA, W. BS. MELD score, allocation, and distribution in the United States. Clin Liver Dis 2013;2:148-151.
13. Rockey DC, Caldwell SH, Goodman ZD, Nelson RC, Smith AD (2009) Liver biopsy. Hepatology (Baltimore, Md) 49:1017–1044
14. Yu YY, Ji J, Zhou GW, Shen BY, Chen H, Yan JQ et al (2004) Liver biopsy in evaluation of complications following liver transplantation. World J Gastroenterol 10:1678–1681
15. Geramizadeh B, Motevalli D, Nikeghbalian S, Malek Hosseini SA (2013) Histopathology of post-transplant liver biopsies, the first report from iran. Hepatitis Monthly 13:e9389
16. Kanodia KV, Vanikar AV, Modi PR, Patel RD, Suthar KS, Nigam LK et al (2015) Histological and clinicopathological evaluation of liver allograft biopsy: an initial experience of fifty six biopsies. J Clin Diagn Res 9:EC17–EC20
17. Voigtlander T, Alten TA, Kirstein MM, Lehner F, Manns MP, Schlue J et al (2017) Clinical impact of liver biopsies in liver transplant recipients. Ann Transplant 22:108–114
18. Fonseca F, Kulkarni B, Hastak M, Kumaran V, Varma V, Kapoor S (2018) An overview of liver transplant pathology: data from a tertiary referral centre in Western India. Ann Hepatol 17:426–436

7

Primary squamous cell carcinoma of the liver: an unexpected pathological finding

Fabio Tuminello[1], Davide Castiglione[2], Giuseppe Broggi[3], Giada Maria Vecchio[3], Antonio Basile[2], Stefano Puleo[1] and Antonio Pesce[1*]

Abstract

Background: Primary squamous cell carcinoma of the liver is a very rare cancer requiring a complete diagnostic investigation, as it presents some differences from other primary hepatic malignancies. We describe the case of an elderly patient with primitive squamous cell carcinoma of the liver treated by percutaneous microwave ablation and transarterial chemoembolization.

Case presentation: Although the pathogenesis remains uncertain, a possible transformation of the biliary epithelium caused by chronic inflammation or metaplasia and subsequent malignant transformation of preexisting benign hepatic cysts has been suggested. A critical review of the existing literature was performed by focusing on the pathogenesis, clinical presentation, and the suggested therapeutic strategies.

Conclusion: A multidisciplinary approach is needed to face rare hepatic malignancies where there are no clear guidelines.

Keywords: Squamous cell carcinoma, Liver cyst, Metaplasia, Transarterial embolization, Multidisciplinary approach

Background

Primary squamous cell carcinoma (SCC) of the liver is a very uncommon finding in everyday clinical practice. The most common anatomical areas are represented by the skin, lungs, distal esophagus, anal canal, cervical, or inguinal lymph nodes, in which a squamocellular epithelium may be identified. Primary SCC of the liver has been mostly reported to be sporadic and associated with hepatic cysts, hepatolithiasis, or hepatic teratoma [1–3].

Although the pathogenesis remains uncertain, a possible transformation of the biliary epithelium caused by chronic inflammation or metaplasia and subsequent malignant transformation of preexisting benign hepatic cysts has been suggested [4–6].

Because of its rare prevalence, the histopathological analysis is imperative and it is often a diagnosis of exclusion, after having carefully examined the patient, looking for other possible primary lesions and ruling out the possibility for secondary SCC.

The prognosis of this rare tumor of the liver is extremely poor and only few patients survive more than 12 months even after surgical resection.

Herein, we reported a case of an elderly patient with primitive squamous cell carcinoma of the liver treated by percutaneous microwave ablation and transarterial embolization. A critical review of the existing literature was performed by focusing on the pathogenesis, clinical presentation, and the suggested therapeutic strategies.

Case presentation

A 79-year-old Caucasian man presented with profuse asthenia, unintentional weight loss (around 20 kg) over the last 3 months, and abdominal chronic pain in the right hypochondrium. He denied alcohol abuse and smoking. The past medical history reported essential hypertension

* Correspondence: nino.fish@hotmail.it
This case report was presented at the following Italian Society of Surgical Researches (SIRC) meeting: «*Chirurgia Insieme: Convegno Congiunto delle Società Specialistiche Chirurgiche Italiane*», Genoa 27–28 June 2019
[1]Section of General Surgery, Department of Medical, Surgical Sciences and Advanced Technologies "G.F. Ingrassia", University Hospital "Policlinico-Vittorio Emanuele", 95123 Catania, Italy

under pharmacological treatment, sigmoid diverticulosis, and cholelithiasis. Physical examination revealed a treatable abdomen, aching on the deep palpation in the right hypochondrium, where the inferior margin of the liver was appreciated 5 cm below the costal arch and a hard irregular mass was recognized. No cervical, axillary, or inguinal lymphadenopathy were appreciated. A dermatological counselling excluded skin lesions. Digital rectal examination was negative. Breathing sound was clear without wheezing or crackle. The remaining physical examination was normal.

Blood tests showed ALT 91 U/l, GGT 308 U/l, total bilirubin level 1.7 mg/dl, Ca 19-9 1956 U/ml, AFP 1.6 ng/ml, CEA 12 U/ml.

Upper endoscopy and colonoscopy excluded esophago-gastric and colorectal lesions, respectively. Abdominal computed tomographic scan (CT-scan) showed a large hypodense liver mass in the right lobe (15 cm × 12 cm in size) on both arterial and portal phases involving the IV-V-VI-VII-VIII segments (Fig. 1a,b) which presented colliquative areas of necrosis within the lesion. Mild dilatation of intrahepatic biliary ducts was observed. Multiple isolated liver cysts were described in both lobes. Moreover, the lesion was very close to the gallbladder, which showed wall thickening and enhanced endoluminal tissue of uncertain origin. The cystic duct was enlarged, and focal endoluminal tissue was detected. Some enlarged lymph nodes in the right sub-diaphragmatic space were reported.

The radiologist, based on these findings, hypothesized the suspicion of gallbladder cancer or intrahepatic cholangiocarcinoma mass forming. A liver biopsy was performed under local anesthesia via combined US/CT guidance. The interventional radiologist used core needle biopsy device (Monopty 18G × 16 cm, BARD, Arizona, USA). Two specimens were collected. No complication occurred.

Histopathological analysis of the liver mass showed a well-differentiated squamous cell carcinoma with diffuse necrosis. Immunohistochemical staining was positive for cytokeratins (CK) 7, 19, and p63; anti-hepatocyte, MUC-5, TTF-1 were negative, suggesting the tumor as primary or metastatic squamous cell carcinoma of the liver (Figs. 2a–d and 3).

After the surprising and unexpected pathological report, a PET/CT scan was performed in order to rule out the presence of another primitive unknown tumor. The examination showed a single area of increased uptake in the right lobe of the liver, corresponding to the tumor mass. The uptake was inhomogeneous with the central part of the mass showing weak or no uptake and the peripheral regions showing an intense uptake. This finding could confirm the presence of areas of colliquative necrosis and areas of active neoplasm, as shown in Fig. 4. No other anatomic regions of altered metabolic captation were discovered. Therefore, the diagnosis of primary squamous cell carcinoma of the liver was confirmed.

After a multidisciplinary meeting involving surgeons, radiologists, oncologists, and hepatologists, the case was accurately discussed and the different treatment options were evaluated. The patient was initially scheduled for major liver resection (extended right hepatectomy after portal venous embolization), but he refused it. In consideration of the size of the mass and the paucity of scientific recommendations, a mini-invasive radiological approach was considered appropriate. A combined approach was proposed: percutaneous transhepatic microwave ablation and transarterial chemoembolization (TACE).

On the same day, the interventional radiology team performed microwave ablation via US guidance, with two different probes at 100 W of energy for 9 min (Evident™ MW Ablation System, Medtronic, Minneapolis, MN, USA) and transarterial chemoembolization (TACE). TACE was performed via left radial artery access, using Simmons 1 catheter and hydrophilic guidewire to negotiate the celiac axis and the proper hepatic artery. Unfortunately, celiac axis dissection was observed during angiographic study and the procedure was

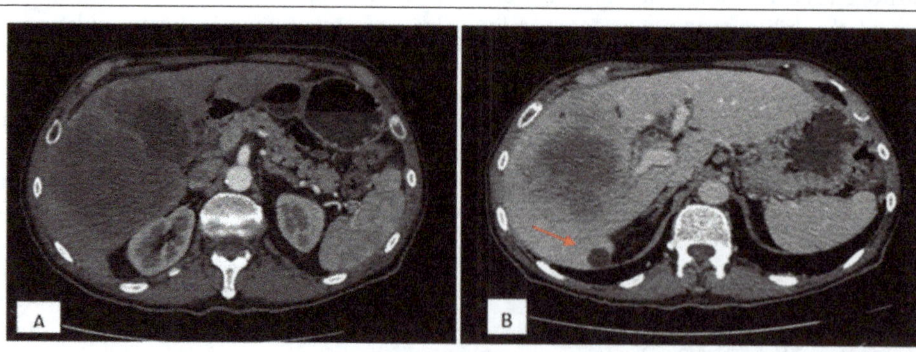

Fig. 1 a Abdominal CT scan, axial view, arterial phase, showing hypodense mass in the right lobe of the liver with weakly enhanced margin. **b** Portal phase, hypodense liver mass and the presence of hepatic cyst (red arrow). Mild dilation of intrahepatic biliary tree

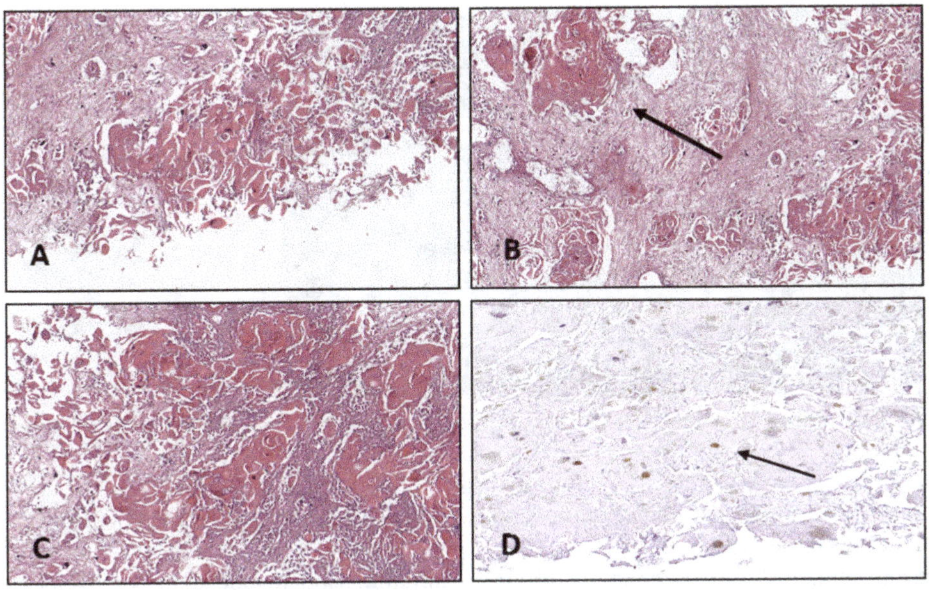

Fig. 2 a Showing a well-differentiated squamous cell carcinoma (H&E, × 100). **b** The tumor shows obvious squamous cell features such as seen here (arrow). **c** Well-differentiated lesion shows prominent keratinization and may form "pearl-like" structures (40 ×). Interposed areas of necrosis and fibrosis are evident. **d** Diffuse nuclear staining (arrow) for p63 in squamous neoplastic cells

completed negotiating the hepatic artery via collateral hypertrophic vessels arising from the superior mesenteric artery. Arteriography of the right hepatic artery showed no relevant hypervascular mass as expected. Some anarchic and tortuous arteries were confirmed as tributaries of the mass (Fig. 5) and then embolized with microparticles (150–300 μm). The immediate post-procedural course was uneventful. The patient presented a global improvement of his quality of life in terms of abdominal pain relief. He was discharged with a poor prognosis.

At 1-month follow-up, an abdominal CT scan did not show significant differences, After the sixth month, the patient developed obstructive jaundice with significant

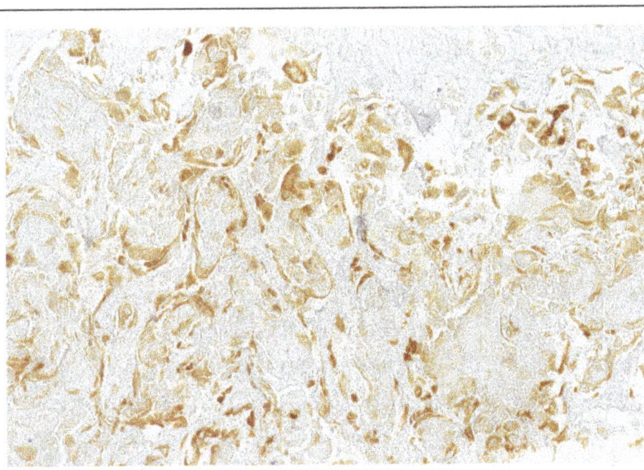

Fig. 3 Showing diffuse positive staining for CK19 in squamous tumor cells

dilatation of intrahepatic biliary system; the liver mass had grown and a percutaneous transhepatic biliary drainage was put in.

He died 9 months later.

Discussion

Primary SCC of the liver is a very rare cancer requiring a complete diagnostic investigation, as it presents some differences from other primary hepatic malignancies [7–9]. In a recent review, Zhang XF et al. [3] reported only 31 cases described in English literature since 1970s and other four patients encountered in their study. The main risk factors associated with the occurrence of SCC of the liver are male sex, hepatic cysts, hepatolithiasis, and liver cirrhosis.

Various etiopathogenetic theories have been proposed to explain the origin of primary squamous cell carcinoma of the liver. Some authors suggest that primary SCC of the liver is often associated with hepatic cysts, but its exact path to carcinoma is not yet proven. Continuous irritation due to chronic inflammation might promote secondary squamous metaplasia and subsequent malignant transformation. In the current case, the patient presented hepatolithiasis and multiple benign liver cysts which may explain the possible trasformation of cyst epithelium to squamocellular carcinoma, but the causes of carcinogenesis need to be further studied. It may be very interesting to establish animal models to mimic the malignant transformation of cyst epithelium to squamous carcinomatous epithelium. In some patients, an

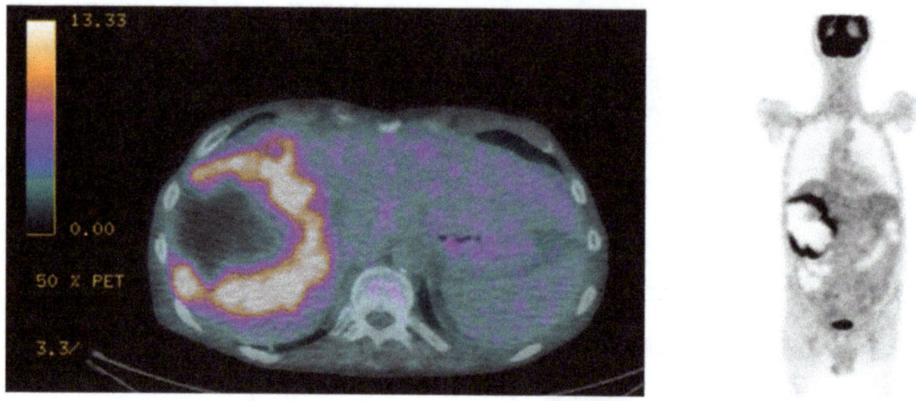

Fig. 4 PET imaging, fusion PET/CT, and PET coronal view showing the high uptake of liver mass. The difference between inner and outer part of the mass are highlighted

association of adenomatous and squamous components has been reported in English literature [10–13].

According to many studies [2–4], patients with primary SCC of the liver may present various symptoms including chronic abdominal pain or general discomfort, anorexia, weight loss, jaundice, and rarely progressive dysphagia. Our patient presented chronic pain in the right hypochondrium, asthenia, remarkable weight loss, and only after a couple of months, he developed obstructive jaundice.

The delayed appearance of jaundice has been an interesting matter of discussion: we considered it as a possible biological characteristic of this particular kind of tumor, with important differences with gallbladder cancer and intrahepatic cholangiocarcinoma, for example.

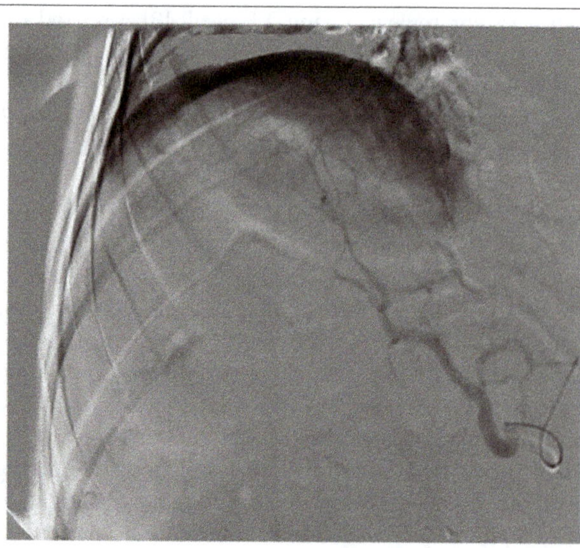

Fig. 5 Digital subtraction angiography (DSA) shows Cobra C2 5Fr catheter in mesenteric artery branch. Accessory right hepatic artery, increased in diameter, acts as anarchic vascularization towards the liver tumor.

Most of these patients may present increased serum levels of ALT, AST, and even bilirubin, due to chronic inflammation in bile ducts or liver cyst and tumor progression. However, there is a lack of specific serum marker of primary liver SCC at the present time.

Sometimes, the clinical and radiological diagnosis is quite hard. Radiological investigations may present important pitfalls. CT seems to be the most valuable preoperative investigation. After systematically examining all anatomical districts from which it can originate, the diagnosis of primary SCC of the liver should only be considered when a suitable biopsy specimen documents the presence of squamous cells. Immunohistochemistry plays an important diagnostic role. The strong positive staining for CK 14 and CK 56 suggest basal cells of keratinized squamous epithelium origin of the cancer cells. Moreover, the positive expression of CK19 confirms the bile ductular ontogeny of the neoplastic cells.

There are still no clear guidelines on the treatment of primary SCC of the liver, unlike other primitive hepatic malignancies in which there are clear scientific recommandations [14–17]. Therapeutic options include surgical resection, chemotherapy, and radiotherapy. Transarterial chemoembolization (TACE) has been reported for treatment of primary SCC of the liver [3]. Like most of the hepatic malignancy, surgical resectability represents the most important factor for improving the prognosis. According to Zhang XF et al. [3], patients undergoing radical surgery had longer overall survival time than those undergoing palliative treatment (median survival 17 vs 5 months, $p = 0.005$). Therefore, complete surgical excision of the tumor is strongly recommended rather than simple drainage or partial excision. Systemic or intra-arterial chemotherapy might be useful in surgically unfit patients [7, 18, 19]. In our specific case, the patient was initially scheduled for major liver resection but after refusing surgical option, a radiological combined approach was preferred to systemic chemotherapy or radiotherapy, with acceptable prognosis in terms of quality of life. The prognosis of squamous cell carcinoma of the liver is extremely poor, with a median overall survival of a few months. However, Kaji R et al. [18] described a case of SCC of the liver that remarkably responded to low-dose intra-hepatoarterial chemotherapy with overall survival of 23 months.

Conclusion

A multidisciplinary approach is needed to face rare hepatic malignancies where there are no clear guidelines in order to choose the best therapeutic option for patients.

Abbreviations

SCC: Primary squamous cell carcinoma; ALT: Alanine aminotransferase; AST: Aspartate aminotransferase; GGT: Gamma-glutamyltransferase; AFP: Alpha fetoprotein; TTF-1: Transcriptional thyroid factor 1; TACE: Transarterial chemoembolization; CEA: Carcinoembryonic antigen; CA 19-9: Cancer antigen 19-9

Acknowledgements

Not applicable.

Authors' contributions

All authors contributed equally to the paper; FT, AP, and SP conceptualized and designed the case report; FT drafted the initial manuscript; DC and AB performed interventional radiology treatment; GB and GMV perfomed histological analysis. All authors reviewed and approved the final version of the manuscript as submitted.

Competing interests

The authors declare that they have no competing interests.

Author details

[1]Section of General Surgery, Department of Medical, Surgical Sciences and Advanced Technologies "G.F. Ingrassia", University Hospital "Policlinico-Vittorio Emanuele", 95123 Catania, Italy. [2]Radiology I Unit, Department of Medical, Surgical Sciences and Advanced Technologies "G.F. Ingrassia", University Hospital "Policlinico-Vittorio Emanuele", 95123 Catania, Italy. [3]Anatomic Pathology, Department of Medical, Surgical Sciences and Advanced Technologies "G.F. Ingrassia", University Hospital "Policlinico-Vittorio Emanuele", 95123 Catania, Italy.

References

1. Bloustein PA, Silverberg SG (1976) Squamous cell carcinoma originating in a hepatic cyst. Case report with a review of the hepatic cystcarcinoma association. Cancer. 38(5):2002–2005
2. Odemiş B, Köksal AS, Yüksel O, Kacar S, Turhan N (2006 Jul) Squamous cell cancer of the liver arising from an epidermoid cyst: case report and review of the literature. Dig Dis Sci. 51(7):1278–1284
3. Zhang XF, Du ZQ, Liu XM, Lv Y (2015 Jul) Primary squamous cell carcinoma of liver - case series and review of literatures. Medicine (Baltimore). 94(28): e868
4. Weimann A, Klempnauer J, Gebel M, Maschek H, Bartels M, Ringe B, Pichlmayr R (1996) Squamous cell carcinoma of the liver originating from a solitary non-parasitic cyst case report and review of the literature. HPB Surg. 10(1):45–49
5. Nakajima T, Kondo Y (1990 Mar 15) A clinicopathologic study of intrahepatic cholangiocarcinoma containing a component of squamous cell carcinoma. Cancer. 65(6):1401–1404
6. Yoo TK, Kim BI, Han EN, Kim DH, Yoo JH, Lee SJ, Cho YK, Kim HJ (2016 Mar) Primary squamous cell carcinoma of the liver: a case report. Clin Mol Hepatol. 22(1):177–182
7. Boscolo G, Jirillo A, Da Pian P (2005 Jan-Feb) Complete remission of poorly differentiated squamous liver carcinoma after systemic chemotherapy and surgery. A case report. Tumori. 91(1):71–72
8. Wilson JM, Groeschl R, George B, Turaga KK, Patel PJ, Saeian K, Gamblin TC (2013) Ciliated hepatic cyst leading to squamous cell carcinoma of the liver - a case report and review of the literature. Int J Surg Case Rep. 4(11):972–975
9. Morito K, Kai K, Miyoshi A, Kubo H, Ide T, Azama S, Irie H, Koga Y, Sumi K, Ikeda O, Kitahara K, Noshiro H (2013 Apr) Primary squamous cell carcinoma of the liver concomitant with primary colon cancer: report of a case. Clin J Gastroenterol. 6(2):134–138
10. Harino T, Tomimaru Y, Noguchi K, Nagase H, Ogino T, Hirota M, Oshima K, Tanida T, Noura S, Imamura H, Akagi K, Iwazawa T, Tamura H, Adachi S, Dono K (2019 Apr) A rare case of adenosquamous carcinoma in the liver with hepatolithiasis. Gan To Kagaku Ryoho. 46(4):772–774
11. Tamaoka K, Tanemura M, Furukawa K, Mikamori M, Saito T, Ohtsuka M, Suzuki Y, Tei M, Kishi K, Yasuoka H, Tsujimoto M, Akamatsu H (2018 Oct 5) Primary intrahepatic squamous cell carcinoma with histological collision of adenocarcinoma and squamous cell carcinoma: a case report. Am J Case Rep. 19:1184–1191
12. Yamao K, Takenaka M, Imai H, Nakai A, Omoto S, Kamata K, Minaga K, Miyata T, Sakurai T, Watanabe T, Nishida N, Matsumoto I, Takeyama Y, Chikugo T, Kudo M (2017) Primary hepatic adenosquamous carcinoma associated with primary sclerosing cholangitis. Oncology. 93(Suppl 1):76–80
13. Gao S, Chen D, Huang L, Wu L, Dai R, Shan Y (2015 Aug 1) Primary adenosquamous carcinoma of the liver: a case report and review of the literature. Int J Clin Exp Pathol. 8(8):9687–9692
14. Trovato MA, Pesce A, Sofia M, Montineri A, Basile A, Palermo F, Fatuzzo F, Nigro L, Puleo S (2013 Oct) Is BCLC algorithm useful in clinical practice? Study on 164 HCC patients. Hepatogastroenterology. 60(127):1742–1745
15. Pesce A, Scilletta R, Branca A, Nigro L, Montineri A, Larocca L, Fatuzzo F, Castaing M, Puleo S (2012 Jun) Does transient elastography (FibroScan®) have a role in decision making in hepatocellular carcinoma? HPB (Oxford). 14(6):403–408
16. Aloia TA, Járufe N, Javle M, Maithel SK, Roa JC, Adsay V, Coimbra FJ, Jarnagin WR (2015 Aug) Gallbladder cancer: expert consensus statement. HPB (Oxford). 17(8):681–690
17. Weber SM, Ribero D, O'Reilly EM, Kokudo N, Miyazaki M, Pawlik TM (2015 Aug) Intrahepatic cholangiocarcinoma: expert consensus statement. HPB (Oxford). 17(8):669–680
18. Kaji R, Sasaki N, Tateishi I, Nagata E, Okabe Y, Yoshida T, Sata M, Ueno T (2003) A case report of primary hepatic squamous cell carcinoma that remarkably responded to low dose arterial injection of anti-cancer drugs. Kurume Med J. 50:71–75
19. Naik S, Waris W, Carmosino L, Mehrishi A, Saif MW (2009) Primary squamous cell carcinoma of the liver. J Gastrointestin Liver Dis. 18:487–489

8

The association between vitamin D status and non-alcoholic fatty liver disease in adults: a hospital-based study

Ahmed Ibrahim Gad[1*], Mohamed Rezk Elmedames[1], Ayman Ramadan Abdelhai[1] and Ayman Mohamed Marei[2]

Abstract

Background: The association between vitamin D levels and non-alcoholic fatty liver disease (NAFLD) has been increasingly determined in recent researches. The aim of this study was to determine the association between vitamin D levels, measured as serum 25-hydroxy vitamin D (25(OH)D) and NAFLD. Serum 25(OH)D was prospectively determined in 80 patients. Of them, 40 subjects had NAFLD, whereas 40 subjects served as healthy control. Vitamin D deficiency was defined as serum 25(OH)D level < 20 ng/ml. Receiver operating characteristic (ROC) and regression analysis methods were used in our analysis.

Results: About 70% of patients with NAFLD had vitamin D deficiency, but only 35% in the control group had. The mean serum 25 (OH)D was significantly lower in patients with NAFLD than the healthy control group (16.13 ± 10.23 versus 27.35 ± 10.58 ng/mL; *P* < 0.001). ROC curve analysis revealed that serum 25(OH)D level of less than 11.2 ng/ml increases the risk of NAFLD with 45% sensitivity and 97.5% specificity (Serum 25(OH)D level ≤ 18.1 ng/ml in males and ≤ 9.4 ng/ml in females increase the risk of NAFLD). Multivariate regression analysis showed that vitamin D deficiency, high age, and high BMI were associated with a significant high risk of NAFLD.

Conclusion: NAFLD patients have low serum vitamin D concentrations, suggesting that vitamin D may have a role in the development of NAFLD. Future studies are recommended to determine the important therapeutic implications of vitamin D for the prophylaxis or the treatment of NAFLD.

Keywords: Non-alcoholic fatty liver disease, Vitamin D, Risk factors

Background

Non-alcoholic fatty liver disease (NAFLD) is a clinico-histopathological entity with histological features that occurs in patients with little or no history of alcohol consumption. Patients with NAFLD have hepatic steatosis, with or without inflammation and fibrosis [1]. NAFLD is classified into non-alcoholic fatty liver (NAFL) and non-alcoholic steatohepatitis (NASH). In NAFL, hepatic steatosis is present without evidence of inflammation; while in NASH, hepatic steatosis is associated with hepatic inflammation [2].

The multiple-hit hypothesis is better framing the variable circumstances implicating the development and progression of NAFLD [3]. However, recent studies show that the progression of NAFLD is not always linear, it is not who is more likely to transform into more advanced stages [4], considered as the hepatic manifestation of NAFLD in most cases associated with type 2 diabetes and dyslipidemia [5].

Fatty liver is the hepatic component of metabolic syndrome. The American Heart Association/National Heart, Lung, and Blood Institute and the International Diabetes Federation considered a patient as having metabolic syndrome if he has at least three abnormal findings of the following: abdominal obesity, low high-density

* Correspondence: ahmedgadmed@yahoo.com
[1]Internal Medicine Department, Faculty of Medicine, Zagazig University, Zagazig, Sharkia 44519, Egypt

lipoprotein, cholesterol, elevated blood pressure, high fasting glucose, or high triglyceride concentration [6].

Vitamin D has been associated with many disease pathogenesis including autoimmune disease, cardiovascular disease, cancers, inflammatory processes, and liver diseases [7–9]. The association between vitamin D levels and NAFLD has been increasingly determined in recent researches [9].

The pathogenesis of the association between NAFLD and low vitamin D levels is still undetermined; however, protective anti-fibrotic and anti-inflammatory function of vitamin D on the hepatic stellate cells has been suggested [10]. Vitamin D reduces free fatty acid-induced insulin resistance in peripheral tissues and in hepatocytes [11]. Therefore, low vitamin D level may lead to intrahepatic lipid accumulation which is responsible for NAFLD pathogenesis [12]. Abramovitch and colleagues confirmed the anti-fibrotic effects of vitamin D through inhibition of hepatic stellate cells proliferation in an in vivo murine model [12].

NHANES III database reviewed more than 6000 patients; of them, about 300 patients showed unexplained elevation in alanine aminotransferase (ALT) and lower vitamin D levels than the control group [13].

Given that vitamin D deficiency and NAFLD have direct and indirect associations with obesity and sedentary lifestyle, it is not unexpected that vitamin D deficiency would be a co-factor in the pathogenesis of NAFLD. Therefore, the aim of this study was to determine the relationship between the serum vitamin D level assessed by 25-hydroxyvitamin D3 (25(OH)D3) and NAFLD in adults.

Methods

Study design

A hospital-based non-interventional cross-sectional controlled study was carried out in the Internal Medicine Department and Immunology Research Lab in Microbiology and Immunology Department at Faculty of Medicine, Zagazig University Hospitals. The institutional review board approved the study (ZU-IRB#3776-30-5-2017). Written informed consent was obtained from all individual participants in the study.

Patients' selection and data collection

Eligible patients had a diagnosis of NAFLD, were aged 18 to 60 years old, and had bright hepatic texture proven with abdominal ultrasound. Matched normal control subjects with normal liver ultrasound /liver chemistry were included. The individual participants in the study were classified into the NAFLD group and healthy control group, were matched in age, gender, residence, the existing comorbidities, and the smoking status.

We excluded patients with chronic viral hepatitis, liver cirrhosis secondary to any cause, primary biliary cirrhosis, primary sclerosing cholangitis, and pregnant women, and patients on calcium or vitamin D supplementation and renal diseases. We also excluded any patients that received vitamin D supply in the previous 2 months.

The following data were collected for each patient eligible for the study: age, gender, residency, smoking status, body mass index (BMI), fasting blood glucose (FBG), hemoglobin A1C (HbA1C), hemoglobin, white blood cells, platelets, total bilirubin, direct bilirubin, alanine transferase (ALT), aspartate transferase (AST), albumin, total plasma protein, alkaline phosphatase, international normalized ratio (INR), creatinine, blood urea nitrogen (BUN), cholesterol, triglyceride, low-density lipoprotein, and high-density lipoprotein. In addition, serum 25(OH)D level was measured for the both groups. Vitamin D deficiency was defined as 25(OH)D levels < 20 ng/ml, while vitamin D insufficiency and sufficiency mean that serum 25(OH)D are equal to 20–30 ng/mL and 30–100 ng/mL, respectively [14–16].

Assessment procedures

Blood samples were obtained from each patient and kept for 30 min for spontaneous clotting. Samples were then centrifuged at 3000 rpm for 5 min and stored for up to 5 days at 2 to 8 °C prior to assaying. Specimens held for a longer time (up to 2 months) and were frozen only once at – 20 °C prior to assay. Serum 25(OH)D level was measured by DBC immunoassay of 25(OH)D enzyme-linked immunosorbent assay (ELISA, DBC Diagnostics Biochem Canada: CAN-VD-510) at the Immunology Research Lab in Microbiology and Immunology Department, Zagazig University Hospitals [17]. All other laboratory tests, including liver and renal function tests, and coagulation tests underwent using the routine laboratory testing methods. Liver ultrasonography (US) was performed to study liver echogenicity, size, cirrhotic changes, or other abnormalities. Liver Ultrasonography (US) scanning was performed to assess the degree of steatosis. Transient elastography (Fibroscan) for measurement of controlled attenuation parameter (CAP) and liver stiffness measurements (LSM) were performed by an experienced radiologist who was blinded to the clinical data of the patients [18, 19].

We used ultrasonographic grading of fatty liver [20] as the following:

Grade 0: normal liver echogenicity.

Grade I: diffusely increased hepatic echogenicity but periportal and diaphragmatic echogenicity are still appreciable.

Grade II: diffusely increased hepatic echogenicity obscuring periportal echogenicity but diaphragmatic echogenicity is still appreciable.

Grade III: diffusely increased hepatic echogenicity obscuring periportal as well as diaphragmatic echogenicity.

Statistical analysis

All categorical variables were presented in frequency and percentage, whereas numerical variables were presented with mean ± standard deviation (SD). Comparative analysis and inferential statistics were performed using parametric independent *t* test that was used for comparison in case of Gaussian distribution, while the Mann-Whitney *U* test was used for non-Gaussian distribution. For categorical variables, the chi-square test (or Fisher's exact test if appropriate) was used. For all statistical tests, P value ≤ 0.05 was considered statistically significant. Spearman's rank correlation coefficient (Spearman's rho) was calculated for 25(OH)D levels and various study parameters. These analyses were performed using the statistical software program, SPSS, for Windows version 25.0 (SPSS; Chicago, IL, USA). Univariate and multivriate logistic regression analysis were used to determine the predictor variables for the presences of NAFLD.

Receiver operating characteristic (ROC) curve analysis was used to identify optimal cutoff values of 25(OH)D levels with maximum sensitivity and specificity for predicting the NAFLD patients. The best cutoff points were the concentration of serum 25(OH)D at the associated criterion of the highest Youden Index from the ROC analysis using the MedCalc software (MedCalc 10 Software bvba, Ostend, Belgium).

Results

Eighty subjects participated in the present study, of whom 40 subjects had NAFLD, whereas 40 subjects served as healthy control. The demographic and baseline characteristics of the subjects based on the groups are presented in Table 1. The two groups were comparable in all demographic data except the BMI, which was significantly higher in the NAFLD Group (30.8 ± 6.3 kg/m^2 versus 34.6 ± 4.3 kg/m^2, P = 0.012). The means CAP and LSM were significantly higher in the NAFLD Group (p < 0.001).

Table 2 shows the results of all laboratory data in the two groups. Blood urea nitrogen (BUN) was lower in the NAFLD Group (14.1 ± 2.3 mg/dL) than the normal control group (17.7 ± 2.4 mg/dL), p = 0.012.

Among the patients with NAFLD, the ultrasonographic grading of fatty liver was as follows: 16 (40%) grade 1, 21 (52.5%) grade 1, and 3 (7.5%) grade 3.

Mean serum 25 (OH)D was significantly lower in the NAFLD group (16.13 ± 10.23 ng/mL) than the control group (27.35 ± 10.58 ng/mL). About 70% of patients with NAFLD had vitamin D deficiency, but only 35% in the control group as seen in Fig. 1.

Table 1 Baseline characteristics of the two study groups at baseline

Variables		Control group	NAFLD group	*P* value
Age (year), mean ± SD		45 ± 10	47 ± 9	0.31
Sex, *N* (%)	Female	27 (67.5%)	27 (67.5%)	1.0
	Male	13 (32.5%)	13 (32.5%)	
Residence, *N* (%)	Rural	23 (57.5%)	22 (55%)	1.0
	Urban	17 (42.5%)	18 (45%)	
Comorbidities, *N* (%)	Diabetes mellitus	6 (15%)	10 (25%)	0.52
	Diabetes/hypertension	5 (12.5%)	7 (17.5%)	
	Gout	1 (2.5%)	1 (2.5%)	
	Hypertension	6 (15%)	7 (17.5%)	
	Hypothyroidism	0 (0.0%)	1 (2.5%)	
	No	22 (55%)	14 (35%)	
Smoking, *N* (%)	No	34 (85%)	35 (87.5%)	1.0
	Yes	6 (15%)	5 (12.5%)	
BMI (kg/m^2), mean ± SD		30.8 ± 6.3	34.6 ± 4.3	**0.012***
Fasting blood glucose (mg/dl), mean ± SD		118.2 ± 32.91	108.7 ± 25.4	0.37
HbA1C (%), mean ± SD		7.77 ± 0.96	7.99 ± 0.43	0.41
CAP (dB/m)		190 ± 37	308 ± 53.3	**< 0.001***
LSM (kPa)		5.2 ± 1.2	6.62 ± 1.5	**< 0.001***

HCV hepatitis C virus, *HBV* hepatitis D virus, *BMI* body mass index, *HbA1C* hemoglobin A1C, *CAP* controlled attenuation parameter, *LSM* liver stiffness measurement

Table 2 Laboratory investigations of the two study groups at baseline

Variables	Control group(mean ± SD)	NAFLD group(mean ± SD)	*P* value
Serum 25 (OH)D (ng/mL)	27.35 ± 10.58	16.13 ± 10.23	**< 0.001***
White blood cells (10^9/L)	6.8 ± 1.8	7.4 ± 1.9	0.44
Hemoglobin (g/dL)	12.5 ± 1.4	12.2 ± 1.3	0.19
Platelets (10^9/L)	258 ± 51	258 ± 57	0.21
Total bilirubin (mg/dL)	0.75 ± 0.20	0.75 ± 0.20	0.96
Direct bilirubin (mg/dL)	0.20 ± 0.14	0.20 ± 0.13	0.94
ALT (U/L)	41 ± 19	43 ± 18	0.63
AST (U/L)	35 ± 26	37 ± 28	0.74
Albumin (g/dL)	4.1 ± 0.4	4.1 ± 0.3	0.71
Total plasma protein (g/dL)	7.36 ± 0.38	7.37 ± 0.37	0.93
Alkaline phosphatase (U/L)	86 ± 20	90 ± 20	0.35
INR	0.99 ± 0.19	1 ± 0.08	0.71
Creatinine (mg/dL)	0.83 ± 0.20	0.78 ± 0.16	0.26
BUN (mg/dL)	17.7 ± 2.4	14.1 ± 2.3	**< 0.001***
Cholesterol (mg/dL)	206.3 ± 32.6	213.2 ± 37.6	0.38
Triglyceride (mg/dL)	161.2 ± 65.6	167.1 ± 69.6	0.69
Low-density lipoprotein (mg/dL)	130 ± 36	130 ± 36	0.98
High-density lipoprotein (mg/dL)	45.9 ± 6.6	45.6 ± 6.6	0.81

INR international normalized ratio, *BUN* blood urea nitrogen, *ALT* alanine aminotransferase, *AST* aspartate aminotransferase

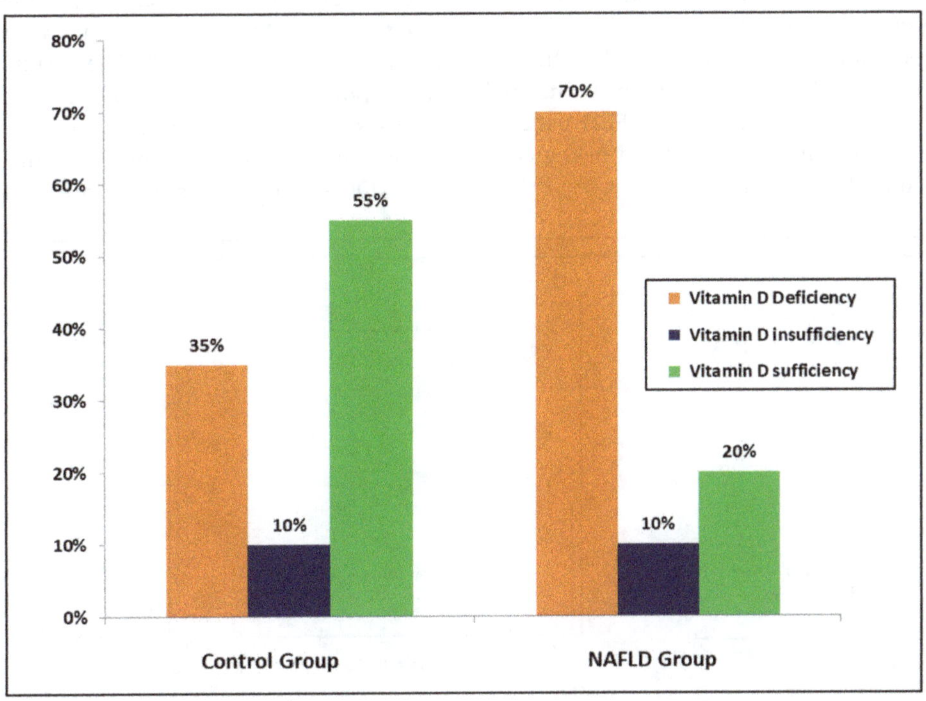

Fig. 1 Comparison of the vitamin D status (serum 25(OH)D) between the study groups

ROC curve analysis reveals that serum 25(OH)D level of ≤ 11.2 ng/ml can predict the presence of NAFLD with 45% sensitivity and 97.5% specificity (Fig. 2a). Furthermore, in male patients, the cut of level of serum 25(OH)D ≤ 18.1 ng/ml can predict the presence of NAFLD with 76.92% sensitivity and 76.92% specificity (Fig. 2b), while in female patients with 25(OH)D level of ≤ 9.4 ng/ml can predict the presence of NAFLD with 44.4% sensitivity and 99.9% specificity (Fig. 2c). The areas under the curve were 0.78, 0.81, and 0.78 respectively.

In the univariate logistic regression analysis model, by considering the vitamin D sufficiency as the reference, the risk of NAFLD for the groups with vitamin D deficiency and insufficiency obtained about 5.15 (95% CI 1.78: 14.9) and 2.51 (95% CI 0.46: 13.6), respectively. In addition, patients with high age and BMI were significantly associated with a high risk of NAFLD [OR = 2.08 (95% CI 1.09: 2.17)] and [OR = 2.82 (95% CI 1.71: 5.94)]. In a multivariate logistic regression analysis model, vitamin D deficiency, high age, and high BMI were associated with a significant high risk of NAFLD as presented in Table 3.

Discussion

Low vitamin D is prevalent in chronic liver disease patients. Even patients with mild liver disease are affected, although patients with liver cirrhosis are more commonly have severe deficiency [21]. Low serum levels of vitamin D have been observed in chronic liver diseases, especially with liver cirrhosis [8, 22], while in patients with NAFLD, the data are still scanty.

Our study demonstrates that the serum 25 (OH)D was significantly lower in the NAFLD group than the normal control group. More than two thirds of NAFLD patients had vitamin D deficiency, but only one third of the control group had vitamin D deficiency.

The recent systematic review of Pacifico and colleagues [23] included 45 studies exploring the association between vitamin D status and NAFLD/NASH. Of them, 29 studies reported an inverse association between vitamin D status and NAFLD, while 16 studies did not support this association.

On the other hand, the meta-analysis on the relationship between serum vitamin D and NAFLD histologic severity found no association between serum vitamin D levels and disease severity as assessed by NAS and fibrosis score among patients with NAFLD [24].

Using the NHANES III database, Liangpunsakul and Chalasani screened 6800 patients. They found 308 patients with unexplained elevation in ALT and compared their serum vitamin D concentrations with 979 matched controls. Patients with elevated ALT were found to have lower vitamin D levels than the control group, even when controlling for metabolic syndrome and serum triglyceride level [13]. Furthermore, Targher et al. confirmed the association between NAFLD and vitamin D deficiency. In addition, vitamin D concentrations were lower in NASH patients when compared to those with isolated fatty liver [25].

Mean serum 25 (OH)D of 16.13 ± 10.23 ng/mL in the NAFLD group was significantly lower than in the normal control group (27.35 ± 10.58 ng/mL). The results of systematic review [23] showed that the median level of vitamin D in the control group is 27.7 ± 8.75 ng/mL, while the mean level in the NAFLD group is 25.7 ± 8.74.

In the cross-sectional study of Ehrampoush and colleagues [26], the mean serum vitamin D was 26.77 ± 8.26 ng/mL in the healthy group, while in the NAFLD group, it was 15.84 ± 5.50. The results showed that the cutoff point for vitamin D in men and women, vitamin D levels lower than 18 nmol/L for women and 21 nmol/L for men, significantly increases the risk of NAFLD. The ROC curve analysis of the present study reveals that

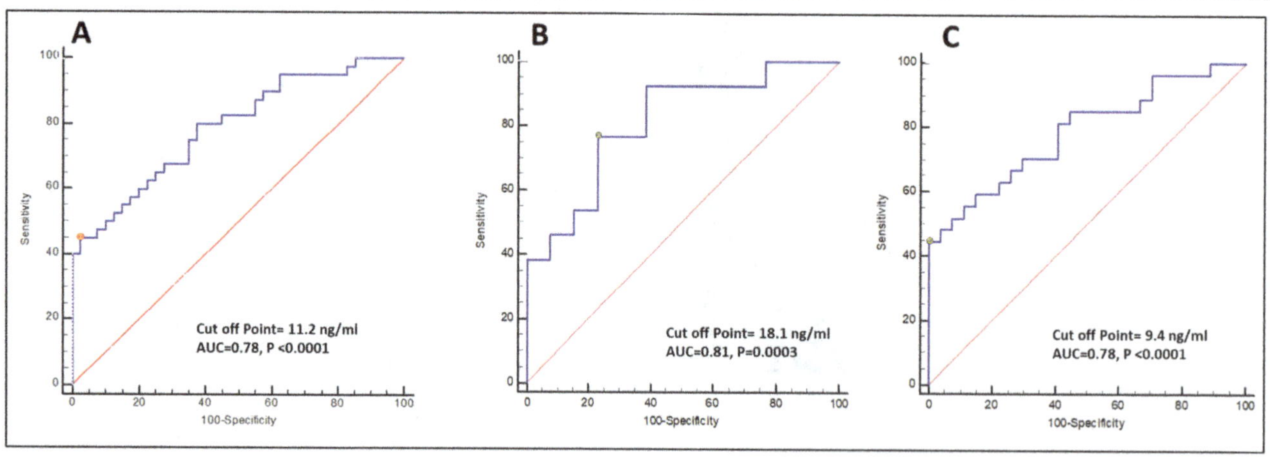

Fig. 2 ROC curve analysis of serum 25(OH)D level that can predict the NAFLD in **a** all patients, **b** male patients, and **c** female patients

Table 3 Binary logistic regression analysis for factors predicting the NAFLD

	Wald	*P* value	OR	95% CI for OR	
				Lower	Upper
Univariate analysis model					
Age	3.046	**0.041**	2.075	1.091	1.167
Gender (ref: male)	0.575	0.448	0.644	0.206	2.010
Diabetes (ref: No.)	1.574	**0.021**	1.913	1.095	5.266
Smoking (ref: No.)	.581	0.446	0.562	0.128	2.472
25(OH)D3 deficiency (ref: sufficiency)	9.151	**0.002**	5.152	1.781	14.905
25(OH)D3 insufficiency (ref: sufficiency)	1.140	0.286	2.511	0.463	13.602
BMI (kg/m2)	8.283	**0.004**	2.815	1.709	5.937
Fasting blood glucose (mg/dl)	0.114	0.735	0.996	0.973	1.020
White blood cells (10^9/L)	0.004	0.949	1.013	0.688	1.491
Hemoglobin (g/dL)	0.106	0.744	0.910	0.517	1.602
Platelets (10^9/L)	0.757	0.384	1.006	0.993	1.018
AST (U/L)	2.380	0.123	1.059	0.985	1.138
ALT(U/L)	1.513	0.219	0.964	0.910	1.022
Albumin (g/dL)	0.007	0.933	0.918	0.126	6.688
Total plasma protein (g/dL)	0.410	0.522	0.499	0.060	4.187
Alkaline phosphatase (U/L)	1.501	0.220	1.022	0.987	1.059
Cholesterol (mg/dL)	0.123	0.726	0.994	0.961	1.028
Triglyceride (mg/dL)	0.313	0.576	1.004	0.990	1.018
Low-density lipoprotein (mg/dL)	0.109	0.741	0.995	0.966	1.025
High-density lipoprotein (mg/dL)	1.223	0.269	0.936	0.833	1.052
Multivariate analysis model					
Age	4.344	**0.037**	1.080	1.005	1.160
BMI (kg/m2)	5.888	**0.015**	2.862	1.764	3.972
25(OH)D3 deficiency (ref: sufficiency)	9.151	**0.002**	4.171	1.345	12.872

serum 25(OH)D level ≤ 11.2 ng/ml can predict the presence of NAFLD; in male patients, the cut of level of vitamin D ≤ 18.1 ng/ml can predict the presence of NAFLD, while in female patients, it was ≤ 9.4 ng/ml.

In our study, we observed nearly normal levels of liver enzymes in patients with NAFLD. This observation was supported by the recent meta-analysis that conducted to determine the proportion of NAFLD patients with normal ALT value in the overall NAFLD patients [27]. They reported that the proportion of NAFLD patients with normal ALT value in overall NAFLD patients was 25% (95% CI 20–31%).

Many of the epidemiological studies linking low serum vitamin D levels with NAFLD is that the two conditions are associated with obesity (high BMI) [25, 28, 29]. Vitamin D is fat soluble and stored in adipose tissue that increases the sequestration of vitamin D in obese individuals who are also prone to NAFLD [30]. Our study showed that patients with high BMI were significantly associated with a high risk of NAFLD.

The main limitation of our study is the small sample size, which might limit the generalizability of the result. We included only adult's patients, while the study by Manco et al. [31] reported that low levels of 25(OH)D in children with NAFLD correlated with histological severity regardless the metabolic characteristics.

In conclusion, our results showed a significant relationship between vitamin D levels and the risk of NAFLD. Particularly, our study suggests that serum 25(OH)D level less than 9.4 ng/ml for females and 18.1 ng/ml for males can increase the risk of NAFLD. It is important to maintain the appropriate serum level of vitamin D for protecting against NAFLD. Determination of a main role of low vitamin D in NAFLD development might have important therapeutic implications in future studies. In addition, conducting future studies comparing the vitamin D levels in different liver disease is highly recommended. Finally, the association between vitamin D deficiency with prognosis of liver diseases as progression to NASH or development of HCC should be addressed through a prospective studies.

Abbreviations

ALT: Alanine aminotransferase; INR: International normalized ratio; AST: Aspartate aminotransferase; BMI: Body mass index; BUN: Blood urea nitrogen; FBG: Fasting blood glucose; HbA1C: Hemoglobin A1C; NAFLD: Non-alcoholic fatty liver disease; NASH: Non-alcoholic steatohepatitis; ROC: Receiver operating characteristic; SD: Standard deviation

Acknowledgements

Authors would like to thank Dr. Hussien Ahmed for the great help in statistics and editorial support. All patients were acknowledged for participations in this research.

Authors' contributions

AG generates the research idea. AG and ME perform the clinical examination. AM performs the laboratory analysis. All authors shared in analyzing and interpreting the patient data and in writing the manuscript. All authors read and approved the final manuscript.

Competing interests

The authors declare that they have no competing interests.

Author details

[1]Internal Medicine Department, Faculty of Medicine, Zagazig University, Zagazig, Sharkia 44519, Egypt. [2]Microbiology and Immunology Department, Faculty of Medicine, Zagazig University, Zagazig, Egypt.

References

1. Younossi ZM, Loomba R, Rinella ME, Bugianesi E, Marchesini G, Neuschwander-Tetri BA, Serfaty L, Negro F, Caldwell SH, Ratziu V, Corey KE, Friedman SL, Abdelmalek MF, Harrison SA, Sanyal AJ, Lavine JE, Mathurin P, Charlton MR, Chalasani NP, Anstee QM, Kowdley KV, George J, Goodman ZD, Lindor K (2018) Current and future therapeutic regimens for nonalcoholic fatty liver disease and nonalcoholic steatohepatitis. Hepatology 68:361–371
2. Sheth SG, Gordon FD, Chopra S (1997) Nonalcoholic steatohepatitis. Ann Intern Med 126:137–145
3. Buzzetti E, Pinzani M, Tsochatzis EA (2016) The multiple-hit pathogenesis of non-alcoholic fatty liver disease (NAFLD). Metabolism 65:1038–1048
4. Younossi ZM, Loomba R, Anstee QM, Rinella ME, Bugianesi E, Marchesini G, Neuschwander-Tetri BA, Serfaty L, Negro F, Caldwell SH, Ratziu V, Corey KE, Friedman SL, Abdelmalek MF, Harrison SA, Sanyal AJ, Lavine JE, Mathurin P, Charlton MR, Goodman ZD, Chalasani NP, Kowdley KV, George J, Lindor K (2018) Diagnostic modalities for nonalcoholic fatty liver disease, nonalcoholic steatohepatitis, and associated fibrosis. Hepatology 68:349–360
5. Angulo P (2008) Obesity and nonalcoholic fatty liver disease. Nutr Rev 65: S57–S63
6. Gastaldelli A (2010) Fatty liver disease: the hepatic manifestation of metabolic syndrome. Hypertens Res 33:546–547
7. Guillot X, Semerano L, Saidenberg-Kermanac'h N, Falgarone G, Boissier M-C (2010) Vitamin D and inflammation. Jt Bone Spine 77:552–557
8. Kitson MT, Roberts SK (2012) D-livering the message: the importance of vitamin D status in chronic liver disease. J Hepatol 57:897–909
9. Kwok RM, Torres DM, Harrison SA (2013) Vitamin D and nonalcoholic fatty liver disease (NAFLD): is it more than just an association? Hepatology 58: 1166–1174
10. Abramovitch S, Dahan-Bachar L, Sharvit E, Weisman Y, Tov AB, Brazowski E, Reif S (2011) Vitamin D inhibits proliferation and profibrotic marker expression in hepatic stellate cells and decreases thioacetamide-induced liver fibrosis in rats. Gut 60:1728–1737
11. Zhou QG, Hou FF, Guo ZJ, Liang M, Wang GB, Zhang X (2008) 1,25-Dihydroxyvitamin D improved the free fatty-acid-induced insulin resistance in cultured C2C12 cells. Diabetes Metab Res Rev 24:459–464
12. Konstantakis C (2016). Vitamin D deficiency in patients with liver cirrhosis. Ann Gastroenterol.
13. Liangpunsakul S, Chalasani N (2011) Serum vitamin D concentrations and unexplained elevation in ALT among US adults. Dig Dis Sci 56:2124–2129
14. Holick MF (2006) High prevalence of vitamin D inadequacy and implications for health. Mayo Clin Proc 81:353–373
15. Bischoff-Ferrari HA, Giovannucci E, Willett WC, Dietrich T, Dawson-Hughes B (2006) Estimation of optimal serum concentrations of 25-hydroxyvitamin D for multiple health outcomes. Am J Clin Nutr 84:18–28
16. Dawson-Hughes B, Heaney RP, Holick MF, Lips P, Meunier PJ, Vieth R (2005) Estimates of optimal vitamin D status. Osteoporos Int 16:713–716
17. Yousif MM, Sadek AMEM, Farrag HA, Selim FO, Hamed EF, Salama RI (2019) Associated vitamin D deficiency is a risk factor for the complication of HCV-related liver cirrhosis including hepatic encephalopathy and spontaneous bacterial peritonitis. Intern Emerg Med 14:753–761
18. Angulo P, Hui JM, Marchesini G, Bugianesi E, George J, Farrell GC, Enders F, Saksena S, Burt AD, Bida JP, Lindor K, Sanderson SO, Lenzi M, Adams LA, Kench J, Therneau TM, Day CP (2007) The NAFLD fibrosis score: a noninvasive system that identifies liver fibrosis in patients with NAFLD. Hepatology 45:846–854
19. Sterling RK, Lissen E, Clumeck N, Sola R, Correa MC, Montaner J, Sulkowski MS, Torriani FJ, Dieterich DT, Thomas DL, Messinger D, Nelson M (2006) Development of a simple noninvasive index to predict significant fibrosis in patients with HIV/HCV coinfection. Hepatology 43:1317–1325
20. Das C, Baruah M, Singh D (2013) Imaging of non alcoholic fatty liver disease: A road less travelled. Indian J Endocrinol Metab 17:990
21. Arteh J, Narra S, Nair S (2010) Prevalence of vitamin D deficiency in chronic liver disease. Dig Dis Sci 55:2624–2628
22. Lange CM, Bojunga J, Ramos-Lopez E, von Wagner M, Hassler A, Vermehren J, Herrmann E, Badenhoop K, Zeuzem S, Sarrazin C (2011) Vitamin D deficiency and a CYP27B1-1260 promoter polymorphism are associated with chronic hepatitis C and poor response to interferon-alfa based therapy. J Hepatol 54:887–893
23. Pacifico L, Osborn JF, Bonci E, Pierimarchi P, Chiesa C (2019) Association between vitamin D levels and nonalcoholic fatty liver disease: potential confounding variables. Mini-Reviews Med Chem 19:310–332
24. Jaruvongvanich V, Ahuja W, Sanguankeo A, Wijarnpreecha K, Upala S (2017) Vitamin D and histologic severity of nonalcoholic fatty liver disease: a systematic review and meta-analysis. Dig Liver Dis 49:618–622
25. Targher G, Bertolini L, Scala L, Cigolini M, Zenari L, Falezza G, Arcaro G (2007) Associations between serum 25-hydroxyvitamin D3 concentrations and liver histology in patients with non-alcoholic fatty liver disease. Nutr Metab Cardiovasc Dis 17:517–524
26. Ehrampoush E, Ghaemi A, Osati S, Maleki M, Raeisi Shahraki H, Honarvar B, Bahmanyar M, Homayounfar R (2019) The association between serum vitamin D level and nonalcoholic fatty liver disease. Hepat Mon 19(9): e92992
27. Ma X, Liu S, Zhang J, Dong M, Wang Y, Wang M, Xin Y (2020) Proportion of NAFLD patients with normal ALT value in overall NAFLD patients: a systematic review and meta-analysis. BMC Gastroenterol 14(1):20
28. Bhatt SP, Nigam P, Misra A, Guleria R, Qadar Pasha MA (2013) Independent associations of low 25 hydroxy vitamin D and high parathyroid hormonal levels with nonalcoholic fatty liver disease in Asian Indians residing in north India. Atherosclerosis 230:157–163
29. Black LJ, Jacoby P, She Ping-Delfos WC, Mori TA, Beilin LJ, Olynyk JK, Ayonrinde OT, Huang RC, Holt PG, Hart PH, Oddy WH, Adams LA (2014) Low serum 25-hydroxyvitamin D concentrations associate with non-alcoholic fatty liver disease in adolescents independent of adiposity. J Gastroenterol Hepatol 29:1215–1222
30. Wortsman J, Matsuoka LY, Chen TC, Lu Z, Holick MF (2000) Decreased bioavailability of vitamin D in obesity. Am J Clin Nutr 72:690–693
31. Manco M, Ciampalini P, Nobili V (2010) Low levels of 25-hydroxyvitamin D3 in children with biopsy-proven nonalcoholic fatty liver disease. Hepatology 51:2229–2229

9

Is the laparoscopic choledochal cyst excision and Roux-En-Y hepaticojejunostomy in adults as safe as that in children?

Nguyen Thanh Xuan[1], Nguyen Huu Son[2] and Ho Huu Thien[1*]

Abstract

Background: Laparoscopic cyst excision and Roux-en-Y hepaticojejunostomy for treating congenital choledochal cysts has been proven to be efficacious in children, but its safety and efficacy in adult patients remain uncertain. This study aims to investigate the safety and effectiveness of laparoscopic choledochal cyst excision and Roux-en-Y hepaticojejunostomy in adults compared to those in children patients.

Results: There was no conversion to open surgery in both groups. The mean operative time and hospital duration stay in adults (253.4 min and 11.7 days, respectively) were longer in than those in children (214.7 min and 9.3 days, respectively). Intraoperative blood transfusion was required in one adult and two children. There was not reoperation due to bile leakage in adults compared to those in 2 children. The time from surgery to drainage removal was longer in adults (3.6 vs. 2.9 days). The outcome within three months of discharge was classified as good in 88.2 % of adults and 90.5% for children. There were no statistically significant differences in early postoperative complications or treatment outcomes between the two groups.

Conclusions: Laparoscopic choledochal cyst excision followed by Roux-en-Y hepaticojejunostomy was safe and efficient in both adults and children. Operative time was longer in adults than in children.

Keywords: Laparoscopic excision, Roux-en-Y hepaticojejunostomy, Choledochal cyst

Background

Choledochal cysts consist of focal or diffuse dilatation of intra- and/or extra-hepatic bile ducts, a congenital abnormality first described by Vater and Ezler in 1723 [1], and later, in 1852 by Douglas. Biliary cysts are usually diagnosed in children. Some studies showed the excellent outcomes of laparoscopic choledochal cyst excision and Roux-en-Y in children [2, 3]. Nowadays, choledochal cyst excision and Roux-en-Y hepaticojejunostomy have become the technique of choice in children in our hospital [4], but its safety and efficacy in adult patients remain uncertain.

However, approximately 20 to 25% of cases is found in adults; the incidence of detection is on the rise, mainly because of improved imaging techniques [5]. The majority of patients are female and of far Eastern origin with well-recognized differences in clinical presentation and symptoms between adults and children [6].

In this report, we sought to investigate the safety and effectiveness of laparoscopic choledochal cyst excision and Roux-en-Y hepaticojejunostomy in adults compared to those in children patients.

* Correspondence: thientrangduc@hotmail.com
[1]Department of Pediatric and Abdominal Emergency Surgery, Hue Central Hospital, 16 Le Loi Street, Hue City, Vietnam

Methods

Patients

Seventy consecutive patients (51 under 16 years of age "children" and 19 older than 16 years of age "adults") diagnosed with type I choledochal cysts underwent laparoscopic choledochal cyst excision and Roux-en-Y hepaticojejunostomy between June 2012 and December 2017.

All procedures were performed by the same surgical team, specialists in both pediatric and adult surgery, according to local practice in Hue Central Hospital, Vietnam [4]. Choledochal cysts were classified according to the Todani classification [7] initially based on preoperative ultrasound, computed tomography scan, and/or magnetic resonance imaging, and finally confirmed by intraoperative gross examination.

This study was approved by the Ethics Committee Review board of Hue Central Hospital under the reference number: HCH-05052012. Confidentiality was ensured by not writing the names of patients on proforma in accordance the Helsinki Declaration.

Operative technique

The patient was positioned supine. Full HD Laparoscopy system (4 K laparoscopic system was used from September 2016) is on the patient's right, surgeon and assistant on the patient's left. A 10-mm infraumbilical trocar (supraumbilical in children) was inserted for the camera and 12 mmHg pneumoperitoneum was achieved with carbon dioxide (8–10 mmHg for children). A 10-mm port was inserted in the left side on the midclavicular line, 3 cm above the umbilicus. Two additional trocars of 5 mm in the right hypochondrium. In some cases, a 5-mm trocar was placed in the subxiphoid area to elevate the liver. After observing the common bile duct cyst at the liver hilum, the gallbladder was separated from the cyst (Fig. 1). Then, the cyst was separated from the duodenum, the narrowed retroduodenal bile duct was reached and was transected with a 60 mm endoscopic stapler if the diameter more than 10 mm; otherwise, it was transected between two hemolocks (Fig. 2). Then, the cyst was separated from the duodenum, the narrowed retroduodenal bile duct was reached and was transected with a 60 mm endoscopic stapler if the diameter more than 10 mm, otherwise it was transected between two hemolocks (Fig. 2). The latter method was in children in most cases. The free distal end of the cyst was retracted laterally and towards the abdominal wall and was separated from other structures in the liver hilum (right hepatic artery and portal vein). The cyst was dissected up to the highest level that can be technically achieved. The jejunum was transected with an endoscopic stapler 25–30 cm away from the ligament of Treitz for hepaticojejunostomy. The distal end was advanced in a retrocolic manner, and the Roux loop was brought to the liver hilum. The cyst was transected and extracted out of the umbilical trocar site with the gallbladder at the end of the operation. When the bile duct was opened, it was observed that the biliary bifurcation has been reached (Fig. 3). The hepaticojejunostomy anastomosis was created following an enterotomy with interrupted Vicryl 3/0 sutures (4/0 vicryl in case of children) (Fig. 4). Finally, a side-to-side enteroenterostomy was created by a 60-mm endoscopic stapler between the loop 60 cm distal from the Roux loop and the afferent loop from the Treitz ligament. In children, the transection of the jejunum and the side to side entero-enterostomy were performed through the enlarge umbilical site about 3 cm. A redon suction drain was placed posterior to the hepaticojejunostomy after completion of cholecystectomy which was remove on third day or less than 3 ml/h.

Follow-up and data analysis

Eleven patients (9 children and 2 adults) were lost to follow-up. Clinical outcome was determined according to the Terblanche classification [8]: grade I, no biliary

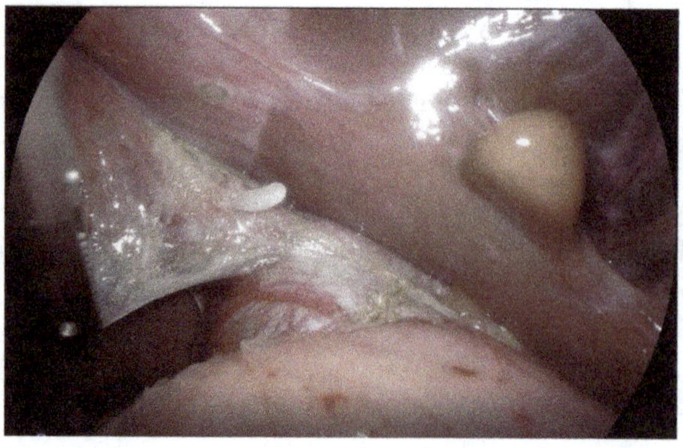

Fig. 1 Transection of the cystic duct

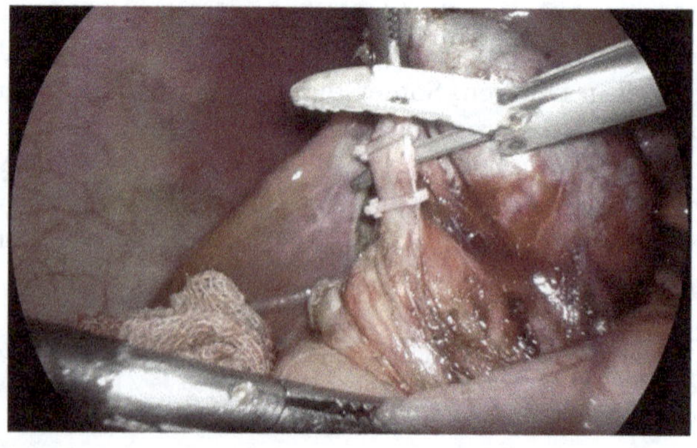

Fig. 2 Distal common bile duct was transected between two hemolocks

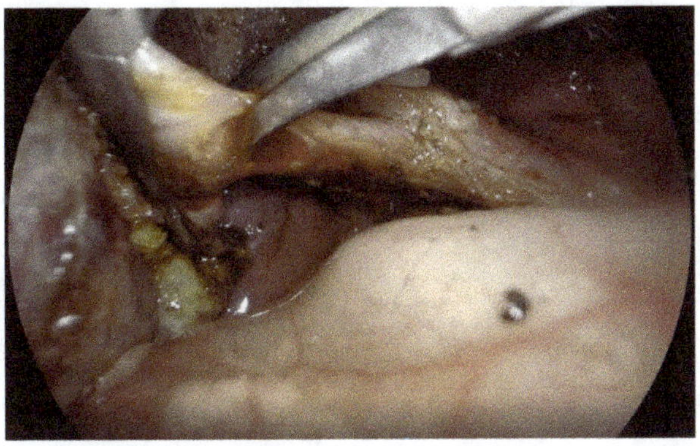

Fig. 3 Common hepatic duct was transected at the hilum

symptoms; grade II, transitory symptoms and no current symptoms; grade III, biliary symptoms requiring medical therapy; and grade IV, recurrent biliary symptoms requiring correction or related to death. Terblanche I, II, and III constituted a clinical success with excellent, good, and fair results, respectively, while Terblanche class IV constituted a poor result.

For comparison between the children and adult groups, we searched the electronic medical records for the following data: patient demographics, operative details, and outcomes such as operation time, need for intraoperative blood transfusion, type of cyst dissection (cyst dissection was considered as standard if the distal part of the cyst was firstly dissected, and non-standard if the cyst was firstly dissected from the proximal part), duration of postoperative hospital stay, and postoperative complications. For descriptive analysis, the frequency or the mean and standard deviation were calculated for each variable. For other continuous variables, independent sample *t* tests were applied to compare the data between children and adults. Their respective *p* values and corresponding confidence intervals were provided by SPSS Version 18.0 (SPSS Inc., Chicago, IL, USA). The statistical significance was set at $p < 0.05$.

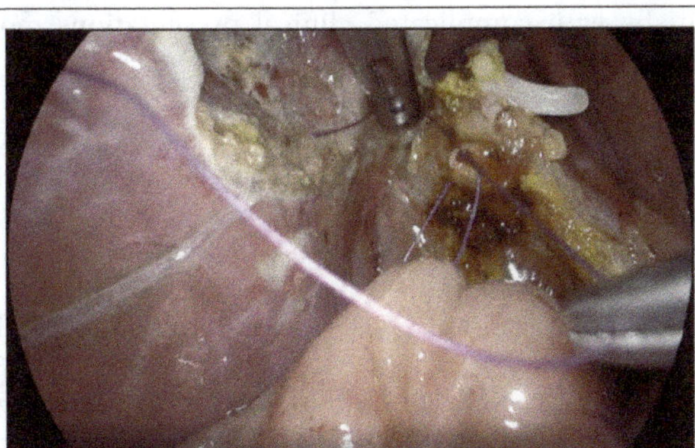

Fig. 4 Hepato-jejuno anastomosis with interrupted suture

Results

Of the 70 patients, 57 were females and 13 were males, 19 were adults, and 51 were children. The mean age at the time of surgery was 12.8 years (range, 2.5 months ~ 75 years), 37.5 years for adults vs. 3.6 years for children. Abdominal pain, fever, and leukocytosis were noted with a significantly higher in adults than those in children, respectively. Conversely, the rate of patients presenting with nausea, vomiting, and jaundice was significantly lower for adults compared to children (Table 1).

For the other laboratory investigation in Table 1, the increasing level of serum bilirubin and hepatic enzyme was significantly lower in adults than in children, respectively.

There was not any conversion to open procedure in both groups.

Table 2 shows the surgical outcomes of laparoscopic choledochal cyst excision and Roux-en-Y hepaticojejunostomy. The mean operative time was 219.8 ± 64.9 min (range, 100~360 min. For adults, the mean operative time was 253.4 ± 55.1 min, range, 120~360 min, statistically significantly longer than in children (214.7 ± 67.9 min (range, 100~360 min).

Intraoperative blood transfusion was required in one adult and two children. The study showed 7 cases of bile leakage, in which 1 adult and 6 children. Conservative treatment was initially implemented for complications, which resulted in complete resolution in 5 cases. Reoperation was required in two children who had persistent bile leakage (accounted for 3.9% of all children patients). From April 2016, 12 children and 3 adults were performed the operations with 4 K laparoscopic system, and we did not recognize any bile leakage postoperatively.

Table 1 Patient characteristics and laboratory findings

Variables	Children (n = 51)	Adults (n = 19)	p value
Gender			
Female	41 (80.4%)	16 (84.2%)	0.9842
Male	10 (19.6%)	3 (15.8%)	
Age (mean)	3.6	37.5	
Symptoms			
Abdominal pain	26 (51.0%)	16 (84.2%)	0.0246
Jaundice	17 (33.3%)	1 (5.3%)	0.0378
Fever	18 (35.3%)	13 (68.4%)	0.0272
Nausea, vomiting	25 (49.0%)	3 (15.8%)	0.0246
Abdominal mass	3 (5.9%)	1 (5.3%)	0.6299
Laboratory findings			
Increased serum AST/ALT	25 (49.0%)	3 (15.8%)	0.0246
Increased total bilirubin	45 (88.2%)	2 (10.5%)	< 0.0001
Leukocytosis	17 (33.3%)	12 (63.2%)	0.0471

Table 2 Surgical outcomes of laparoscopic choledochal cyst excision and Roux-en-Y hepaticojejunostomy

Variables	Children group (n = 51)	Adult group (n = 19)	p value
Operating time (min)	214.7 ± 67.9	253.4 ± 55.1	0.0295
Number of patient requiring blood transusion	2 (3.9%)	1 (5.2%)	0.6699
Blood transfusion volume	125.0 ± 35.4	250	–
Non-standard cyst dissection	3 (5.9%)	5 (26.3%)	0.0177
Time to first flatus (h)	40.3 ± 28.5	45.5 ± 31.3	0.5108
Time to drain removal (days)	2.9 ± 1.0	3.6 ± 1.9	0.0492
Hospital stay (days)	9.3 ± 3.4	11.7 ± 5.5	0.0314
Complications			
Biliary leakage	6 (11.8%)	1 (5.3%)	0.7206
Pancreatitis	2 (3.9%)	1 (5.3%)	0.6843
Outcome classification according to Terreblanche*	n = 42	n = 17	
Good	38 (90.5%)	15 (88.2%)	0.8277
Fair	4 (9.5%)	2 (11.8%)	

*Eleven patients (9 children and 2 adults) were lost to follow-up

Postoperative follow-up results after hospital discharge to 3 months were classified as good in 88.2% of adults and 90.5% for children. There was no malignancy found in both adults and children.

The only statistically significant differences were also found in time to drain removal (3.6 ± 1.9 vs. 2.9 ± 1.0, p = 0.0492) and duration of hospital stay (11.7 ± 5.5 vs. 9.3 ± 3.4, p = 0.0314) in adults and children, respectively.

Conservative treatment was initially implemented for complications, which resulted in complete resolution in seven cases. Reoperation was required in two patients who had persistent bile leakage. Postoperative follow-up results after hospital discharge to 3 months were classified as good in 90.5% of children and 88.2% for adults. There was not malignancy found in both children and adult.

Discussion

Congenital bile duct cysts, although a pediatric disease, can be detected in adults. It is more common in far eastern countries such as China, Korea, Japan, and Vietnam. Although there are various classifications, the most common type (78%) is fusiform dilatation of the extrahepatic bile ducts (Todani Type I) [9]. Laparoscopic choledochal cyst excision and hepaticojejunostomy in children is widely accepted, and several studies have described the advantages of laparoscopic surgery [10, 11]. Liem NT et al. reported laparoscopic choledochal cyst excision and reconstruction of the biliary-digestive system as safe and effective with cases of a large number of choledochal cyst patients [10, 12].

Our results confirm that choledochal cysts, essentially a congenital disease, can be silent until adulthood. While certain differences have been described in the symptomology, and clinicopathology laparoscopic choledochal cyst excision and hepaticojejunostomy is safe and effective in adults as well as in children.

Several authors have indicated that the signs and symptoms of patients with choledochal cysts as well as the clinicopathological characteristics differ between children and adults [5, 13, 14]. The classical triad of jaundice, right upper quadrant pain, and a palpable mass has been reported to occur more often in children compared to adults in whom cholangitis, liver abscess, biliary cirrhosis, pancreatitis, cholangiocarcinoma, and antecedent biliary tract disease have been observed more commonly [14]. While choledochal cysts may remain asymptomatic for many years and be diagnosed incidentally, when asymptomatic patients undergo imaging studies for a seemingly unrelated reason, many patients have a long history of digestive tract disorders [13]. Thus, the differences in circumstances of discovery are more of a diagnostic nature than disease related. This may also explain why adult patients are seen initially with complicated clinical presentations more often than children in our study (Table 1) as well as other authors [5, 13, 14].

One of the main complications of laparoscopic choledochal cyst excision is bleeding that can potentially require intraoperative or post-operative blood transfusion. We met the severe inflammation of the cyst more often in adults than children, but careful dissection with surgical energy device the bleeding could be avoided. Both Liem et al [10]. and Tang et al [15]. mentioned the need for intraoperative blood transfusion. In our study, one adult and two children required blood transfusion, and the difference was not significantly seen.

Concerning postoperative complications, several authors have reported post-operative complications after cyst excision and anastomosis, including postoperative bile leakage [11, 16, 17] and pancreatitis (said to be more frequent in patients with preoperative pancreatitis) [18]. Compared to other studies, the rates of early complications of our study were low. We noted three cases of pancreatitis and seven cases of bile leakage (1 adult and 6 children), which resulted in complete resolution in 5 cases. The rate of bile leakage was not significantly different in adults compared to children (Table 2). However, reoperation was required in two children with persistent bile leakage. Besides, the rate of pancreatitis was not significantly different between the two groups.

No postoperative complications have been observed within 3 months in our study, but our follow-up was far from ideal. This is one of the limitations of our study. Postoperative follow-up after hospital discharge to 3 months, the outcome was classified as good in 88.2% of adults and 90.5% of children. There were no significant differences between the two groups ($p = 0.8277$).

During the study, several tips have been suggested to reduce the rate of bile leakage. Firstly, electrical dissection should not be overused, and scissors should be used to cut the hepatic duct. Secondly, the anastomosis should be carefully checked before the end of the operation. Thirdly, a bowel loop with a good arterial arcade with sufficient length should be chosen to construct a tension-free anastomosis. Finally, the using of 4 K laparoscopic system with good images help us a lot in cyst dissection as well as hepaticojejunostomy, which was shown in our later study.

Conclusions

In our series of 70 patients, 27% ($n = 19$) were adults. Laparoscopic choledochal cyst excision and Roux-en-Y hepaticojejunostomy in adults was as safe and effective as that in children. Operative time and hospital duration stay were longer in adults than in children. The rate of bile leakage was not significantly higher in adults compared to that in children.

Acknowledgements
The authors thank A. Fingerhut for his assistance.

Authors' contributions
HHT and NTX has contributed to format the design of the study and revised the collected data. NTX and NHS has done the main work of the statistical data analysis. HHT and HTX has shared the operational work of the study and writing works. HHT and NTX has recruited the participants, contributed to the operational works, interpretation, and analysis of the results. Finally, all authors have read and approved the manuscript.

Competing interests
The authors declare that they have no competing interests.

Author details
[1]Department of Pediatric and Abdominal Emergency Surgery, Hue Central Hospital, 16 Le Loi Street, Hue City, Vietnam. [2]Pediatric Center, Hue Central Hospital, Hue City, Vietnam.

References

1. Soares KC, Arnaoutakis DJ, Kamel I, Rastegar N, Anders R, Maithel S, Pawlik TM (2014) Choledochal cysts: presentation, clinical differentiation, and management. J Am Coll Surg. 219:1167–1180
2. Liem NT (2013) Laparoscopic surgery for choledochal cysts. J Hepatobiliary Pancreat Sci. 20:487–491
3. Song G, Jiang X, Wang J, Li A (2017) Comparative clinical study of laparoscopic and open surgery in children with choledochal cysts. Saudi Med J. 38:476–481
4. Xuan NT, Hiep PN, Thien HH, Vu PA, Thanh PH, Khanh LD, Chau DLM (2013) Laparoscopic excision of choledochal cyst in Hue Central Hospital. Vietnam Laparoscopic surgery and Endoscopy Journal. 1:22–25
5. Woon CY, Tan YM, Oei CL, Chung AY, Chow PK, Ooi LL (2006) Adult choledochal cysts: an audit of surgical management. ANZ J Surg. 76:981–986
6. Huang CS, Huang CC, Chen DF (2010) Choledochal cysts: differences between pediatric and adult patients. J Gastrointest Surg. 14:1105–1110
7. Dumitrascu T, Lupescu I, Ionescu M (2012) The Todani classification for bile duct cysts: an overview. Acta Chir Belg. 112:340–345
8. Terblanche J, Worthley CS, Spence RA, Krige JE (1990) High or low hepaticojejunostomy for bile duct strictures? Surgery. 108:828–834
9. Soreide K, Korner H, Havnen J, Soreide JA (2004) Bile duct cysts in adults. Br J Surg. 91:1538–1548
10. Liem NT, Pham HD, Dung le A, Son TN, Vu HM (2012). Early and intermediate outcomes of laparoscopic surgery for choledochal cysts with 400 patients. J Laparoendosc Adv Surg Tech A. 22: 599-603.
11. Qiao G, Li L, Li S, Tang S, Wang B, Xi H, Gao Z, Sun Q (2015) Laparoscopic cyst excision and Roux-Y hepaticojejunostomy for children with choledochal cysts in China: a multicenter study. Surg Endosc. 29:140–144
12. Nguyen Thanh L, Hien PD, Dung le A, Son TN (2010). Laparoscopic repair for choledochal cyst: lessons learned from 190 cases. J Pediatr Surg. 45: 540-544.
13. Lenriot JP, Gigot JF, Segol P, Fagniez PL, Fingerhut A, Adloff M (1998) Bile duct cysts in adults: a multi-institutional retrospective study. French Associations for Surgical Research. Ann Surg. 228:159–166
14. Mabrut JY, Bozio G, Hubert C, Gigot JF (2010) Management of congenital bile duct cysts. Dig Surg. 27:12–18
15. Tang ST, Yang Y, Wang Y, Mao YZ, Li SW, Tong QS, Cao GQ, Zhao ZX (2011) Laparoscopic choledochal cyst excision, hepaticojejunostomy, and extracorporeal Roux-en-Y anastomosis: a technical skill and intermediate-term report in 62 cases. Surg Endosc. 25:416–422
16. Ono S, Fumino S, Shimadera S, Iwai N (2010) Long-term outcomes after hepaticojejunostomy for choledochal cyst: a 10- to 27-year follow-up. J Pediatr Surg. 45:376–378
17. Sheng Q, Lv Z, Xu W, Xiao X, Liu J, Wu Y (2017) Reoperation After Cyst Excision with Hepaticojejunostomy for Choledochal Cysts: Our Experience in 18 Cases. Med Sci Monit. 23:1371–1377
18. Acker SN, Bruny JL, Narkewicz MR, Roach JP, Rogers A, Karrer FM (2013) Preoperative imaging does not predict intrahepatic involvement in choledochal cysts. J Pediatr Surg. 48:2378–2382

10

The association between character of portal blood flow and post-TIPS incidence of hepatic encephalopathy

Helmy El-Shazly[1], Mohamed Abdel-Samiee[1,3*], El-Sayed Tharwa[1], Hassan Zaghla[1], Shrief Abass[1], Mohamed El-Warraky[2] and El-Sayed Ibrahim[1]

Abstract

Background: Hepatic encephalopathy (HE) is one of the serious complications observed post-TIPS operations in patients with different complications of portal hypertension such as refractory ascites, refractory hydrothorax, bleeding varices, and hepato-renal syndrome. Herein, we aimed to clarify predisposing factors for post-TIPS incidence of HE according to pre-TIPS hemodynamics.

Results: Fifty patients were enrolled in this study with different complications of portal hypertension; most of them have Child A and B scores. Patients were evaluated by ultrasound Doppler for the flow inside the portal vein and clinically recorded into two groups: group 1, 31 patients with hepatopetal flow; and group 2, 19 patients with hepatofugal flow. Then, TIPS was performed and patients were reassessed 1 month later to detect HE. Multiple variables such as age, gender, etiology of liver disease, and indication for TIPS had no significant differences. The incidence of HE post-TIPS was observed more at group 1 more than at group 2 ($P = 0.02$).

Conclusions: Post-TIPS incidence of HE was interestingly related to pre-TIPS flow in the portal vein (hepatopetal group more than hepatofugal group). Patients with hepatofugal flow in the portal vein are perfect candidate for TIPS than patients with hepatopetal flow in the portal vein. Patients with previous history of HE are contraindicated for TIPS except as a bridge for liver transplantation.

Keywords: Portal hypertension, Ultrasound Doppler, Flow inside the portal vein, TIPS, HE

Background

In 1980, the transjugular intrahepatic portosystemic shunt (TIPS) was developed to reduce complications of portal hypertension. Therefore, TIPS was rapidly applied to the treatment of many of the complications of portal hypertension when the shunt could be placed with relative ease. These complications include active bleeding of gastro-esophageal varices, control of refractory cirrhotic ascites and hepatic hydrothorax, and treatment of hepatorenal failure and hepato-pulmonary syndrome [1, 2]. Hepatic encephalopathy (HE) is a well-known complication of patients with liver cirrhosis after TIPS; its pathogenesis is not well understood [3, 4]. In the last decade, substantial progress has been made in the treatment of portal hypertension and its associated complications. TIPS has been considered as a minimally invasive therapy for portal hypertension complications [5–7]. From the clinical point of view, TIPS resembles a surgical side to side shunt leading to an increased rate of HE which can be seen after TIPS. The incidence of HE after TIPS varies from 18 to 45% [8–10].

This high rate attracts researchers in investigating the causative factors for HE besides predicting factors of HE after TIPS which had been much controversial. The

* Correspondence: Drmohammed100@yahoo.com
[1]Hepatology and Gastroenterology Department, National Liver Institute, Menoufia University, Yassin Abdel-Ghafar street, Shebeen El-Kom, Menoufia 32511, Egypt
[3]National Liver Institute, Menoufia University, Shebeen El-Kom, Egypt

study aimed to verify the relationship between pre-transjagular intrahepatic portosystemic shunt intrahepatic hemodynamics and the incidence of post-transjagular intrahepatic portosystemic shunt hepatic enchephalopathy.

Methods

Fifty patients were included in this prospective single-center study with different causes of portal hypertension; patients underwent TIPS in the National Liver Institute, Menoufia University, from 2015 to 2017. Patients were divided into two groups according to the flow inside the portal vein by Doppler: group I—31 patients with hepatopetal flow (Toward the Liver), and group II—19 patients with hepato-fugal flow (away from the liver).

The day before the procedure, a basal evaluation of HE including examination and grading of the patients' mental state, asterixis, and psychometric performance (trail-making test-A, TMT-A), as well as their venous blood ammonia determination, were carried out. The evaluation of the degree of HE was based on the alteration of the patient's mental state using modifications of the West Haven criteria. The mental state was assessed in each patient by the same investigator using standardized tests and questions.

TIPS

A catheter was inserted via the jugular vein past the right atrium and into the hepatic veins. A needle was then inserted into the hepatic parenchyma, and contrast was injected as the needle was slowly withdrawn. When a branch of the portal vein was identified, a wire was inserted into the vein followed by a catheter. Pressures were obtained, and portography was performed. Before shunt placement, the pressure gradient is measured by calculating the difference in pressure between the wedged catheter and after placing the catheter freely in the hepatic vein. After shunt placement, the pressure gradient is measured by calculating the difference in pressure measured directly while the catheter is in the portal vein and after withdrawal of the catheter to the hepatic vein. A tract within the hepatic parenchyma was then created using a balloon and stent deployed. The used stents were self-expanding.

Follow-up

Patients were followed up at the hospital for 1 week then discharged and followed up for another 3 weeks for the incidence of HE. Hepatic encephalopathy was diagnosed and graded according to the "West Haven criteria" as moderate (grades I–II) and severe (grades III–IV). Episodic hepatic encephalopathy was defined as the sporadic occurrence of alteration in the neuropsychiatric function that develops over a short period of time.

Statistical analysis

The data collected were tabulated and analyzed by SPSS (Statistical Package for Social Sciences) version 22.0 on IBM compatible computer.

Two types of statistics were done:

Descriptive statistics:

- For example, percentage (%), mean, and standard deviation (SD).

Analytic statistics:

- For example, chi-square test (χ^2) was used to study the association between two qualitative variables.
- Fischer exact test for 2 × 2 tables when expected cell count of more than 25% of cases was less than 5 and p value < 0.05 was considered significant.
- Student t test is a test of significance used for comparison between two groups having quantitative variables.
- Mann-Whitney test (nonparametric test) is a test of significance used for comparison between two groups not normally distributed having quantitative variables.
- Paired t test is a test of significance used for comparison between two related groups having quantitative variables.

Results

The etiology of portal hypertension was more in post-HCV (70%), HBV (4%), HCV, and HBV (8%), then Bilharizial periportal fibrosis (18%) [11, 12]. There are 20 males and 30 females with no significant difference in the incidence of post-TIPS; there was no statistically significant difference as regards gender (p value 0.41) (Table 1). The liver function has no significant difference except in calculating the Child score. The kidney function is important; the more increase in creatinine level and HRS, the more the post-TIPS (p value 0.14; this indicates the more cirrhosis and portal hypertension and ascites in these patients only, with no clinical importance in post-TIPS HE).

The most common indication of TIPS is refractory ascites (64%) then refractory, hydrothorax (20%) then refractory, and bleeding varices (12%) then HRS (4%), respectively, as shown in (Table 2). Patients who underwent TIPS with previous history of HE had HE post-TIPS (100%), and this shows that pre-TIPS HE is a significant predictor for post-TIPS HE as in Table 3. Thus, TIPS seems useful for the management of severe PHT-related complications.

The higher the Child score, the more the post-TIPS incidence of HE, none of Child A (0%), 9 patient of Child B (20%), and two patients of Child C (100%); this

Table 1 Clinical characteristics of the studied groups before TIPS

	Hepatofugal group (no. = 19)		Hepatopetal group (no. = 31)		χ^2 test	*P* value
	No.	%	No.	%		
Gender						
Male	9	47.4	11	35.5	0.69	0.41 (> 0.05)
Female	10	52.6	20	64.5		
Ascites						
Negative	1	5.3	1	3.2	0.43	0.94 (> 0.05)
Mild	1	5.3	3	9.7		
Moderate	4	21.1	6	19.4		
Severe	13	68.4	21	67.7		
History of paracentesis						
Negative	1	5.3	4	12.9	0.83	0.64 (> 0.05)
Positive	18	94.7	27	87.1		
HE before TIPS						
Negative	19	100	29	93.5	1.96	0.52 (> 0.05)
Positive	0	0	2	6.5		
Child score						
A	2	10.5	2	6.5	1.48	0.48 (> 0.05)
B	17	89.5	27	87.1		
C	0	0	2	6.5		

HE hepatic encephalopathy, *TIPS* transjagular intrahepatic portosystemic shunts, *No.* number

relationship can tell us that patients with Child score less than C are fit for TIPS with fewer predictors for post-TIPS HE.

All patients with hepatopetal flow or hepatofugal flow had their mean arterial blood pressure decreased post-TIPS especially in hepatopetal flow, and this indicates the change in the heamodynamics post-TIPS as shown in Table 3. The hepatic artery RI was more in the hepatofugal group than the hepatopetal group before TIPS. The hepatic artery RI decreased significantly post-TIPS in the hepatofugal group.

The pressure inside the inferior vein cava increased significantly post-TIPS due to shunting of the blood to a new way through the shunt and IVC. The pressure inside the portal vein decreased significantly post-TIPS also due to shunting most of the blood that passes through it to the IVC. The incidence of HE was less in the hepatofugal flow group (10%) than the hepatopetal flow group (29%) (Tables 4, 5, and 6).

Table 2 Comparison between studied groups regarding indication of TIPS

Indication	Hepatofugal group (*n* = 19)		Hepatopetal group (*n* = 31)		χ^2 test	*P* value
	No.	%	No.	%		
Refractory ascites	14	73.7	18	58.1	2.002	0.57
Refractory pleural effusion	3	15.8	7	22.6		
Refractory bleeding varices	2	10.5	4	12.9		
Hepatorenal syndrome	0	0.0	2	6.5		

TIPS transjagular intrahepatic portosystemic shunts

Discussion

Transjugular intrahepatic portosystemic stent-shunts (TIPS) have been increasingly used for the treatment of the complications of portal hypertension. A meta-analysis of randomized controlled trials confirms the superiority of TIPS over the endoscopic treatments in the prevention of variceal rebleeding but without any improvement in mortality [13]. Additionally, TIPS is effective in the resolution of refractory ascites in some patients [13]. But it remains unclear as to whether there is any survival advantage [14]. Hepatic encephalopathy is thought to result from intestinally derived toxins that bypass the normal metabolic pathways of the liver, either because of shunting of portal vein blood flow away from

Table 3 Comparison between the studied groups regarding post-HE

		Hepatofugal group (no. = 19)		Hepatopetal group (no. = 30)		Fisher exact test	*P* value
		No.	%	No.	%		
Post HE	Negative	17	89.5	22	71.0	2.55	0.02
	Positive	2	10.5	9	29.0		

HE hepatic encephalopathy, *No.* number

Table 4 Comparison between the studied groups regarding MAP before and after

	Hepatofugal group (no. = 19)	Hepatopetal group (no. = 30)	*t* test	P value
	Mean ± SD	Mean ± SD		
MAP before	76.8 ± 7.1	80.9 ± 7.5	1.91	0.06
MAP after	76.4 ± 6.2	79.7 ± 6.1	1.85	0.07
MELD	11.7 ± 3.3	12.8 ± 4.8	0.46	0.64

MAP mean arterial blood pressure, *No.* number, *MELD* model of end-stage liver disease

the liver parenchyma as in TIPS patients or because of the inability of the liver to handle such substances because of chronic hepatocellular disease. Certainly, both of these factors may play a role in patients with cirrhosis, with either one being more important [15].

Many studies have focused on the relevant factors of HE, but the effects of pre-/post-TIPS factors were found to be contradictory. The factors include pre-TIPS, age, liver function, pre-TIPS HE, Child score, and the direction of flow in the portal vein. In this study, we found that the occurrence of post-TIPS HE was closely related to the pre-TIPS portal blood flow direction; the low incidence of post-TIPS HE was observed in patients with hepatofugal portal blood flow (n = 2) 10%, but high incidence in those with prograde (hepatopetal) portal blood flow (n = 9) 29%, indicating that the pre-TIPS pattern of blood flow may greatly affect the occurrence of post-TIPS HE [16].

In the study done by Zuckerman et al. [17], the occurrence of HE after TIPS was independent of central venous pressures; portosystemic gradients (before and after TIPS); the direction of blood flow (before and after TIPS) in the right, left, and main portal veins; and the presence of encephalopathy after TIPS, and this is contrary to our results [17].

In a similar study done by Deng et al., the incidence of post-TIPS HE in the hepatofugal group 16% was lower than that in hepatopetal group 37%, which agrees with our study [18].

Many studies agree that age more than 60 years old increases the incidence of post-TIPS HE. Sanyal et al. [19] stated that increasing age was significantly associated with encephalopathy, which agrees with our study [20].

In this study, we found that Child score was very important in the post-TIPS incidence of HE, with the Child score increasing, the more the post-TIPS incidence of HE. In this study, 4 patients had Child score A, none of them had post-TIPS HE; 44 patients had Child score B, 9 had post-TIPS HE; and 2 patients had Child score C, two had post-TIPS HE.

In a similar study by Sanyal et al., increasing Child class is significantly associated with post-TIPS HE, which agrees with our study [19].

Careful selection of patients for elective TIPS insertion is crucial, as is the experience of the center performing this procedure. TIPS is not recommended in patients with serum bilirubin > 3 mg/dl and low platelet count, current hepatic encephalopathy or chronic hepatic encephalopathy, concomitant active infection, progressive renal failure, severe systolic or diastolic dysfunction, or pulmonary hypertension.

In another study by Somberg et al., post-TIPS HE is associated with multivariate like hypoalbuminemia (albumin is one of the main variables in assessing Child score) [21].

In this study, we found that pre-TIPS incidence of HE is associated with post-TIPS incidence of HE as two patients had pre-TIPS HE and the two patients had post-TIPS HE. In another study, those patients who developed clinically evident HE were significantly more likely to have a past history of encephalopathy and tended to be male [8, 22].

Past history of encephalopathy along with increasing age has previously been identified as important variables

Table 5 Comparison between the studied groups regarding liver functions before TIPS

	Hepatofugal group (no. = 19)	Hepatopetal group (no. = 31)	Mann-Whitney test	*P* value
	Mean ± SD	Mean ± SD		
ALT (IU/L)	57.2 ± 51.7	40.5 ± 35.1	1.22	0.22 (> 0.05)
AST (IU/L)	57.6 ± 50.3	52.5 ± 37.3	0.62	0.54 (> 0.05)
ALP (IU/L)	136 ± 66.4	129.7 ± 40.9	0.09	0.93 (> 0.05)
Albumin(g/dL)	2.5 ± 0.56	2.8 ± 1.03	1.33	0.18 (> 0.05)
T. Bilirubin (mg/dL)	1.5 ± 0.58	1.6 ± 0.53	0.62	0.54 (> 0.05)
D. Bilirubin (mg/dL)	0.95 ± 0.77	0.98 ± 1.03	0.22	0.83 (> 0.05)
INR	1.46 ± 0.22	1.45 ± 0.23	0.23#	0.82 (> 0.05)
Na^+	132.1 ± 3.1	130.2 ± 4.2	1.79#	0.08 (> 0.05)
K^+	3.8 ± 0.47	3.7 ± 0.57	0.31#	0.76 (> 0.05)

TIPS transjagular intrahepatic portosystemic shunts, *No.* number, *ALT* alanine aminotransferase, *AST* aspartate aminotransferase, *INR* international normalized ratio, *ALP* alkaline phosphatase, *Na* sodium, *K* potassium

Table 6 Comparison of the studied variables in relation to post-TIPS incidence of hepatic encephalopathy

Variables	Post TIPS hepatic encephalopathy		*P*-value
	Negative	Positive	
Age in years (mean ± SD)	44.67 ± 7.38	47.36 ± 6.36	0.372 (> 0.05)
MAP (mean ± SD)	79.10 ± 7.96	80.18 ± 5.96	0.663 (> 0.05)
MELD score	11.72 ± 2.98	14.73 ± 7.16	0.304 (> 0.05)
HARI (mean ± SD)	0.58 ± 0.10	0.61 ± 0.05	0.459 (> 0.05)
IVC pressure mmHg (mean ± SD)	5.18 ± 0.89	5.37 ± 0.84	0.403 (> 0.05)
PVP mmHg (mean ± SD)	33.90 ± 11.10	34.45 ± 5.66	0.934 (> 0.05)

MAP mean arterial blood pressure, *IVC* inferior vena cava, *MELD* model of end-stage liver disease, *HARI* hepatic artery resistive index, *PVP* portal vein pulsatility

increasing the risk of post-TIPS HE [19] that goes with our study.

In another study, the mean age difference between patients with TIPS-related encephalopathy and other patients was not statistically significant ($P = 0.11$ (> 0.05)). The statistical power of this test was only 0.35; therefore, we cannot guarantee that TIPS-related encephalopathy is independent of age, and a large sample would be required [23].

In this study, we found that there was no any significant difference between causes of TIPS in patients with portal hypertension and post-TIPS incidence of HE, except in HRS cases; we had 2 cases, and the two cases developed post-TIPS HE.

In a similar study by Zuckerman et al., the cause of liver disease had no interrelationship with patients with TIPS-related HE, which agrees with our study in general [17].

In another study by Oliviero et al., serum creatinine level was the only variable related to the development of refractory HE at the logistic multivariate analysis. That agrees also with our study in the HRS cases, but we think that this issue needs more studies with more cases for more accurate results [24].

According to the hepatic artery RI, normally, when portal perfusion decreases, hepatic arterial blood may increase to maintain the relative invariableness of liver blood supply. This mechanism is called hepatic arterial buffer response (HABR). In this study, we found that before TIPS, the hepatic artery RI of patients of hepatopetal flow (0.61 ± 0.11) was significantly lower than that of hepatofugal group (0.75 ± 0.79) (*P* value 0.005).

In a similar study by Deng et al., the hepatic artery RI of the patients before TIPS was lower than that of the patients with prograde flow, indicating the difference of post-TIPS intrahepatic hemodynamics, and this agree with our study [18].

Also, we found in this study that the hepatic artery RI in the hepatopetal group decreases after TIPS (0.6 ± 0.11 before to 0.59 ± 0.07 after) but less than that in the hepatofugal group (0.75 ± 0.79 before to 0.57 ± 0.07 after) ($P =$ 002); this indicates that there is a great change in the hemodynamics in the patient of the hepatofugal group after TIPS.

In a similar study by Deng et al. [18], hepatic hemodynamics of patients with hepatofugal portal flow only changed a little after TIPS and was still dependent on the hepatic artery perfusion. Therefore, the RI of the hepatic artery was changed a little before and after TIPS, and this contrary to our study; although in patients with hepatofugal flow, large spontaneous portosystemic anastomosis could be found, and more importantly, the long-term existence of small to large pre-TIPS spontaneous portosystemic anastomoses might enable the cerebrum to adapt to some neurotoxic substances in the blood, which causes HE [18]. The lack of control subjects, however, does limit the ability to evaluate this approach.

According to post-TIPS hemodynamics and mean arterial blood pressure (MAP) before and after in this study, we found that MAP of patients with hepatofugal flow (76.8 ± 7.1) was less than those with hepatopetal flow (80.9 ± 7.5); also, we found that the MAP decreased after TIPS, and the decrease was more in patients with hepatopetal flow more than that of hepatofugal flow. All these results indicate that there is an alteration in the hemodynamic in patients post-TIPS more in patients with hepatopetal flow, and this may explain the high rate of post-TIPS HE.

Another study showed that the average MAP was (92 mmHg) before TIPS; a tendency of MAP to increase after TIPS replacement was noted (100 mmHg), but the difference was not significant. Two months later, it decreased to a value lower than the baseline (85 mmHg), and this agrees with our study [25].

HE is a well-known complication of patients with liver cirrhosis after portosystemic shunt. In recent years, TIPS has been accepted as minimally invasive therapy for complications of portal hypertension recurrent bleeding from varices, refractory ascites, and liver failure due to Budd-Chiari syndrome. Because TIPS resembles a surgical side-to-side shunt, an increased rate of HE can be seen after TIPS; the higher incidence of HE after TIPS has attracted the interest of researches in investigating the causative factors for HE. Besides, predicting factors of HE after TIPS have been much controversial.

Conclusion

Patients with hepatofugal flow in the portal vein are perfect candidates for TIPS than patients with hepatopetal flow in the portal vein.

Recommendation

Further research should be done to analyze the efficacy of TIPS in HRS cases. Further research should be done to standardize the use of Child score and pre-TTPS HE as good predictors of post-TIPS HE.

Abbreviations

HE: Hepatic encephalopathy; TIPS: Transjugular intrahepatic portosystemic shunt; HCV: Hepatitis C virus; HBV: Hepatitis B virus; SD: Standard deviation

Acknowledgements

No grant or other financial support was received for this study.
Forms of support received by each author for this study included a good selection of cases, instructive supervision, continuous guidance, valuable suggestions, and good instructions.
Our paper is an extended version of the selected abstract by the Committee of the 29th Asian Pacific Association for the Study of the Liver (APASL) 2020 in Bali, Indonesia, to be presented as a part of the Scientific Program under the theme of "Golden Ages of Hepatology" (abstract submission no.: APASL2020-ABS477).

Authors' contributions

All authors have read and approved the manuscript. All authors have agreed both to be personally accountable for the author's own contributions and to ensure that questions related to the accuracy or integrity of any part of the work, even the ones in which the author was not personally involved, are appropriately investigated, resolved, and the resolution documented in the literature. HE was responsible for provision of study materials, patients, analysis, and acquisition of the financial support for the project leading to this publication and application of statistical, mathematical, computational, or other formal techniques to analyze or synthesize study data. MA performed the design of the work, managed activities to annotate (produce metadata), for initial use and later reuse plus ideas, and contributed to the formulation or evolution of overarching research goals and aims and acquisition of the financial support for the project leading to this publication. ET contributed to the management and coordination responsibility for the research activity planning and execution plus conception, verification, whether as a part of the activity or separate, of the overall replication/ reproducibility of results/experiments and other research outputs, and acquisition of the financial support for the project leading to this publication. HZ created and/or presented the published work, specifically in writing the initial draft (including substantive translation), and is responsible for the oversight and leadership responsibility for the research activity planning and execution, including mentorship external to the core team. He revised the work and contributed to the acquisition of the financial support for the project leading to this publication. SA was responsible for the programming, software development, designing computer programs, implementing the computer code and supporting algorithms, testing of existing code components, creating new software, and acquiring financial support for the project leading to this publication. ME conducted the research and investigation process, specifically performing the experiments or data/ evidence collection, conception, management, and coordination and is responsible for the research activity planning and execution and provision of study materials, instrumentation, or other analysis tools. El shared creation, presentation of the published work, specifically writing the initial draft (including substantive translation), interpretation of data and acquisition of the financial support for the project leading to this publication.

Competing interests

The authors declare that there is no conflict of interest regarding the publication of this paper.

Author details

[1]Hepatology and Gastroenterology Department, National Liver Institute, Menoufia University, Yassin Abdel-Ghafar street, Shebeen El-Kom, Menoufia 32511, Egypt. [2]Radiology Department, National Liver Institute, Menoufia University, Shebeen El-Kom, Egypt. [3]National Liver Institute, Menoufia University, Shebeen El-Kom, Egypt.

References

1. Thomas D. Boyer, Conn HO, et al, Hepatology: a textbook of liver disease (4ail Philadelphia: Saunders (2003) 21:627-628.
2. Ibrahim ES, Alsebaey A, Zaghla H, Moawad Abdelmageed S, Gameel K, Abdelsameea E (2017) Long term rifaximin therapy as a primary prevention of hepatorenal syndrome. Eur J Gastroenterol Hepatol 29(11):1247–1250
3. Bonnel AR, Bunchorntavakul C, Rajender RK (2014) Transjugular intrahepatic portosystemic shunts in liver transplant recipients. Liver Transpl 20:130–139
4. Butteworth RF (2001) Neurotransmitter dysfunction in hepatic encephalopathy: new approaches and new findings. Metab Brain Dis 16:55–65
5. Gerber TSH (2000) Hepatic encephalopathy in liver cirrhosis; pathogenesis. Diagnosis and management. Drugs 60:1353–1370
6. Berry K, Lerrigo R, Liou IW, Ioannou GN (2016) Association between transjugular intrahepatic portosystemic shunt and survival in patients with cirrhosis. Clin Gastroenterol Hepatol 14:118–123
7. Stefankova J, Fejfar T, Safka V, Hulek P, Krajina A, Fendrichova M (2002) Hepatic encephalopathy after TIPS retrospective study. Vnitriek 48:390–395
8. Tripathi D, Helmy A, Macbeth K, Balata S, Lui HF, Stanley AJ et al (2004) Ten years' follow-up of 472 patients following transjugular intrahepatic portosystemic stent-shunt insertion at a single centre. Eur J GastroenterolHepatol 16:9–18
9. Gaba RC, Parvinian A, Casadaban LC, Couture PM, Zivin SP, Lakhoo J et al (2015) Survival benefit of TIPS vs. serial paracentesis in patients with refractory ascites: a single institution case-control propensity score analysis. Clin Radiol 70:e51–e57
10. Khan S, Tudur SC, Williamson P, Sutton R (2006) Porto systemic shunts versus endoscopic therapy for varicealrebleeding in patients with cirrhosis. Cochrane Database Syst Rev:CD000553
11. Galal IF, Zakaria Z, Allam WR, Mahmoud MA, Ezzat AR, Osman A, Waked I, Strickland GT, Abdelwahab SF (2014) Cross reactive cellular immune response to HCV genotype 1 and 4 antigens among genotype 4 exposed subjects. PLoS One 9(6):e101264. https://doi.org/10.1371/journal.pone.0101264 eCollection 2014
12. Abdelwahab SF, Zakaria Z, Sobhy M, Hamdy S, Mahmoud MA, Mikhail N, Allam WR, Rewisha E, Waked I (2015) Differential distribution of IL28B. rs12979860 single-nucleotide polymorphism among Egyptian healthcare workers with and without a hepatitis C virus-specific cellular immune response. Arch Virol 160(7):1741–1750. https://doi.org/10.1007/s00705-015-2446-7 Epub 2015 May 15
13. Salerno F, Camma C, Enea M, Rossle M, Wong F (2007) Transjugular intrahepatic portosystemic shunt for refractory ascites: a meta-analysis of individual patient data. Gastroenterology 133:825–834
14. Saab S, Nieto JM, Lewis SK, Runyon BA (2006) TIPS versus paracentesis for cirrhotic patients with refractory ascites. Cochrane Database Syst Rev: CD004889
15. Spiro H (1993) Clinical gastroenterology, 4thed. McGraw-Hill, New York, pp 1184–1188
16. Kramer L, Bauer E, Gendo A, Funk G, Madi C, Pidlich J et al (2002) Neurophysio logical evidence of cognitive impairment in patients without hepatic encephalopathy after transjagular intrahepatic portosystemic shunts. Am J Gastroenterol 97:162–166
17. Darryl A. Zuckerman, Michael D. Darcyi, Thomas P. Bocchini, Charles F. Hildebolt, AJR 1997; 169:1727-1731.
18. Dan Deng, Ming-Song Liao, Jian-Ping Qin and Xiao-An Li. Hepatobiliarypancreat Dis Int 2006; 5:232-236.
19. Sanyal AJ, Freedman AM, Shiffman ML, Purdum PP 3rd, Luketic VA, Cheatham AK (1994) Portosystemic encephalopathy after transjugular intrahepatic portosystemic shunt: results of a prospective controlled study. HEPATOLOGY 20:46–55
20. Sanyal AJ, Freedman AM, Luketic VA, Purdum P III, Shiffman M, Cole P, Tisnado J, Simmons S (1997) Transjugular intrahepatic portosystemic shunts

compared with endoscopic sclerotherapy for the prevention of recurrent variceal hemorrhage. A randomized, controlled trial. Ann Intern Med 126: 849–857

21. Somberg KA, Riegler JL, LaBerge JM, Doherty-Simor MM, Bachetti P, Roberts J, Lake JR (1995) Hepatic encephalopathy after transjugular intrahepatic portosystemic shunts: incidence and risk factors. Am J Gastroenterol 90:549–555
22. Schemmer P, Radeleff B, Flechtenmacher C, Mehrabi A, Richter GM, Buchler MW, Schmidt J (2006) TIPSS for variceal hemorrhage after living related liver transplantation: a dangerous indication. World J Gastroenterol 12:493–495
23. Ward TJ, Techasith T, Louie JD, Hwang GL, Hofmann LV, Sze DY (2015) Emergent salvage direct intrahepatic portocaval shunt procedure for acute variceal hemorrhage. J Vasc Interv Radiol 26:829–834
24. Oliviero R, Stefania A, Filippo S, Adriano D, Federica C, Alessin F, Adolfo F, Manuela M, AJG 2008:2738-2746.
25. Salem R, Vouche M, Baker T, Herrero JI, Caicedo JC, Fryer J et al (2015) Pretransplant portal vein recanalization-transjugular intrahepatic portosystemic shunt in patients with complete obliterative portal vein thrombosis. Transplantation 99:2347–2355

11

Large subcapsular hematoma of the liver due to faja corset: a rare case report

Sheharyar Minhas[1,2*], Ahmed Minhas[3], Maira Malik[3] and Phaniram Sumanam[1]

Abstract

Background: Subcapsular hematoma of the liver is a potentially life-threatening but extremely rare condition. It is often caused by a blunt trauma or other predisposing conditions such as a liver tumor, intra-tumor hemorrhage, surgery, preeclampsia, liver biopsy, and hemodialysis. Predisposing causes of liver hematoma include its large size and proximity to fixed structures. To date, there have been no reported cases of subcapsular liver hematoma caused by tight clothing such as corsets. Our case report is about an extremely rare case of subcapsular hematoma of the liver caused by wearing a tight faja corset in a young healthy female.

Case presentation: A forty-five-year-old Spanish female without any underlying health problems presented with sudden onset epigastric and right upper quadrant abdominal pain after wearing a faja corset the night prior to the hospital presentation. CT abdomen was noted for subcapsular hematoma of the liver. Her symptoms persisted and repeat CT abdomen showing worsening of the liver hematoma. Patient had interventional radiology (IR) guided drainage and was subsequently discharged home.

Conclusions: Subscapular liver hematomas need to be considered in patients presenting with acute onset abdominal pain after wearing certain tight clothing. The necessity of an early and accurate diagnosis is vital for management as hemodynamically stable patients can be managed conservatively. Our patient was managed with IR-guided aspiration drainage of the hematoma. Surgery can be considered a last resort in case of life-threatening hemodynamic instability, peritoneal signs, free abdominal fluid, and failure of arterial embolization. Our case highlights the importance of early recognition of traumatic subcapsular hematomas to prevent life-threatening complications.

Keywords: Subcapsular hematoma, Corset, Liver, Baja, Surgical intervention, Case report

Background

Subcapsular hematoma of the liver is an extremely rare but potentially life-threatening condition. It is most commonly associated with blunt abdominal trauma, with the liver after spleen being the second most common abdominal organ injured during blunt trauma. Predisposing causes of liver hematoma include its large size and proximity to fixed structures. Other predisposing causes of liver hematoma include pregnancy, preeclampsia, hemodialysis, intra-tumor hemorrhage, surgery, and liver biopsy. To date, no cases have been reported of subscapular liver hematoma associated with tight clothing such as corsets. Here, we report the first case of a subcapsular hematoma of the liver in a young healthy female secondary to use of faja without any apparent anatomical lesion and in the absence of coagulopathy.

Case presentation

A forty-five-year-old Hispanic female without any significant past medical history was admitted to a community hospital with sudden onset of epigastric and right upper quadrant abdominal pain radiating to the back. She denied any nausea, vomiting, fever, or chills. Further

* Correspondence: sminhas7@yahoo.com
[1]Department of Internal Medicine, Nazareth Hospital, 2601 Holme Avenue, Philadelphia, PA 19152, USA
[2]Rollins School of Public Health, Emory University, Atlanta, GA, USA

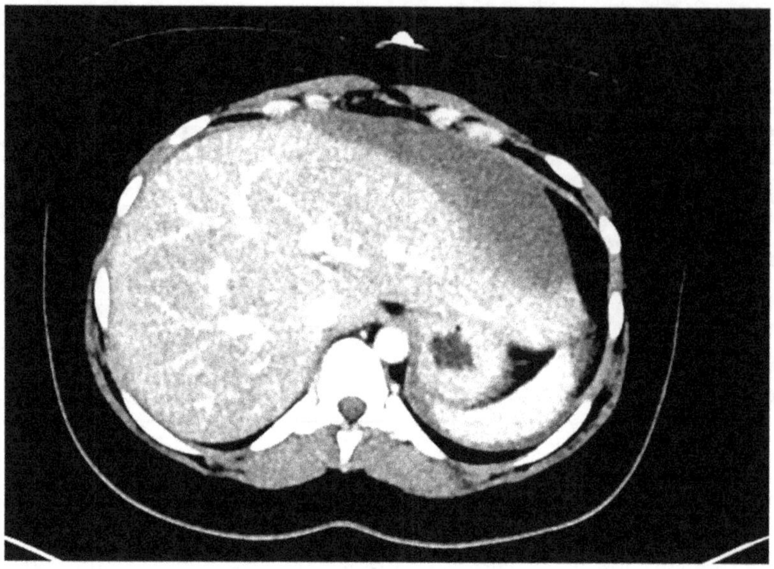

Fig. 1 Initial CT abdomen/pelvis (cross-sectional view)

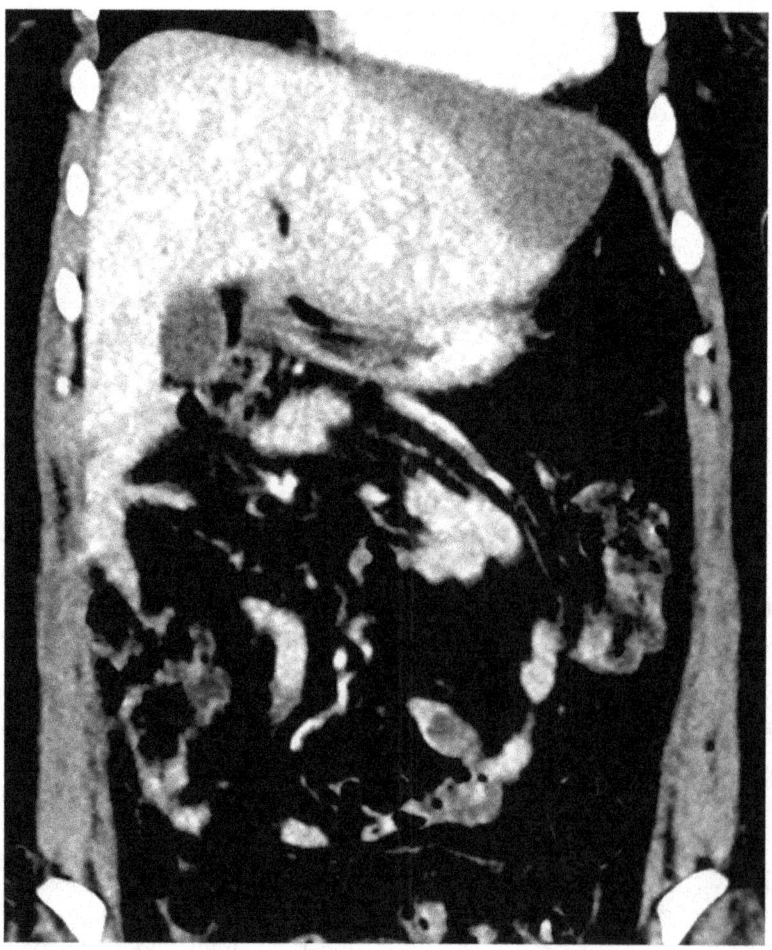

Fig. 2 Initial CT abdomen/pelvis (coronal view)

history revealed that she wore a faja corset for a cultural event the night prior to hospital presentation. Patient did not report any other signs of trauma, fall, or history of abdominal surgery. She denied any trauma, fall, or history of abdominal surgery. Initial vitals were normal with temperature 36.8 °C, pulse 93, blood pressure 115/67, and saturation 98% on room air. Urine drug screen was negative. Beta-human chorionic gonadotropin (β-HCG) was negative. Laboratory workup was unremarkable with hemoglobin 12.3. Physical exam was noted for a hyposthenic body habitus. Abdominal exam findings were unremarkable except for some mild right upper quadrant tenderness and the liver was noted to be higher in the abdominal cavity. CT abdomen with contrast revealed a 5.5 × 4.2 × 14.2 cm subcapsular liver hematoma along the anterior aspect of the lateral left hepatic lobe (Figs. 1 and 2). It was also noted for an elongated cartilaginous tip of the xiphoid process (Fig. 3). Surgery team evaluated the patient and no intervention was recommended. She was subsequently discharged home. The next day, the patient presented again with worsening epigastric abdominal pain. Vitals were stable and hemoglobin was 10.0. CT abdomen with contrast showed worsening of subcapsular liver hematoma in the left hepatic lobe measuring 13.7 × 5.6 × 9.5 cm (Figs. 3 and 4). The liver otherwise showed normal enhancement without any fatty changes. Surgery recommended non-operative evacuation and patient subsequently underwent percutaneous IR-guided aspiration of enlarging liver hematoma to drain the fluid. Patient's symptoms improved and repeat abdominal ultrasound showed decrease in size of liver hematoma. Patient was subsequently discharged home the following day (Fig. 5).

Discussion

A subcapsular hematoma of the liver is an accumulation of blood between the liver parenchyma and Glisson's capsule. It has a 75% mortality rate if it ruptures into the peritoneal cavity [1]. In 75% of patients, it is located around the right lobe of the liver and only 25% of patients have involvement of the left lobe of the liver. Symptoms manifest as abdominal pain, anemia, hypotension, fever, and peritonism. Risk factors include blunt trauma, iatrogenic injuries following endoscopic retrograde cholangiopancreatography, anticoagulation treatment, liver tumors, hepatic adenomatosis, peliosis

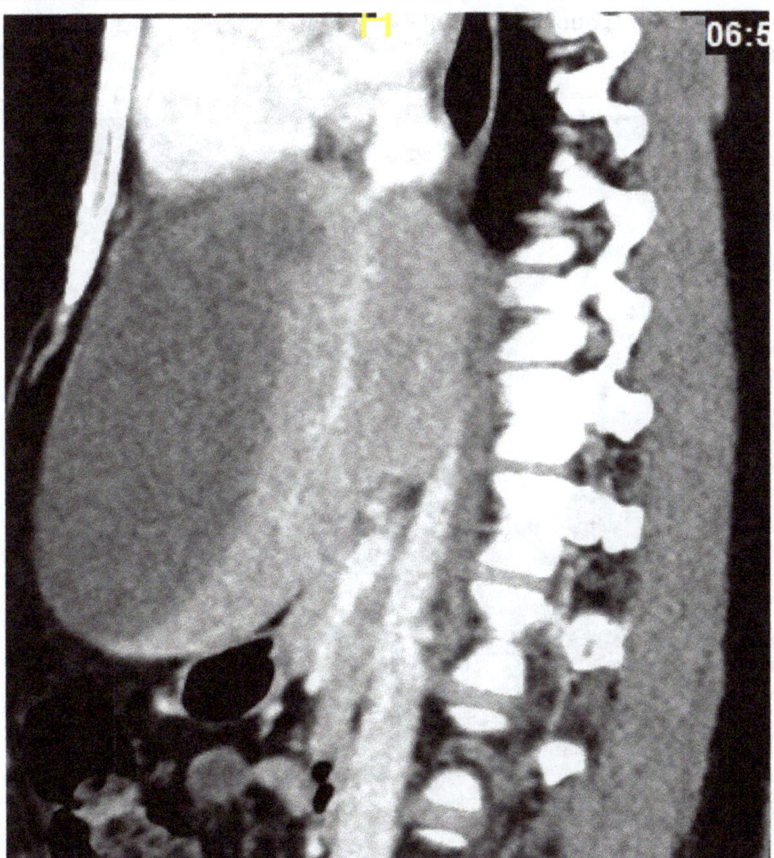

Fig. 3 Initial CT abdomen/pelvis (sagittal view)

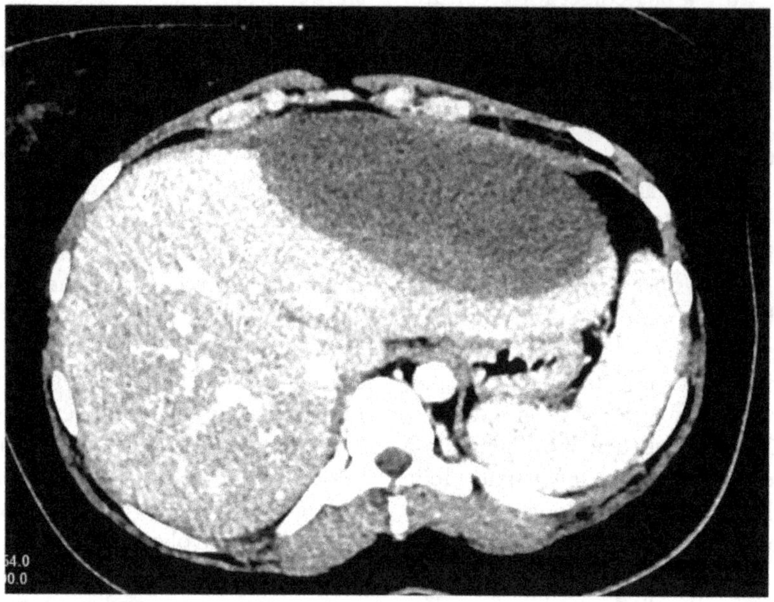

Fig. 4 Repeat CT abdomen/pelvis (cross-sectional view)

hepatis, hemodialysis, preeclampsia, and the HELLP syndrome [2, 3].

Our case is unique without any of the above risk factors commonly associated with hepatic subcapsular hematoma. One possible mechanism of hepatic hematoma in our patient is that an increase in intraabdominal pressure associated with tight clothing compresses the xiphoid process and results in bony trauma. The necessity of an early and accurate diagnosis in subcapsular hepatic hematomas derives its importance as

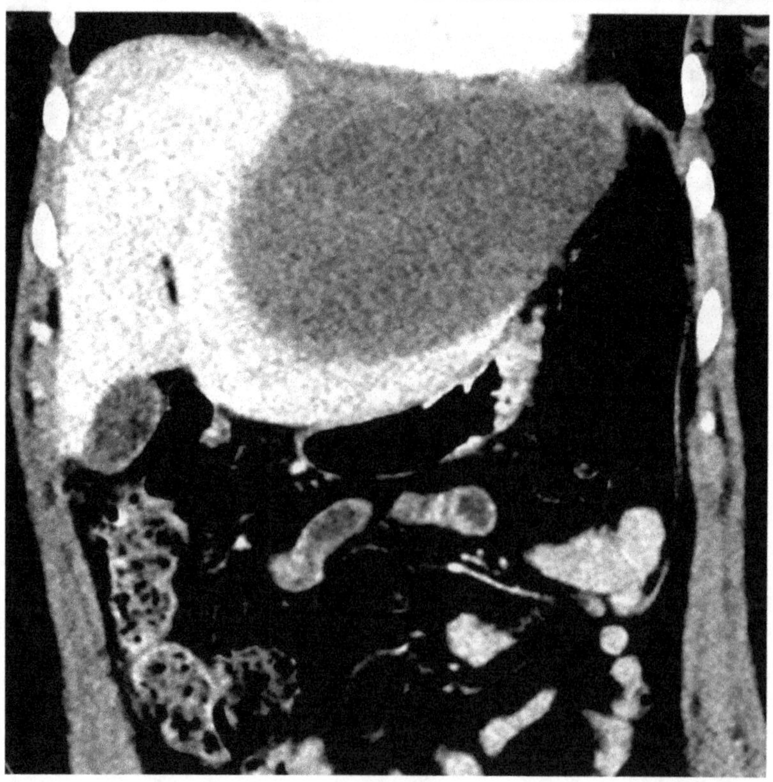

Fig. 5 Repeat CT abdomen/pelvis (coronal view)

patients who are hemodynamically stable can be managed conservatively. These patients are stable with a limited, peripheral, and non-compressive hematoma. Our patient was initially managed conservatively and discharged home after an observation period of 24 h. She presented to the hospital the following day with worsening symptoms and enlarging size of hepatic hematoma.

CT abdomen is the imaging of choice for diagnosing subcapsular hematoma of the liver. On CT imaging, the acute hematoma looks like a lenticular, ellipsoid, perihepatic collection that is typically, hyperdense (40–60 HU) due to its high protein content [4]. Although rare, these hepatic hematomas have potential to rupture that can rapidly lead to hemodynamic instability and death [5]. Therefore, these need close monitoring in an acute care setting. Patients can be safely discharged home if hemodynamically stable after a close period of observation.

Subcapsular hematomas of the liver associated with hemodynamic compromise, significant drop in hemoglobin, and in the presence of rapid expansion in size should have a low threshold for radiological or surgical intervention. Our patient was readmitted with worsening abdominal pain in the presence of increase in size of the hematoma. She subsequently underwent IR-guided drainage procedure of the hematoma. If IR-guided drainage does not result in resolution of the hematoma, then an arterial embolization performed by interventional radiology should be attempted. Surgery should be considered a last resort in case of life-threatening hemodynamic instability, peritoneal signs, free abdominal fluid, and failure of arterial embolization.

Conclusions

Subscapular liver hematomas can be observed in patients presenting with an acute onset abdominal pain after wearing certain tight clothing such as corsets. The necessity of an early and accurate diagnosis is vital for management as hemodynamically stable patients can be managed conservatively. Surgical intervention is necessary for subscapular hematomas of the liver associated with hemodynamic instability. Traumatic liver subscapular hematomas can be observed in hemodynamically stable patients and it is a real challenge for surgeons.

Acknowledgements
None

Disclosures
There is no relationship with any industry

Authors' contributions
All authors have read and approved the manuscript. SM: leading author, supervised, implemented study, and final review. AM: worked on introduction. MM: worked on conclusion. PS: working on clinical case and provided review/editing

Authors' information
None

Competing interests
The authors declare that they have no competing interests.

Author details
[1]Department of Internal Medicine, Nazareth Hospital, 2601 Holme Avenue, Philadelphia, PA 19152, USA. [2]Rollins School of Public Health, Emory University, Atlanta, GA, USA. [3]Department of Internal Medicine, East Tennessee State University, Johnson City, TN, USA.

References

1. Orea JG, Gavino I, Cardenas JL, Cuanalo A, Brachet S (1984) Rupture of the liver and subcapsular hematoma caused by toxemia. A case successfully treated by left lobectomy. Ann Chir. 38:19–22
2. Behranwala KA, Tisdall M, Habib NH, Canelo R (2004) Spontaneous bilobar subcapsular hematoma of the liver while undergoing anticoagulation therapy: our experience and review of the literature. Int Surg. 89:212–216
3. Ulu EM, Uyusur A, Ekici Y, Hunca Ç, Coşkun M (2009) Multidetector CT findings of spontaneous rupture of hepatic adenoma in a patient with hepatic adenomatosis. Diagn Interv Radiol. 15:135–138
4. Badea R, Chiorean L, Mitre C, Botar-Jid C, Caraiani C (2013) Spontaneous retroperitoneal and subcapsular liver hematoma: the diagnostic contribution of CT, US and CEUS, Case report. Medical Ultrasonography. 15(2):157–160
5. González-López R, García-Cano E, Espinosa-González O, Cruz-Salgado Á, Montiel-Jarquin ÁJ, Hernández-Zamora V (2015) Surgical treatment for liver haematoma following endoscopic retrograde cholangiopancreatography; an unusual case. Cir Cir. 83:506–509

12

Recent advances in non-invasive diagnosis and medical management of non-alcoholic fatty liver disease in adult

Jayanta Paul

Abstract

Background: Number of non-alcoholic fatty liver disease (NAFLD) cases is increasing over time due to alteration of food habit, increase incidence of metabolic syndrome, and lack of exercise. Liver biopsy is the test for diagnosis and staging of NAFLD, but nowadays several biochemical markers, scoring systems, and imaging studies are available to diagnose and stage NAFLD which is linked to end-stage liver disease, hepatocellular cancer, and elevated cardiovascular- and cancer-related morbidity and mortality. Therefore urgent diagnosis and management are required to avoid complications related to NAFLD. This review summarizes recent advances in diagnosis and medical management of non-alcoholic fatty liver disease.

Main text: Recently published studies from PubMed, Red Cross, Copernicus, and also various previous studies were reviewed. We have discussed various non-invasive methods for detection of non-alcoholic fatty liver disease, non-alcoholic steatohepatitis (NASH), and hepatic fibrosis. Non pharmacological therapies for NAFLD, indications, and approved medications for NAFLD and other commonly used non-approved medications have been discussed in this review article.

Conclusions: Multiple non-invasive tests are available for diagnosis of NAFLD, and its different stages however gold standard test is liver biopsy. NALFD without NASH and significant fibrosis is treated by lifestyle modifications which include moderate to vigorous exercise and diet modification. To improve hepatic steatosis, minimum of 3–5% of body weight loss is necessary, but > 7–10% weight reductions is required for histological improvement in NASH and fibrosis. Pharmacotherapy is indicated when patient is having NASH with significant fibrosis.

Keywords: NAFLD, NASH, Hepatic fibrosis, Recent advances in NAFLD, Non-invasive diagnosis of NAFLD, Medical management of NAFLD

Background

Incidence and prevalence of "Non-alcoholic fatty liver disease" (NAFLD) is increasing over time mainly due to bad food habit, weight gain, and sedentary lifestyle. NAFLD is the most common cause of abnormal liver function tests (LFTs) in the UK [1]. In the USA, prevalence of NAFLD is in between 10 and 30%, which is similar to Asia and Europe [2, 3]. Singh et al. in 2004 [4] showed that 24.5% of healthy attendants had evidence of fatty liver on abdominal ultrasound. NAFLD is commonly associated with one or more component of metabolic syndrome such as obesity, diabetes mellitus, and dyslipidemia and is defined as the presence of ≥ 5% hepatic steatosis in histological examination without evidence of hepatocellular injury such as hepatocyte ballooning [5]. Around 20% of patients with NAFLD develop non-alcoholic steatohepatitis (NASH) which may progress to cirrhosis [6], however most common cause of death in NAFLD patients is cardiovascular disease,

Correspondence: dr.jayantapaul@gmail.com
Consultant Gastroenterologist and Liver Specialist, Department of Gastroenterology, Desun Hospital and Heart Institute, Kolkata 700124, India

and NAFLD is the third most common cause of hepatocellular carcinoma [5]. "Burned out" NAFLD can be a hidden cause of cryptogenic cirrhosis. So, early diagnosis, and treatment of NAFLD and underlying predisposing factors are important to avoid liver damage which may progress to liver failure.

Diagnosis

Liver biopsy is the gold standard test for diagnosis, grading, and histological assessment of NAFLD, and a four-point histopathologic grading system is used to assess severity of steatosis that ranges from 0 to 3, depending on presence of the percentage of fat-containing hepatocytes (Table 1) [7]. But the value of a liver biopsy for the diagnosis of NAFLD in routine clinical practice is controversial, especially in the presence of a generally good prognosis for most patients with NAFLD, the lack of an established form of effective therapy, and the risks and costs associated with the liver biopsy.

Before considering the diagnosis of NAFLD, alcoholic fatty liver has to be excluded. Significant alcohol intake is considered when alcohol consumption > 7 standard drinks/week (70 g ethanol) in women and > 14 (140 g ethanol) in men (according to Asia-Pacific Guidelines) or > 21 standard drink on average per week in men and > 14 standard drink per week in women (according to AASLD guidelines) or > 30 g/day in men and > 20 g/day in women (according to EASL guideline). One standard drink in Asia specific area and Europe is roughly 10 gms of pure alcohol, however in USA it is 14 gms of pure alcohol. Therefore, patient should not take significant alcohol before diagnosis of NAFLD.

Non-invasive tests for diagnosis of hepatic steatosis

Imagings for diagnosis of hepatic steatosis

Table 1 Histological and ultrasonographic grading of hepatic steatosis

Grading of hepatic steatosis	Histological findings	Ultrasonographic findings
Grade 0 steatosis	Less than 5% of hepatocytes contain fat	
Grade 1 steatosis	6–33% of hepatocytes contain fat	Hepatic echogenicity is more than the renal cortex.
Grade 2 steatosis	34–66% of hepatocytes contain fat	Liver echogenicity obscures echogenic wall of portal venous branches.
Grade 3 steatosis	> 66% of hepatocytes contain fat	Diaphragmatic wall and portal venous walls are not visible due to increased hepatic echogenicity.

A. Abdominal ultrasonography: Usually, "Hepatic steatosis" is diagnosed incidentally by abdominal ultrasonography (USG) which detect the increased echogenicity of the liver and divides fatty liver into three grades (Table 1) [8]. To identify hepatic steatosis, USG has sensitivity from 60 to 94% and specificity from 84 to 95% [9], and sensitivity is more than 90% when liver biopsy shows > 20% steatosis [10] (Fig. 1). Hepatorenal index of 1.34 or higher has sensitivity of 92% and specificity of 85% for identifying steatosis > 5% [11]. Another semi-quantitative score (ultrasonographic fatty liver indicator) which requires the presence of liver/kidney contrast (brighter liver than kidney) among other parameters can detect NAFLD when score ≥ 2 [12]. USG has several advantages (non-invasive test, widely available, low cost, quick diagnosis) and disadvantages (degree of fibrosis cannot be detected, low sensitivity when steatosis is less than 20%, and limited use in obese individuals) for detection of fatty liver.
B. Controlled attenuation parameter: Transient elastography is an ultrasound-based study and also known as vibration-controlled transient elastography or Fibroscan which can measure controlled attenuation parameter (CAP). CAP which ranges from 100 to 400 decibels per meter (dB/m) can detect significant hepatic steatosis, but it is less accurate to distinguish between the different grades of hepatic steatosis [13]. However other studies indicate that CAP score is well correlated with steatosis grades in real-world clinical practice [14–16]. The optimal cut-off values of CAP for estimation of hepatic steatosis grades such as S1, S2, and S3 are ≥ 263dB/m, ≥ 281dB/m and ≥ 283dB/m respectively [13]. Another study also graded hepatic steatosis depending on CAP value into S1 ≥ 238 dB/m, S2 ≥ 260 dB/m, and S3 ≥ 293 dB/m [17]. It does not predict liver-related events, non-hepatocellular carcinoma cancers, and cardiovascular events [18]. CAP showed excellent diagnostic performance for differentiating presence and absence of hepatic steatosis by using a cutoff value of 241 dB/m in children with NAFLD but has limited value in evaluating grades of steatosis, especially in children with high BMI (> 30 kg/m^2) [19]. Before recommendation for hepatic steatosis measurement, CAP needs further validation.
C. Computed tomography (CT scan): Decreased attenuation of hepatic parenchyma compared to intrahepatic vessels, spleen, and kidney is detected in NAFLD by both contrast-enhanced and non-contrast CT scan. When hepatic density is higher than spleen, hepatic steatosis can be excluded.

Non Invasive tests for diagnosis of Hepatic steatosis	
Imagings	**Scoring Systems**
Abdominal ultrasonography	**NAFLD liver fat score (NLFS)**
1. USG has sensitivity from 60 to 94% and specificity from 84 to 95%. 2. Sensitivity is > 90% when liver biopsy shows > 20% steatosis. 3. Hepatorenal index of 1.34 or higher has sensitivity of 92% and specificity of 85% for identifying steatosis ≥ 5%. 4. Ultrasonographic Fatty Liver Indicator score ≥ 2 indicates NAFLD.	1. NLFS value > - 0.640 has a sensitivity of 86% and specificity of 71% to identify hepatic steatosis > 5.56%. 2. Different stages of NAFLD cannot be distinguished. 3. Higher NLFS is associated with increased liver disease mortality.
Controlled Attenuation Parameter	**Fatty liver index (FLI)**
The optimal cut-off value of CAP to estimate hepatic steatosis grades: 1. CAP value ≥238 dB/m : S1 (Grade 1) 2. CAP value ≥260 dB/m : S2 (Grade 2) 3. CAP value ≥293 dB/m : S3 (Grade 3)	1. Fatty liver index: < 30 rules out fatty liver and value ≥ 60 rules in fatty liver (sensitivity: 86% and specificity 87%)
Computed tomography scan (CT Scan)	**Hepatic steatosis Index (HSI)**
Moderate-to-severe hepatic steatosis can be identified when-- 1. liver attenuation value <40-42 HU or 2. Hepatic-spleenic attenuation ratio is < 0.8.	1. HSI (value < 30) excludes hepatic steatosis with 93.1% sensitivity or 3. HSI (value > 36) detects hepatic steatosis with a specificity of 92.4%.
Magnetic resonance imaging (MRI)	**Lipid accumulation product (LPA)**
1. MRI to detect histologically confirmed hepatic steatosis: Sensitivity (76.7 to 90.0%) and Specificity (87.1 to 91%) 2. Can detect liver fat as low as 5%-10%. 3. Hydrogen-1 MR spectroscopy (H-MHS) is a non-invasive technique which can diagnose and quantify hepatic steatosis into three grades. 4. Proton density fat fraction (PDFF) with MRI: It is an accurate biomarker of hepatic steatosis and can discriminate different grades of hepatic steatosis with a good diagnostic accuracy. 5. Hepatic phosphorus-31 MRS (31P MRS) shows promise in the differentiation of NAFLD stages.	1. Cut-off value of LAP for detection of hepatic steatosis in men is 30.5 (sensitivity: 77%, specificity: 75%). 2. Cut-off value of LAP for detection of hepatic steatosis in women is 23.0 (sensitivity: 82%, specificity: 79%).
Xenon-133 liver scan	**SteatoTest**
1. It is superior to ultrasound with a sensitivity of 94.3% and specificity of 87.5%. 2. More accurate to detect mild grade of steatosis. 3. It is not expected to distinguish between different subtypes of NAFLD. 4. It does not provide information of liver morphology.	1. A cut-off value of 0.30 has 90% sensitivity to detect hepatic steatosis. 2. A cut-off of 0.72 has 90% specificity to diagnose hepatic steatosis
	NAFL screening score
	1. The lower cut-off value with a sensitivity of 92% and negative predictive value of 95% is 0.24 2. The high cut-off value with 90% specificity and positive predictive value of 84% is 0.44

Fig. 1 Non invasive tests for diagnosis of hepatic steatosis

Hepatic steatosis can be detected in CT scan of the abdomen when spleen attenuation > liver attenuation or when liver attenuation value < 48 Hounsfield units (HU) [20]. Moderate-to-severe hepatic steatosis can be identified with a specificity of 100% when liver attenuation value is < 40–42 HU and hepatic-spleenic attenuation ratio is < 0.8 [21]. Qualitative evaluation of the liver on a portal venous phase contrast-enhanced CT is highly specific to detect hepatic steatosis, but sensitivity (around 60%) is low. CT scan has several limitations such as limited accuracy to detect mild degree hepatic steatosis, risk of radiation exposure, high cost, and availability. CT scan is commonly used to detect hepatic steatosis for living liver donor candidate [22]. Dual energy CT (DECT) findings are strongly correlated with histopathologic findings in cases of steatosis and can allow rapid, accurate evaluations of hepatic steatosis.

D. *Magnetic resonance* imaging (MRI): MRI is considered as the most definitive imaging study for qualitative and quantitative assessment of hepatic steatosis. The sensitivity and specificity of MRI to detect histologically confirmed hepatic steatosis are 76.7 to 90.0% and 87.1 to 91%, respectively [7, 23]. Frequency-selective MRI, chemical-shift-encoded MRI, MR spectroscopy, and magnetic resonance elastography techniques are usually used to assess hepatic fat content [24]. In MRI, both in-phase (IP) and out-of-phase (OOP) imaging to be adequately assessed to detect fatty liver (FL), and in out-of-phase image FL appears as hyper intense (in T1 image), mildly hyper intense (in T2 image), and signal droop out (signal loss is demonstrated when there is 10–15% fat fraction with maximum signal loss occurring when there is 50% fatty infiltration of the liver). Advantages of MRI-based detection of fatty liver are no radiation exposure; high diagnostic accuracy; can detect fat as low as 5–10%; operator independent; highly responsive to changes in steatosis throughout parenchyma; and not significantly impacted by demographics, histologic activity, or co-existing hepatic conditions. It has the following disadvantages: high cost and taking long time.
Hydrogen-1 MR spectroscopy (1H-MRS) is a non-invasive technique which can diagnose and quantify hepatic steatosis into three grades, and H-MHS thresholds correspond with histopathologic grading of steatosis and may obviate liver biopsy (Table 2) [25]. 1H-MRS allows the direct measurement of the area under the lipid resonance peak. This test result is not modified by the presence of confounding factors such as fibrosis, iron overload, and glycogen. Main drawbacks of H-MHS are high cost, less availability, complex technique requiring patient co-operation, samples only a small portion of the entire liver, and not well validated and still considered a research tool.
Proton density fat fraction (PDFF) in MRI is also used for quantifying hepatic steatosis. PDFF is an accurate marker of hepatic steatosis and allows discriminating with a good diagnostic accuracy between different grades of hepatic steatosis [26]. The accuracy of PDFF measurement using chemical shift-encoded methods is similar to that of MRS. Recently, hepatic phosphorus-31 MRS (31P-MRS) is proposed in different studies as a potential marker to detect distinct biochemical changes in different NAFLD states. It shows promise in the differentiation of NAFLD stages [27].

Table 2 Hydrogen-1 MR spectroscopy grading of fatty liver

Grading of fatty liver	Hydrogen-1 MR spectroscopy findings
Grade 0 steatosis	Proton density fat fraction threshold of less than 17.0%
Grade 1 steatosis	Proton density fat fraction threshold of 17.0–38.6%
Grade 2 or greater steatosis	Proton density fat fraction threshold greater than 38.6%

E. Xenon–133 liver scan: Xe-133 liver scan is a safe, reliable, non-invasive method with low radiation exposure to detect and quantify hepatic steatosis, and is superior to ultrasound with a sensitivity of 94.3% and specificity of 87.5% [28]. Compared with other imaging investigations, Xe-133 scan is more accurate to detect mild grade of steatosis [28]. One major limitation of Xe-133 scan is that it only detects fat; therefore, it is not expected to distinguish between different subtypes of NAFLD and does not provide information of liver morphology. The usefulness of Xe-133 scan in the diagnosis of NAFLD has not been well studied till now (Fig. 1).

Non-invasive scoring systems for diagnosis of hepatic steatosis

There is no single laboratory marker that can be used for the diagnosis of NAFLD. Gamma-glutamyltransferase (GGT) in the serum is frequently elevated in NAFLD patients and associated with increased mortality [29], however does not help in diagnosis of NAFLD. Alanine aminotransferase (ALT) and aspartate aminotransferase (AST) levels are not sensitive for diagnosis of NAFLD. Following scoring systems are available to identify NAFLD.

A. NAFLD liver fat score (NLFS): The NAFLD liver fat score is estimated by using the presence of the metabolic syndrome, type 2 diabetes, fasting serum insulin level, fasting serum AST, and the AST/ALT ratio [30]. NLFS value > − 0.640 has a sensitivity of 86% and specificity of 71% to identify hepatic steatosis > 5.56% [30]. However, by this scoring system, different stages of NAFLD cannot be distinguished. This score provide simple and non-invasive tool to predict NAFLD and liver fat content. Higher NLFS is associated with increased liver disease mortality but not with other mortality outcomes [31].

B. Fatty liver index (FLI): Fatty liver index is a suitable and simple predictor for hepatic steatosis. FLI is calculated by measuring waist circumference, body mass index, serum triglyceride, and gamma-glutamyltransferase [32]. Score varies from zero to 100. Fatty liver index < 30 rules out fatty liver, but value ≥ 60 rules in fatty liver with a sensitivity and specificity of 86% and 87%, respectively [32]. FLI independently associates with overall, cardiovascular and cancer-related mortality. FLI can serve as a surrogate marker for hepatic steatosis and metabolic syndrome in type 1 diabetes [33].

C. Hepatic steatosis index (HSI): It is a simple, effective NAFLD screening tool derived by a logistic regression model. It includes gender, history of T2DM, body mass index (BMI), alanine transaminase (ALT), and aspartate transaminase (AST). HSI is calculated by the following formula: 8 × (ALT/AST ratio) + BMI (addition of +2 if female; +2 if diabetes mellitus) [33]. HSI value < 30 excludes NAFLD with 93.1% sensitivity and value > 36 detects NAFLD with a specificity of 92.4% [23]. It may be utilized for selecting individuals for hepatic USG and for determining the need of lifestyle modifications.

D. Lipid accumulation product (LAP): It is significantly associated with the presence of liver steatosis and has a high diagnostic accuracy to identify NAFLD in the general population, and diagnostic accuracy is higher in young age group individuals [34, 35]. Following calculation is used to measure LAP: [waist circumference (cm) − 65] × triglyceride concentration (mmol//L) in men and [waist circumference (cm) − 58] × triglyceride concentration (mmol/L) in women [35]. Cutoff values of LAP in men and women are 30.5 (sensitivity 77%, specificity 75%) and 23.0 (sensitivity 82%, specificity 79%), respectively [35]. Although this is a very simple and low cost test, it needs further validation before recommendation. Lipid accumulation product can also predict metabolic syndrome in individuals without fatty liver disease [36].

E. SteatoTest: SteatoTest includes ten components such as serum α2-macroglobulin, apo A1, haptoglobin, total bilirubin, GGT, ALT, body mass index, serum cholesterol, triglycerides, and glucose adjusted for age and gender. It is a simple and non-invasive method to identify liver steatosis and may reduce the need for liver biopsy, particularly in patients with component of metabolic syndrome [37]. A cutoff of 0.30 has 90% sensitivity, and a cutoff of 0.72 has 90% specificity to diagnose hepatic steatosis [37]. It needs further validation before recommendation.

F. NAFL screening score: It is a model to detect NAFLD with the following six components: age, fasting blood glucose, BMI, triglyceride, ALT/AST, and uric acid. The lower cutoff value with a sensitivity of 92% and negative predictive value of 95% is 0.24, and the high cutoff value with 90% specificity and 84% positive predictive value is 0.44 [38].

Non-invasive tests for diagnosis of non-alcoholic steatohepatitis (NASH)

NASH can progress to cirrhosis and its complications such as portal hypertension, liver failure, and hepatocellular carcinoma. Cirrhosis develops in 21 to 28% of NASH patients compared to only 3% of patients with non-alcoholic fatty liver. The gold standard for diagnosis of NASH is liver biopsy. But liver biopsy is an invasive procedure and has several complications, non-invasive tests has been developed for diagnosis of NASH (Fig. 2).

Serum biomarkers

A. Serum cytokeratin (CK)-18: It is a marker of hepatocyte apoptosis, most widely investigated for diagnosis of NASH and is the most consistent single parameter for differentiating steatosis from NASH [39]. Cutoff value of CK-18 > 240 U/L has a sensitivity of 76.7% and specificity of 95.0% for diagnosis of NASH [40]. Another study showed that optimal cutoff point of serum CK-18-fragments for definite NASH was 270 U/L with sensitivity and specificity of 64% and 76%, respectively [41].

B. Serum aminotransferases: It is commonly used in clinical practice as a surrogate marker for liver inflammation but has poor predictive value for diagnosis of NASH [5]. Serum alanine aminotransferase (ALT) value > 2 times the upper limit of normal (> 70 U/L) has a sensitivity of 50% and specificity of 61% for NASH detection [42], but ~ 80% of patients with fatty liver have shown ALT levels within normal limits [43]. Aminotransferase levels do not correlate with the degree of hepatic fibrosis. Liver enzymes should not be used for detection of NASH. Further studies are required to

Non invasive tests for diagnosis of steatohepatitis (NASH)

Serum Biomarkers

Serum cytokeratin (CK)-18

1. Cut-off value of CK-18 is >240 U/L for diagnosis of NASH (sensitivity: 76.7% and specificity: 95.0%).
2. Most consistent single parameter for differentiating steatosis from NASH.

Serum aminotransferases

1. Serum alanine aminotransferase (ALT) value > 2 times the upper limit of normal (>70 U/L) has a sensitivity of 50% and specificity of 61% for NASH detection.
2. ~ 80% of patients with fatty liver have shown ALT levels within normal limits.
3. Aminotransferase levels do not correlate with the degree of hepatic fibrosis.
4. Liver enzymes should not be used for detection of NASH

Serum Adiponectin

1. Cut-off negative predictor for NASH is 29.16 μg /L.

Fibroblast growth factor 21 (FGF21)

1. Its level correlates with severity of steatohepatitis in patients with NASH.
2. FGF21 level may help to identify patients who is having highest risk of disease progression.

Proprotein convertase subtilisin/kexin type 9 (PCSK9)

1. Circulating PCSK9 increases with hepatic fat accumulation.
2. Correlates with the severity of steatosis.

Plasma pentraxin 3(PTX3)

1. Higher serum concentration is seen in patients with more advanced stages of NAFLD.

Malondialdehyde (MDA)

1. High serum level is seen in patients with NASH than without NASH

Tumor Necrosis Factor Alpha (TNF-α)

1. It is elevated in patients with NASH.
2. High level of TNF-α has increased higher adverse hepatic events risk compared to patients with low level of TNF-α

Interleukin-6 (IL-6)

1. IL-6 is positively correlated with severity of hepatocyte inflammation, stage of fibrosis in patients with NASH.

Non-invasive scoring systems

NASH test

It divides NASH into three categories:
1. NASH (AUROC of 0.79),
2. Borderline NASH (AUROC of 0.69)
3. No-NASH (AUROC of 0.77-0.83)

NASH diagnostic index (NDI)

1. NDI value ≥22 has a specificity of 82% for identifying a diagnosis of simple steatosis
2. NDI value ≥50 has a specificity of 86% for diagnosing histologically confirmed NASH

HAIR score

1. The presence of ≥ 2 parameters predict NASH (sensitivity of 80% and specificity of 89%)

Nice model

1. Cut off value is 0.14 for diagnosis of NASH (84% sensitivity, 86% specificity)

Palekar score

1. ≥ 3 risk factors distinguishes NASH from steatosis (73.7% sensitivity, 65.7% specificity)

NASH ClinLipMet score

1. The sensitivity of this scoring system is 75%.
2. This test is usually is used in research because of high cost.

NASH predictive index (NPI)

1. Predicting the presence of NASH, this index is promising (AUROC of 0.87 to 0.90)

NAFIC score

1. This score includes ferritin, fasting insulin, and type IV collagen 7S.

Gholam score

NASH Score

oxNASH score

1. Score > 72 were 10 times more likely to have NASH

Imagings

Proton magnetic resonance (1H-MRS)

1. This method is studied in detecting NASH with a sensitivity of 87.4% and specificity of 74.3%

Magnetic resonance elastography (MRE)

1. Can accurately identify NASH prior to fibrosis.
2. Differentiate NASH from NAFL with a sensitivity of 94% and specificity 73% by using a threshold of 2.74 kPa

Breath test

1. Analyzing three volatile organic compounds (n-tridecane, 3-methyl-butanonitrile, and 1-propanol) in the exhaled breath
2. Distinguishes patients with NASH from without NASH
3. Negative predictive value of 82% and positive predictive value81%

Fig. 2 Non invasive tests for diagnosis of non alcoholic steatohepatitis

find out cutoff value of liver enzymes to prevent unnecessary diagnostic work-ups and early detection of NASH.

C. Serum adiponectin: Adiponectin is exclusively synthesized by adipose tissue and involves in glucose and lipid metabolism. It is a negative predictor of NASH in fatty liver patients with a cutoff value 29.16 μg/L [44].

D. Fibroblast growth factor 21 (FGF21): Serum FGF21 level correlates with severity of steatohepatitis in patients with NASH, and its level may help to identify patients who are having highest risk of disease progression. Plasma FGF21 was higher in patients with NASH with mean value of 453 ± 262 pg/mL when compared to patients without NASH [45]. To improve the positive predictive value (PPV) and negative predictive value (NPV) of FGF21, CK-18 is combined with FGF21, which improves the PPV to 82% and NPV to 74% [46].

E. Proprotein convertase subtilisin/kexin type 9 (PCSK9): Hepatocytes secrete PCSK9 which inhibits the uptake of low-density lipoproteins by targeting the receptor for degradation and possibly lipogenesis. In a recent study, Paquette et al. described strong association between PCSK9 and liver biomarkers as well as hepatic steatosis [47]. Circulating PCSK9 increases with hepatic fat accumulation and also correlates with the severity of steatosis [48].

F. Plasma pentraxin 3(PTX3): Higher serum concentration of pentraxin 3 protein is seen in patients with more advanced stages of NAFLD, and higher values are correlated with advanced stages of the hepatic fibrosis. Therefore, serum PTX3 level could be used as a marker to assess severity of hepatic fibrosis [49].

G. Malondialdehyde (MDA): High serum level of malondialdehyde is seen in type 2 diabetes patients with NASH than without NASH [50]. MDA can stimulate hepatic stellate cells and result in fibrosis.

H. Tumor necrosis factor alpha (TNF-α): Tilg et al. described that TNF-α is elevated in serum of those with NASH [51]. Patients with high level of TNF-α have increased burden of NAFLD and higher adverse hepatic event risk compared to patients with low level of TNF-α [51].

I. Interleukin-6 (IL-6): Elevated serum IL-6 is associated with an increased likelihood of exhibiting NAFLD. IL-6 is positively correlated with severity of hepatocyte inflammation, stage of fibrosis in patients with NASH [52]. However, Yoneda et al. in their study did not find any increase in expression of IL-6 in patients with steatohepatitis as compared to patients with simple hepatic steatosis [53].

Non-invasive scoring systems for diagnosis of steatohepatitis (NASH)

A. NASH test: NASH test is a simple and non-invasive scoring system to predict the presence or absence of NASH in patients with non-alcoholic fatty liver disease [54]. It includes 13 components (age, sex, height, weight, serum levels of triglycerides, cholesterol, a2-macroglobulin, apolipoprotein A1, haptoglobin, g-glutamyltransferase, aminotransferases ALT, AST, and total bilirubin) to identify NASH and divide NASH into three categories: NASH (AUROC of 0.79), Borderline NASH (AUROC of 0.69), and No-NASH (AUROC of 0.77–0.83) [55].

B. HAIR score: This score depends on the following parameters: hypertension, alanine aminotransferase [ALT] level, and insulin resistance. The presence of at least two of the three parameters provides the best combination of sensitivity of 80% and specificity of 89% for predicting NASH especially in severely obese individuals [56].

C. NASH diagnostic index (NDI): This index is calculated by serum insulin, glucose, triglycerides, ALT, and waist-to-hip ratio. By using a value ≥ 22, NDI has a specificity of 82% for establishing a diagnosis of simple steatosis, and NDI has a specificity of 86% for diagnosing NASH when value is ≥ 50 [57].

D. NICE model: A simple and non-invasive composite model includes metabolic syndrome (MS), CK-18, and serum ALT level. This model is designed to diagnose NASH in morbidly obese patients. The equation of "Nice model" is: – 5.654 + 3.780E–02 × ALT (IU/L) + 2.215E–03 × CK18 fragment levels (IU/L) + 1.825 × (presence of MS = 1) [58]. The best cutoff value is 0.14 for diagnosis of NASH and this value is associated with 84% sensitivity, 86% specificity, 44% positive predictive value, and 98% negative predictive value.

E. Palekar score: It was proposed to distinguish NASH from steatosis. This scoring system includes the following risk factors: age ≥ 50 years, female gender, AST ≥ 45 IU/L, body mass index (BMI) ≥ 30 mg/kg2, AST/ALT ratio ≥ 0.80, and hyaluronic acid ≥ 55 μg/L. The presence of three or more risk factors has 73.7% sensitivity and 65.7% specificity to distinguish NASH from steatosis [59].

F. NAFIC score: This score is used by using ferritin, fasting insulin, and type IV collagen 7S for predicting non-alcoholic steatohepatitis in NAFLD patients [60].

G. NASH ClinLipMet score: This test is used by utilizing serum AST value, fasting insulin value, PNPLA3 genotype, glutamate, isoleucine, glycine, lysophosphatidylcholine 16:0, and phosphoethanolamine 40:6. The sensitivity of this scoring system is 75% [55]. This test is usually used in research because of high cost.

H. NASH predictive index (NPI): This index is used by using age, female gender, body mass index (BMI), homeostatic model assessment (HOMA) of insulin resistance, and log [aspartate aminotransferase (AST) × ALT]. For predicting the presence of NASH, this index is promising (AUROC of 0.87 to 0.90) but lacks external validation [61].

I. Other scoring systems: Gholam score (AST and diabetes mellitus) [62] and oxNASH (13-hydroxyl-octadecadienoic acid/linoleic acid ratio, age, BMI, and AST) score > 72 were 10 times more likely to have NASH compared to those with oxNASH score < 47 [63], and a clinical score by Chunming et al. [64] including ALT, gamma-glutamyl transpeptidase, C-reactive protein, and ApoB/ApoA1 ratio, NASH Score [65] (AST, PNPLA3 genotype and fasting insulin) were studied for identification of NASH.

Breath test for diagnosis of non-alcoholic steatohepatitis

A study showed that analyzing three volatile organic compounds (n-tridecane, 3-methyl-butanonitrile, and 1-propanol) in the exhaled breath were sufficient to distinguish patients with NASH from without NASH with negative and positive predictive values of 82% and 81%, respectively [66].

Imagings for diagnosis of non-alcoholic steatohepatitis

Routine imaging techniques (Ultrasonography, CT, or MRI) are unable to differentiate NASH from simple steatosis.

A. Proton magnetic resonance (1H-MRS): This method is studied in detecting NASH with a sensitivity of 87.4% and specificity of 74.3% [67].

B. Magnetic resonance elastography (MRE): MRE can accurately identify NASH prior to fibrosis and differentiate NASH from NAFL with a sensitivity of 94% and specificity 73% by using a threshold of 2.74 kPa [68]. But it needs further validation.

Non-invasive tests for diagnosis of hepatic fibrosis:

Stages of liver fibrosis are the most important factor for the prognosis of NAFLD and predicting the risk of progression to cirrhosis and its complications. There are several predictive models available to identify hepatic fibrosis (Fig. 3).

Non-invasive scoring systems for diagnosis of hepatic fibrosis

A. AST/platelet ratio index (APRI): This is measured by using the patient's AST level, upper limit of normal AST value, and platelet count. APRI cutoff of ≥ 0.7 has a sensitivity of 77% and specificity of 72% to detect significant hepatic fibrosis (≥ F2 by Metavir) and a cutoff score of at least 1.0 has a sensitivity of 61 to 76% and specificity of 64 to 72% for detection of severe fibrosis/cirrhosis (F3 to F4 by Metavir) [69]. APRI has a good negative predictive value to exclude advanced fibrosis but does not accurately differentiate intermediate fibrosis from mild or severe fibrosis.

B. FIB-4: It is a simple, accurate, and inexpensive method for assessing liver fibrosis and includes the following components: age, platelet count, AST, and ALT. It is calculated by using [age (years) × AST (U/L)]/[number of platelets (10^9/L) × ALT (U/L) (1/2)] formula. An FIB-4 score > 3.25 has a positive predictive value of 82.1% with a specificity of 98.2% to confirm the existence of a significant fibrosis (F3-F4 by Metavir) [70]. FIB-4 has high negative predictive value (> 90%) for ruling out advanced fibrosis when score is < 1.45.

C. BARD score: This is calculated by using the sum of 3 variables (BMI ≥ 28 = 1 point, AST-to-ALT Ratio ≥ 0.8 = 2 points, the presence of diabetes = 1 point), and score ≥ 2 is associated with advanced fibrosis [71]. Due to its simplicity, it is popular among general practitioners, However due to its low positive predictive value (< 42%) it includes many patients without NASH/ fibrosis into high risk group and limits its utility in clinical practice.

D. NAFLD fibrosis score (NFS): A simple scoring system accurately separates NAFLD with and without advanced fibrosis. It includes age, hyperglycemia, body mass index, platelet count, albumin, and AST/ALT ratio as variables. By using low cutoff score of − 1.455, advanced hepatic fibrosis could be excluded with high negative predictive value of 93%, and by applying the high cutoff score of 0.676, advanced hepatic fibrosis could be diagnosed with high positive predictive value of 90% [72]. Advantages of the NFS are as follows: (1) its ability to provide prognostic information and (2) identify NAFLD patients who are at increased risk for liver-related complications such as ascites and gastroesophageal varices or death.

E. King's score: The King's score is a simple index for predicting cirrhosis and calculated by the following formula: age × AST (U/L) × INR/platelet count

Non invasive tests for diagnosis of Hepatic fibrosis

Scoring systems

AST/Platelet Ratio Index (APRI)

1. Cut-off value is ≥ 0.7 to detect significant hepatic fibrosis (≥ F2 by Metavir)
2. Has an sensitivity of 77% and specificity of 72%

FIB-4 score

1. Score > 3.25 has a positive predictive value of 82.1% with a specificity of 98.2% to confirm the existence of a significant fibrosis (F3-F4 by Metavir)

BARD score

1. Score ≥ 2 is associated with advanced fibrosis
2. Low positive predictive value (42%) limits its utility in clinical practice

NAFLD fibrosis score (NFS)

1. By using low cut-off score of -1.455, advanced hepatic fibrosis could be excluded with high negative predictive value of 93%
2. By applying the high cut-off score of 0.676, advanced hepatic fibrosis could be diagnosed with high positive predictive value of 90%

King's score

1. Score ≥ 16.7 predicts cirrhosis with sensitivity 86%, specificity 80% and a high negative predictive value of 96%

Fibrosis Index score (FI)

1. Sensitivity and positive predictive value of FI score ≥ 3.30 for the prediction of F4 is 70.8% and 81.0% respectively

Enhanced Liver Fibrosis (ELF) panel

1. It has 3 cut-off values:
   (1) value 7.7 for exclusion of fibrosis,
   (2) value 9.8 for identification of fibrosis with sensitivity of 69%, specificity of 98% for moderate fibrosis,
   (3) value 11.3 to discriminate cirrhosis with 83% sensitivity and specificity of 97%

FibroTest

1. Cut-off value of 0.30 has 90% negative predictive value for advanced fibrosis with sensitivity of 77%
2. Cut-off value of 0.70 has a 73% positive predictive value for advanced fibrosis with specificity of 98%.

Fibroindex

Forns Index

Fibrospect II

1. Score > 0.42 indicates presence of stage F2 to F4 fibrosis with sensitivity of 80.6% and specificity of 71.4%

Imagings

Transient Elastography (Fibroscan)

1. Cut-off value of < 8 kPa has a 94%–100% negative predictive value to exclude significant hepatic fibrosis
2. Cut-off values used to identify stages of hepatic fibrosis
   F ≥ 2: 7.1 kPa
   F ≥ 3: 9.5 kPa
   F4: 12.5 kPa

Acoustic Radiation Force Impulse (ARFI) elastography

1. Using a predictive shear stiffness of 4.24kpa, it distinguishes low (fibrosis stage 0-2) from high (fibrosis stage 3-4) fibrosis stages (sensitivity of 90% and a specificity of 90%)

Shear wave elastography (SWE)

1. In healthy population, liver stiffness value ranges in between 4.5-5.5 kPa
2. By using cut-off values of 7.10kpa and 9.1kpa to detect F ≥ 2 and F ≥ 3 have sensitivity and specificity of 93.8% and 52%, and 93.1% and 80.8% respectively
3. When 13kpa and 15.73 kpa are used to detect F4 fibrosis, the sensitivity and specificity are 75.3 and 87.8, and 100% and 82 % respectively

Magnetic Resonance Elastography (MRE)

1. Cut-off value of > 3.63 kPa has a sensitivity of 86%, specificity of 91%, NPV of 97% and PPV of 68% to discriminate advanced fibrosis (F3–F4) from stage F0–F2 fibrosis.

Fig. 3 Non invasive tests for diagnosis of hepatic fibrosis

(10^9/L). Score of ≥ 16.7 predicts cirrhosis with sensitivity 86%, specificity 80%, and a high negative predictive value of 96% [73]. This score was initially evaluated for diagnosis of cirrhosis in patients with hepatitis C infection.

F. Fibrosis index score (FI): This is a simple index to detect hepatic fibrosis noninvasively and measured by "8 − 0.01 × number of platelets (10^9/L) − albumin (g/dL)" formula. Sensitivity and positive predictive value of FI score ≥ 3.30 for the prediction of F4 is 70.8% and 81.0%, respectively [74].

G. Cao et al. published a score by measuring CK-18, ALT, platelets, and triglycerides that had significant positive correlation with staging hepatic fibrosis [75].

H. Egy-Score: This score is a useful non-invasive panel of surrogate biomarkers that can accurately predict stages of hepatic fibrosis. Egy-Score was calculated by the following formula: 3.52 + 0.0063 × CA19-9 + 0.0203 × age + 0.4485 × alpha-2-macroglobulin + 0.0303 × bilirubin − 0.0048 × platelet − 0.0462 × albumin [76].

I. Enhanced liver fibrosis (ELF) panel: It includes three variables: hyaluronic acid, tissue inhibitor of metalloproteinase 1, and aminoterminal peptide of procollagen III. It has 3 cutoff values: (1) value 7.7 for exclusion of fibrosis, (2) value 9.8 for identification of fibrosis with sensitivity of 69% and specificity of 98% for moderate fibrosis, and (3) value 11.3 to discriminate cirrhosis with 83% sensitivity and specificity of 97% [77].

J. FibroTest: This is calculated by using five biomarkers: haptoglobin, α2-macroglobulin, apolipoprotein A1, total bilirubin, and GGT. Cutoff value of 0.30 has 90% negative predictive value for advanced fibrosis with sensitivity of 77%, and a cutoff value of 0.70 has a 73% positive predictive value for advanced fibrosis with specificity of 98%. False positive result is seen in Gilbert's syndrome, cholestasis, acute hemolysis, renal insufficiency, on medications that may cause unconjugated hyperbilirubinemia, and acute liver inflammation [78].

K. Fibroindex: This simple scoring system is measured by using the following three biochemical markers: AST, platelet count, and gamma globulin. It has good specificity for mild or significant fibrosis (94% and 97% respectively) but has low sensitivity (40% and 36% respectively) [79]. Due to its low sensitivity, it is not an adequate tool to be used alone for detection of hepatic fibrosis.

L. HepaScore: Age, sex, total bilirubin, GGT, alpha-2-macroglobulin, and hyaluronic acid levels are used to calculate HepaScore. Score ≤ 0.2 has 98% negative predictive value to exclude fibrosis and ≥ 0.8 has a positive predictive value of 62% to predict cirrhosis [80].

M. Forns index: It has the following components: age, gamma-glutamyltransferase (GGT), cholesterol, and platelet count. Score < 4.25 has a negative predictive value of 96% to exclude significant fibrosis and value > 6.9 has positive predictive value of 66% for diagnosis of significant fibrosis [81].

N. Fibrospect II: This test (including hyaluronic acid, tissue inhibitor of a metalloproteinase-1 (TIMP-1), and alpha-2-macroglobulin as variables) can be used to predict stages of hepatic fibrosis (F2 to F4). Score > 0.42 indicates presence of stage F2 to F4 fibrosis with sensitivity of 80.6% and specificity of 71.4% [82].

Imagings for diagnosis of hepatic fibrosis

A. Transient elastography (Fibroscan): This is an easy-to-perform, non-invasive, day care procedure which takes about 5 to 10 min and measures the velocity of 50 MHz shear wave that is emitted by ultrasound transducer probe and transmitted through hepatic tissue. This velocity of share wave in the liver is positively related to liver stiffness, and value ranges from 1.5 to 75 kPa. Fibroscan examines a larger area of liver tissue (1 cm diameter × 5 cm in length) than liver biopsy and provides a more representative assessment of the entire hepatic parenchyma. Two types of probe are available to measure hepatic stiffness: "M" probe is the most commonly used to measure shear wave velocity, and "XL" probe is usually used in obese people to reduce the failure rate. Cutoff value of < 8 kPa has a 94–100% negative predictive value to exclude significant hepatic fibrosis [83], and cutoff values used to identify stages of hepatic fibrosis are as follow: 7.1 kPa for F ≥ 2, 9.5 kPa for F ≥ 3, and 12.5 kPa for F4 [84]. Conditions which increase liver stiffness without fibrosis are acute hepatitis, hepatic congestion (e.g., in heart failure), mass lesions within the liver, and cholestasis. Failure or unreliable to take readings are seen more frequently in the following patients: obesity (BMI > 30–35 kg/m^2), older age, and presence of ascites. There are no absolute contraindications for this test, however manufacturer also advises against the use of this device in pregnancy and in patients with a pacemaker and implantable defibrillators. Despite these limitations, Fibroscan is one of the more reliable non-invasive methods to estimate liver fibrosis and is recommended during the management of NAFLD in the current guidelines [5].

B. Acoustic radiation force impulse (ARFI) elastography: ARFI uses a conventional B-mode ultrasonography probe which produces an acoustic pulse. Hepatic stiffness is expressed as shear wave velocity in meter per second (m/s) after calculating the median for 10 successful measures. Using a predictive shear stiffness of 4.24 kPa, it distinguishes low (fibrosis stage 0–2) from high (fibrosis stage 3–4) fibrosis stages with a sensitivity of 90% and a specificity of 90% [85]. The advantages of ARFI are as follows: (1) the acoustic energy pulse is not affected by obesity or ascitic fluid, (2) specific regions of interest can be focused during procedure to measure varying depths in specific areas of the liver, (3) at the same time whole liver can be evaluated by ultrasonography which is not possible with Fbroscan. However, the presence of severe steatosis can affect accuracy of ARFI [86].
C. Shear wave elastography (SWE): By using conventional ultrasonography machine, SWE estimates liver stiffness in the right lobe and positively correlated with liver fibrosis severity and can potentially differentiate intermediate degrees of liver fibrosis in patients with NAFLD. Shear waves produced by a conventional ultrasound beam are directly related to the hepatic stiffness and are reported to be more accurate than transient elastography in assessing significant fibrosis of the liver (LS) (≥ F2) [87]. Hepatic stiffness is measured in the right lobe of the liver, and measurement of LS in the left lobe is inappropriate because it is affected by cardiac pulsation. In healthy population, liver stiffness value ranges in between 4.5 and 5.5 kPa [88]. Food intake increases LS value and results in falsely high fibrosis stages, and usually 180 min after food intake, value comes to the normal range; therefore, it is recommended to measure hepatic stiffness at least 4 h after food intake [89]. By using cut-off values of 7.10 kPa and 9.1 kPa to detect, F ≥ 2 and F ≥ 3 have sensitivity and specificity of 93.8% and 52%, and 93.1% and 80.8% respectively[85]. When 13 kPa and 15.73 kPa are used to detect F4 fibrosis, the sensitivity and specificity are 75.3 and 87.8, and 100% and 82 % respectively [90, 91].
D. Magnetic resonance elastography (MRE): It can assess a larger surface area of the liver or the entire liver than US-based modalities and is not limited by ascites and obesity. MRE has a sensitivity of 94% and specificity of 95% to differentiate F0 to F1 from F2 to F4, and 98% sensitivity and 94% specificity in differentiating F0 to F3 from F4 [92]. A cutoff value of > 3.63 kPa has a sensitivity of 86%, specificity of 91%, NPV of 97%, and PPV of 68% to discriminate advanced fibrosis (F3–F4) from stage F0 to F2 fibrosis [93]. Limitations of MRE are as follows: (1) it cannot be applied to individuals with hepatic iron overload due to the interfering signal intensity, (2) high cost of MRE, (3) needs further validations.

Emerging genetic biomarkers for diagnosis of different stages of NAFLD

Several genetic biomarkers were studied to diagnose or identify different stages of NAFLD. However, it needs further research before recommendations on emerging genetic biomarkers.

A. Lipidomic serum tests: These tests distinguish NAFLD from normal liver (NL) and NASH from non-alcoholic fatty liver (NAFL) with high accuracy. The diagnostic performances of the validated tests for discrimination between NAFLD and NL show sensitivity and specificity of 0.94 and 0.57, respectively and sensitivity of 0.70 and specificity of 0.81, respectively for the discrimination between NASH and NAFL [94]
B. Proteomic analysis: This analysis can be used to differentiate simple steatosis from NASH with significant fibrosis (F3/F4 group), and the NASH with significant fibrosis (F3/F4 group) and without significant fibrosis [95]. Complement component C7 was three-fold higher in the NASH group with significant/advanced fibrosis (F2–F4) compared with the early NASH (F0–F1). Complement component C7 and Fibulin-1 are positively correlated with liver stiffness, whereas complement component C8 γ chain is negatively correlated. High levels of complement C7 are associated with NASH with significant/advanced fibrosis [96].
C. Gut microbiome-based metagenomic signature: Gut microbiome compositions using whole-genome shotgun sequencing of DNA extracted from stool can be used to identify advanced hepatic fibrosis in NAFLD patients. The gut microbiomes in NAFLD are dominated by members of Bacteroidetes and Firmicutes followed by Actinobacteria and Proteobacteria in much lower amount. Proteobacteria phylum has a statistically significant increase in amount (while the Firmicutes phylum decrease) as the disease progresses from mild/moderate NAFLD to advanced fibrosis [97].

Management of NAFLD (Fig. 4)

NALFD patients without NASH and hepatic fibrosis are treated by lifestyle changes which include diet modification and moderate physical exercise along with treatment of underlying causes. Pharmacotherapy is available in presence of NASH and fibrosis (≥ 2). NAFLD patients with an advanced liver fibrosis (ELF

Non alcoholic fatty liver disease (NAFLD)

↓

Treatment of underlying causes (Diabetes mellitus, Obesity, Dyslipidemia, etc)

↓

NAFLD without non alcoholic steatohepatitis (NASH) and significant fibrosis

↓

Lifestyle modification:

A] Diet modification-

1. Energy restriction
2. Low calorie, low fat, and low carbohydrate diet
3. 500-1000 kcal deficit diet to induce a weight loss of 500-1000 gram/week
4. Coffee intake ≥2 cups/day improves NAFLD by inhibiting proliferation of hepatic stellate cell
5. Fructose-containing beverages and foods should be avoided
6. Avoid alcohol consumption
7. Omega-3 fatty acid supplementation may be a new treatment option for NAFLD but Omega-3 fatty acid should not be used as a specific treatment of NAFLD or NASH, but it can be used to treat hypertriglyceridemia in NAFLD patients

Plus

B] Physical exercise-

1. Both moderate- vigorous aerobic exercise

At least 3%-5% of body weight loss is necessary to improve hepatic steatosis, but > 7% weight loss is required for histological improvement in NASH and fibrosis

NASH with significant fibrosis (fibrosis stage ≥2 or fibroscan value > 10.51)

↓

Lifestyle modifications

Plus

Physical exercise

Plus

One or more of the following medications:

1. Pioglitazone:
   - Indicated in biopsy-proven NASH patients with and without type 2 diabetes mellitus
   - 15-30mg daily dose of Pioglitazone is recommended
   - Treatment should be stopped if there is no reduction in aminotransferases after 6 months of therapy and in patients with normal ALT at baseline, no recommendations can be made
2. Vitamin E:
   - Vitamin E may be considered at a daily dose of 800 IU/day in nondiabetic adults with biopsy-proven NASH
3. Ursodeoxycholic acid (UDCA):
   - According to NICE, EASL, Asia-pacific and AASLD guidelines, UDCA is not recommended for treatment of NAFLD, NASH or hepatic fibrosis
   - But few recent studies showed (1) (Parikh P et al (2016) UDCA is an effective and safe alternative to Vitamin E in nondiabetic–non-cirrhotic Indian NAFLD patients

     (2) (Mappala H, 2019) UDCA is a frontline therapeutic option for NASH and thereby preventing its progression to cirrhosis and liver cancer

Fig. 4 Medical management of non-alcoholic fatty liver disease

test > 10.51) a indication for pharmacotherapy in the NICE guideline [98]. Patients with NASH should be the main target of treatment due to higher risk of mortality related to the disease. A weight loss of at least 7% is required for histological improvement in obese NASH patients.

A. Lifestyle modification: It is an effective therapy to downgrade hepatic injury in NAFLD patients [99].

Diet modification: Energy restriction with a low calorie, low fat, and low carbohydrate or high-protein

Mediterranean diet is advised in NAFLD patients. 500–1000 kcal deficit diet per day to induce a weight loss of 500–1000 g/week is usually recommended (according to EASL, Asia-Pacific and AASLD guidelines). According to the Italian Association for the Study of the Liver (IASL), amount of fat and carbohydrate should be < 30% and < 50% of total calories respectively.

Coffee drinking is protective in NAFLD by reducing histological severity and liver-related outcomes and inversely related to the steatohepatitis severity [100]. Therefore daily coffee consumption should be encouraged in NAFLD patients. Coffee intake ≥ 2 cups/day improves NAFLD and reduces liver-related morbidities [101]. Caffeine inhibits proliferation of hepatic stellate cell, thus exerting an anti-fibrogenic effect via adenosine receptor blockade [102].

Fructose-containing beverages and foods should be avoided because it appears as one major factor for initiation of hepatic steatosis and also its progression to NASH and more severe stages of the liver fibrosis [103, 104].

Alcohol intake should be < 30 g/day for men and < 20 g/day for women but better to avoid alcohol consumption of any type or amount in individuals with NAFLD [105].

Omega-3 fatty acid supplementation reduces hepatic steatosis and improves serum gamma-glutamyltransferase, triglyceride, and high-density lipoprotein in patients with NAFLD; therefore, omega-3 fatty acid supplementation may be a new treatment option for NAFLD [106, 107]. But according to AASLD guideline (2018), omega-3 fatty acid should not be used as a specific treatment of NAFLD or NASH, but it can be used to treat hypertriglyceridemia in NAFLD patients [5].

Physical exercise: Both moderate and vigorous aerobic exercise (e.g., brisk walking, stationery cycling) and resistance training (150–200 min/week in 3–5 sessions) is effective to reduce hepatic steatosis by reducing weight , and choice of exercise should be based on patients' preference [108]. In general, 5 to 10% reduction in body weight in obese or overweight people over 6 to 12 months has been advocated through diet modification and physical exercise.

At least 3–5% of body weight loss is necessary to improve hepatic steatosis, but > 7% weight loss is required for histological improvement in NASH and fibrosis [5].

Therefore, the first line intervention in the management of NAFLD is lifestyle modification which includes (1) at least 7–10% weight loss by a combination of low-calorie diet with discourage of high fructose and saturated fat in foods. Diet with omega-3 fatty acid supplement may be advised, and (2) moderate to vigorous physical activity.

B. Pharmacotherapy: Only few drugs are recommended in the treatment of biopsy-proven NASH and fibrosis stage ≥ 2 or Fibroscan value > 10.51.

Pioglitazone: It is a peroxisome proliferator-activated receptor (PPAR) gamma agonist which improves histological features in biopsy-proven NASH patients with and without type 2 diabetes mellitus. Fifteen to thirty milligrams daily dose of Pioglitazone is recommended in the above indication. The optimal duration of therapy is unknown, but according to EASL guideline [107], treatment should be stopped if there is no reduction in aminotransferases after 6 months of therapy, and in patients with normal ALT at baseline, no recommendations can be made. Bone loss in women and weight gain are common side effect associated with use of Pioglitazone. Bladder cancer has been a concern during use of Pioglitazone, but another study found that there is no statistically significant association between use of Pioglitazone and risk of bladder cancer [109].

Vitamin E: It is superior to placebo for the treatment of NASH in adults without diabetes, and compared with placebo, vitamin E use is associated with significantly higher rate of improvement in non-alcoholic steatohepatitis (43% vs. 19%). It reduces hepatic steatosis and lobular inflammation, but no improvement in hepatic fibrosis scores [110]. According to AASLD and NICE guidelines, vitamin E may be considered at a dose of 800 IU/day in nondiabetic adults with biopsy-proven NASH [5]. But according to Asia-Pacific guideline, vitamin E therapy is not beneficial for NASH management [111].

Saroglitazar: Saroglitazar (dual PPAR α/γ agonist) at a dose of 4 mg improves ALT value and fatty liver (evaluated by transient elastography) in patients with NALFD and diabetic dyslipidemia [112]. Saroglitazar can be a potential therapeutic option for the management of metabolic syndrome associated NAFLD and NASH [113]. Another study from India with 12 months follow-up showed that Saroglitazar is safe and effective in management of NAFLD patients and is a potential option in the future [114]. But it needs further exploration before recommendation.

Liraglutide: It is a glucagon-like peptide-1 (GLP-1) analog which is safe, well tolerated, and associated with histological improvement of non-alcoholic steatohepatitis with 1.8 mg subcutaneous injections daily [115]. Most common side effects are diarrhea, constipation, and loss of appetite. However, it needs large studies for further evaluation for recommendation for the treatment of NAFLD.

Ursodeoxycholic acid (UDCA): Histological activities of NASH are not improved by using UDCA (13–15 mg/kg/day) alone, but improvements are seen when combination of vitamin E and UDCA is given [116]. High-dose UDCA (23–28 mg/kg/day) also fails to improve the overall histology in patients with NASH [117]. According to NICE, EASL, Asia-pacific, and AASLD guidelines, UDCA is not recommended for treatment of NAFLD, NASH, or hepatic fibrosis however few recent articles showed positive results [118, 119]. Parikh et al. in their study indicated that UDCA is an effective and safe alternative to vitamin E in non-diabetic–non-cirrhotic Indian NAFLD patients [118]. Another systemic review recommended UDCA as a frontline therapeutic option for NASH, thereby preventing its progression to cirrhosis and liver cancer [119].

Obeticholic acid: This synthetic farnesoid X receptor agonist at a dose of 25 mg daily is associated with histological improvement of NASH [120, 121]. Obeticholic acid might become the first approved pharmacotherapy for NASH fibrosis after result of recent multicentre, randomized, placebo-controlled phase 3 trial done by Younossi et al. [122]. For long-term safety and tolerability, it requires further studies, as obeticholic acid can increase low density lipoprotein level and pruritus is also extremely common with high dose of obeticholic acid.

Statin and n-3 polyunsaturated fatty acids: There are no data to support their use specifically for NASH.

SGLT-2 inhibitors: These drugs improve the serum liver enzymes value and reduce hepatic steatosis and fibrosis in type 2 diabetes patients with NAFLD [123]. Therefore use of SGLT2-inhibitors in type 2 diabetes patients with NAFLD is promising. Further researches are required to progress in this evolving field.

Others emerging drugs for management of NAFLD:

Elafibranor: It is a peroxisome proliferator-activated receptor-α and peroxisome proliferator-activated receptor-δ agonist and improves insulin sensitivity, glucose homeostasis, and lipid metabolism, and reduces inflammation. Ratziu et al. in their study showed that elafibranor (120 mg/day for 1 year) resolved NASH without fibrosis worsening [124]. It has an effect on the resolution on NASH and improvises two key drivers of NASH progression—insulin resistance and serum lipid normalization [125]. It induces nuclear factor-κB results in inhibition of inflammatory genes and decreases the expression of acute-phase response genes [126]. It causes reversible elevation of serum creatinine level; therefore, its use is potentially limiting in patients with concurrent renal disease. Common side effects are congestive heart failure, peripheral edema, bone fractures, and weight gain.

Lanifibranor (IVA337): It is a pan-peroxisome proliferator-activated receptor (PPAR) agonist with moderate and well-balanced activity on the three PPAR isoforms (α, γ, δ). It inhibits proliferation and activation of hepatic stellate cells which are the key cells driving liver fibrogenesis in NASH. It improves liver histology by decreasing liver steatosis, inflammation, and ballooning. Wettstein et al. in their study indicated that lanifibranor has therapeutic potential in the treatment of NASH [127].

Solithromycin: Solithromycin is a highly potent macrolide antibiotic. A clinical trial is going on (NCT02510599) which showed that there is reduction of NAFLD activity score and ALT level after 90 days treatment with Solithromycin in patients with NASH by targeting intestinal microbiomes and metabolic endotoxemia.

Cenicrivoric: Cenicriviroc is a CCR (C—C chemokine receptor) 2 and CCR5 dual antagonist which is playing an important role in macrophage recruitment and polarization in NASH pathogenesis. One phase 2 trial (2018) showed that there was improvement in fibrosis and no worsening of steatohepatitis compared with placebo [128]. Therefore, the drug is now in phase 3.

Selonsertib: It is an apoptosis signal-regulating kinase 1 (ASK1, involved in response to various stresses) inhibitor. Loomba et al. in their phase 2 trial described that selonsertib may reduce liver fibrosis in patients with non-alcoholic steatohepatitis and stage 2–3 fibrosis [129]. Now this drug is in phase 3 trial.

Emricasan: It is an oral pan-caspase inhibitor. Lipotoxicity leading to excessive caspase-mediated apoptosis and inflammation is responsible of liver damage in NAFLD. Shiffman et al. in their study showed that emricasan (25 mg twice daily) decreases ALT and biomarkers in NAFLD patients after 28 days of treatment [130].

C. Management of underlying diseases: Along with above treatment, underlying causes of NAFLD should be treated adequately like management of each component of metabolic syndrome if present.

Conclusion

Though liver biopsy is the gold standard test to detect NAFLD and to identify different stages of hepatic steatosis and fibrosis, multiple non-invasive tests are also available nowadays. Few of them are FDA approved and others' diagnostic tests need further evaluation before recommendation in clinical practice. The NAFLD fibrosis score, transient elastography are recommended to assess hepatic fibrosis and disease activity [5] however for diagnosis of NASH, liver biopsy is required due to lack of availability of serum cytokeratine 19 fragments test in clinical practice. Further studies are required to find out cutoff values and role of non-invasive markers and tests for NAFLD before giving approval. Liver biopsy should be considered in the following conditions: (1) when a competing etiology of chronic liver disease cannot be excluded just by non-invasive methods, (2) suspect of NAFLD-related advanced liver disease. Treatment of NAFLD can be divided into lifestyle modification (including diet restriction, low calorie diet intake, physical exercise leading to weight loss), pharmacotherapy (restricted to NAFLD patients with NASH and fibrosis), and management of underlying causes of NAFLD. Early diagnosis and proper management are required to avoid longterm complications of NAFLD.

Abbreviations

NAFLD: Non-alcoholic fatty liver disease; LFT: Liver function test; USG: Ultrasonography; CAP: Controlled attenuation parameter; BMI: Body mass index; CT scan: Computed tomography; MRI: *Magnetic resonance* imaging; 1H-MRS: Hydrogen-1 MR spectroscopy; PDFF: Proton density fat fraction; 31P- MRS: Hepatic phosphorus-31 MRS; GGT: Gamma-glutamyltransferase; ALT: Alanine aminotransferase; AST: Aspartate aminotransferase; NLFS: NAFLD liver fat score; FLI: Fatty liver index; HSI: Hepatic steatosis index; T2DM: Type 2 diabetes mellitus; LAP: Lipid accumulation product; NAFL: Non-alcoholic fatty liver; NASH: Non-alcoholic steatohepatitis; CK: Serum cytokeratin; FGF21: Fibroblast growth factor 21; PPV: Positive predictive value; NPV: Negative predictive value; NDI: NASH diagnostic index; MS: Metabolic syndrome; NPI: NASH predictive index; HOMA: Homeostatic model assessment; 1H-MRS: Proton magnetic resonance; MRE: Magnetic resonance elastography; APRI: Aspartate aminotransferase/platelet ratio index; NFS: NAFLD fibrosis score; FI: Fibrosis index score; ELF: Enhanced liver fibrosis; ARFI: Acoustic radiation force impulse; SWE: Shear wave elastography; LS: Liver stiffness; MRE: Magnetic resonance elastography; UDCA: Ursodeoxycholic acid; SGLT-2 inhibitor: Sodium-glucose cotransporter-2 inhibitor; FDA: Food and Drug Administration

Acknowledgements

Not applicable.

Author's contributions

The author contributed in the interpretation of the study data, manuscript writing, and revising. The author read and approved the final manuscript.

Competing interests

The author declares that he has no competing interests.

References

1. Armstrong MJ, Houlihan DD, Bentham L et al (2012) Presence and severity of non-alcoholic fatty liver disease in a large prospective primary care cohort. J Hepatol 56:234–240
2. Farrell GC, Wong VW, Chitturi S (2013) NAFLD in Asia--as common and important as in the West. Nat Rev Gastroenterol Hepatol 10:307–318
3. Younossi ZM, Koenig AB, Abdelatif D et al (2016) Global epidemiology of nonalcoholic fatty liver disease-meta analytic assessment of prevalence, incidence, and outcomes. Hepatology 64:73–84
4. Singh SP, Nayak S, Swain M et al (2004) Prevalence of nonalcoholic fatty liver disease in coastal eastern India: a preliminary ultrasonographic survey. Indian J Gastroenterol. 25:76–79
5. Chalasani N, Younossi Z, Lavine JE et al (2018 Jan) The diagnosis and management of nonalcoholic fatty liver disease: practice guidance from the American Association for the Study of Liver Diseases. Hepatology. 67:328–357
6. Matteoni CA, Younossi ZM, Gramlich T et al (1999) Nonalcoholic fatty liver disease: a spectrum of clinical and pathological severity. Gastroenterology. 116:1413–1419
7. Brunt EM (2001) Nonalcoholic steatohepatitis: definition and pathology. Semin Liver Dis 21:3–16
8. Van Werven JR, Marsman HA, Nederveen AJ et al (2010) Assessment of hepatic steatosis in patients undergoing liver resection: comparison of US, CT, T1-weighted dual-echo MR imaging, and point-resolved 1H MR spectroscopy. Radiology 256:159–168
9. Joseph AE, Saverymuttu SH, al-Sam S, et al. Comparison of liver histology with ultrasonography in assessing diffuse parenchymal liver disease. Clin Radiol 1991; 43:26-31.
10. Dasarathy S, Dasarathy J, Khiyami A et al (2009) Validity of real time ultrasound in the diagnosis of hepatic steatosis: a prospective study. J Hepatol 51:1061–1067
11. Shiralkar K, Johnson S, Bluth EI, Marshall RH, Dornelles A, Gulotta PM (2015) Improved method for calculating hepatic steatosis using the hepatorenal index. *J Ultrasound Med.* 34:1051–1059
12. Ballestri S, Lonardo A, Romagnoli D et al (2012) Ultrasonographic fatty liver indicator, a novel score which rules out NASH and is correlated with metabolic parameters in NAFLD. Liver Int 32:1242–1252
13. Chan WK, Nik Mustapha NR, Mahadeva S (2014) Controlled attenuation parameter for the detection and quantification of hepatic steatosis in nonalcoholic fatty liver disease. J Gastroenterol Hepatol 29:1470–1476
14. Ahn JM, Paik YH, Min SY et al (2016) Relationship between controlled attenuation parameter and hepatic steatosis as assessed by ultrasound in alcoholic or nonalcoholic fatty liver disease. Gut Liver 10:295–302
15. Yen YH, Chen JF, Wu CK et al (2017) The correlation of controlled attenuation parameter results with ultrasound-identified steatosis in real-world clinical practice. J Formos Med Assoc. 116:852–861
16. Machado MV (2017) Controlled attenuation parameter as a noninvasive method to detect and quantify hepatic steatosis in chronic liver disease: what is the clinical relevance? GE Port J Gastroenterol. 24:157–160
17. Sasso M, Beaugrand M, Ledinghen V et al (2010) Controlled attenuation parameter (CAP): a novel VCTE (TM) guided ultrasonic attenuation measurement for the evaluation of hepatic steatosis: preliminary study and validation in a cohort of patients with chronic liver disease from various causes. Ultrasound Med Biol. 36:1825–1835
18. Liu K, Wong VW, Lau K et al (2017) Prognostic value of controlled attenuation parameter by transient elastography. Am J Gastroenterol 112: 1812–1823
19. Shin J, Kim MJ, Shin HJ et al (2019) Quick assessment with controlled attenuation parameter for hepatic steatosis in children based on MRI-PDFF as the gold standard. BMC Pediatr 19:112
20. Valls C, Iannacconne R, Alba E et al (2006) Fat in the liver: diagnosis and characterization. Eur Radiol. 16(10):2292e308
21. Kani KK, Moshiri M, Cuevas C et al (2012) Imaging patterns of hepatic steatosis on multidetector CT: pearls and pitfalls. *Clin Radiol.* 67(4):366–371
22. Lee SW, Park SH, Kim KW et al (2007) Unenhanced CT for assessment of macrovesicular hepatic steatosis in living liver donors: comparison of visual grading with liver attenuation index. Radiology 244:479–485
23. Lee SS, Park SH, Kim HJ et al (2010) Non-invasive assessment of hepatic steatosis: prospective comparison of the accuracy of imaging examinations. J Hepatol 52:579–585
24. Bley TA, Wieben O, François CJ et al (2010) Fat and water magnetic resonance imaging. J Magn Reson Imaging 31:4–18
25. Georgoff P, Thomasson D, Louie A et al (2012) Hydrogen-1 MR spectroscopy for measurement and diagnosis of hepatic steatosis. AJR Am J Roentgenol. 199:2–7

26. Paparo F, Cenderello G, Revelli M et al (2015) Diagnostic value of MRI proton density fat fraction for assessing liver steatosis in chronic viral C hepatitis. Biomed Res Int. 2015:758164
27. Sevastianova K, Hakkarainen A, Kotronen A et al (2010) Nonalcoholic fatty liver disease: detection of elevated nicotinamide adenine dinucleotide phosphate with in vivo 3.0-T 31P MR spectroscopy with proton decoupling. Radiology. 256(2):466–473
28. Al-Busafi SA, Ghali P, Wong P et al (2012) The utility of Xenon-133 liver scan in the diagnosis and management of nonalcoholic fatty liver disease. Can J Gastroenterol 26:155–159
29. Ruhl CE, Everhart JE (2009) Elevated serum alanine aminotransferase and gamma-glutamyltransferase and mortality in the United States population. Gastroenterology 136:477–485
30. Kotronen A, Peltonen M, Hakkarainen A et al (2009) Prediction of non-alcoholic fatty liver disease and liver fat using metabolic and genetic factors. Gastroenterology 137:865–872
31. Unalp-Arida A, Ruhl CE (2018) Liver fat scores predict liver disease mortality in the United States population. Aliment Pharmacol Ther. 48(9):1003–1016
32. Bedogni G, Bellentani S, Miglioli L et al (2006) The fatty liver index: a simple and accurate predictor of hepatic steatosis in the general population. BMC Gastroenterol. 6:33
33. Sviklāne L, Olmane E, Dzērve Z et al (2018) Fatty liver index and hepatic steatosis index for prediction of non-alcoholic fatty liver disease in type 1 diabetes. J Gastroenterol Hepatol 33:270–276
34. Bedogni G, Kahn HS, Bellentani S et al (2010) A simple index of lipid over accumulation is a good marker of liver steatosis. BMC Gastroenterol 10:98
35. Dai H, Wang W, Chen R et al (2017) Lipid accumulation product is a powerful tool to predict non-alcoholic fatty liver disease in Chinese adults. Nutr Metab (Lond) 14:49
36. Cheng YL, Wang YJ, Lan KH et al (2017) Fatty liver index and lipid accumulation product can predict metabolic syndrome in subjects without fatty liver disease. Gastroenterol Res Pract. 2017:9279836
37. Poynard T, Ratziu V, Naveau S et al (2005) The diagnostic value of biomarkers (SteatoTest) for the prediction of liver steatosis. Comp Hepatol. 4:10
38. Zhou YJ, Zhou YF, Zheng JN et al (2017) NAFL screening score: a basic score identifying ultrasound-diagnosed non-alcoholic fatty liver. Clin Chim Acta 475:44–50
39. Machado MV, Cortez-Pinto H (2013) Non-invasive diagnosis of non-alcoholic fatty liver disease. A critical appraisal. J Hepatol. 58:1007–1019
40. Maher MM, Ibrahim WA, Saleh SA et al (2014) Cytokeratin 18 as a non invasive marker in diagnosis of NASH and its usefulness in correlation with disease severity in Egyptian patients. Egypt j med hum Genet 16:41–46
41. Aida Y, Abe H, Tomita Y et al (2014) Serum cytokeratin 18 fragment level as a noninvasive biomarker for non-alcoholic fatty liver disease. Int J Clin Exp Med 7:4191–4198
42. Verma S, Jensen D, Hart J et al (2013) Predictive value of ALT levels for non-alcoholic steatohepatitis (NASH) and advanced fibrosis in nonalcoholic fatty liver disease (NAFLD). Liver Int 33:1398–1405
43. Mofrad P, Contos MJ, Haque M et al (2003) Clinical and histologic spectrum of nonalcoholic fatty liver disease associated with normal ALT values. Hepatology. 37:1286–1292
44. Bechmann LP, Kocabayoglu P, Sowa JP et al (2013) Free fatty acids repress small heterodimer partner (SHP) activation and adiponectin counteracts bile acid-induced liver injury in superobese patients with nonalcoholic steatohepatitis. Hepatology. 57:1394–1406
45. Barb D, Bril F, Kalavalapalli S et al (2019) Plasma fibroblast growth factor 21 is associated with severity of nonalcoholic steatohepatitis in patients with obesity and type 2 diabetes. J Clin Endocrinol Metab. 104:3327–3336
46. Shen J, Chan HL, Wong GL et al (2012) Non-invasive diagnosis of non-alcoholic steatohepatitis by combined serum biomarkers. J Hepatol 56:1363–1370
47. Paquette M, Gauthier D, Chamberland A et al (2020) Circulating PCSK9 is associated with liver biomarkers and hepatic steatosis. Clin Biochem. 77:20–25
48. Ruscica M, Ferri N, Macchi C et al (2016) Liver fat accumulation is associated with circulating PCSK9. Ann Med. 48(5):384–391
49. Yoneda M, Uchiyama T, Kato S et al (2008) Plasma pentraxin3 is a novel marker for nonalcoholic steatohepatitis (NASH). BMC Gastroenterol. 8:53
50. Casoinic F, Sampelean D, Buzoianu AD et al (2016) Serum levels of oxidative stress markers in patients with type 2 diabetes mellitus and non-alcoholic steatohepatitis. Rom J Intern Med. 54(4):228–236
51. Tilg H, Moschen AR, Roden M (2017) NAFLD and diabetes mellitus. Nat Rev Gastroenterol Hepatol. 14(1):32–42
52. Jamali R, Arj A, Razavizade M, Aarabi MH (2016) Prediction of nonalcoholic fatty liver disease via a novel panel of serum adipokines. Medicine (Baltimore). 95(5):e2630
53. Yoneda M, Mawatari H, Fujita K et al (2007) High-sensitivity C-reactive protein is an independent clinical feature of nonalcoholic steatohepatitis (NASH) and also of the severity of fibrosis in NASH. J Gastroenterol. 42(7):573–582
54. Poynard T, Ratziu V, Charlotte F et al (2006) Diagnostic value of biochemical markers (NashTest) for the prediction of non alcoholo steato hepatitis in patients with non-alcoholic fatty liver disease. BMC Gastroenterol 6:34
55. Zhou Y, Orešič M, Leivonen M et al (2016) Noninvasive detection of nonalcoholic steatohepatitis using clinical markers and circulating levels of lipids and metabolites. Clin Gastroenterol Hepatol 14:1463–1472
56. Mauss S, Berg T, Rockstroh J et al (2018) Hepatology – a clinical textbook, 3rd edn, Germany
57. Younossi ZM, Otgonsuren M, Hunt S et al (2013) Development and validation of Nash diagnostic index as a non-invasive model for diagnosing non-alcoholic steatohepatitis (Nash). J Hepatol 58:S409–S566
58. Anty R, Iannelli A, Patouraux S et al (2010) A new composite model including metabolic syndrome, alanine aminotransferase and cytokeratin-18 for the diagnosis of non-alcoholic steatohepatitis in morbidly obese patients. Aliment Pharmacol Ther. 32:1315–1322
59. Palekar NA, Naus R, Larson SP et al (2006) Clinical model for distinguishing non-alcoholic steatohepatitis from simple steatosis in patients with non-alcoholic fatty liver disease. Liver Int. 26:151–156
60. Sumida Y, Yoneda M, Hyogo H et al (2011) A simple clinical scoring system using ferritin, fasting insulin, and type IV collagen 7S for predicting steatohepatitis in nonalcoholic fatty liver disease. J Gastroenterol 46:257–268
61. Zein CO, Edmlson JM, Schluchter M, et al. A NASH predictive index (NPI) for use in patients with nonalcoholic fatty liver disease [abstract] Hepatology. 2007; 46:747A.
62. Gholam PM, Flancbaum L, Machan JT et al (2007) Nonalcoholic fatty liver disease in severely obese subjects. Am J Gastroenterol 102:399–408
63. Alkhouri N, Berk M, Yerian L et al (2014) OxNASH score correlates with histologic features and severity of nonalcoholic fatty liver disease. Digestive diseases and sciences. 59:1617–1624
64. Chunming L, Jianhui S, Hongguang Z et al (2015) The development of a clinical score for the prediction of nonalcoholic steatohepatitis in patients with nonalcoholic fatty liver disease using routine parameters. Turk J Gastroenterol 26:408–416
65. Hyysalo J, Mannisto VT, Zhou Y et al (2014) A population based study on the prevalence of NASH using scores validated against liver histology. J Hepatol 60:839–846
66. Verdam FJ, Dallinga JW, Driessen A et al (2013) Nonalcoholic steatohepatitis: a non-invasive diagnosis by analysis of exhaled breath. Journal of hepatology. 58:543–548
67. Kim TH, Jeong CW, Jun HY et al (2019) Accuracy of proton magnetic resonance for diagnosing non-alcoholic steatohepatitis: a meta-analysis. Scientific Reports 9:15002
68. Chen J, Talwalkar JA, Yin M et al (2011) Early detection of non-alcoholic steatohepatitis in patients with non-alcoholic fatty liver disease by using MR elastography. Radiology. 259:749–756
69. Lin ZH, Xin YN, Dong QJ et al (2011) Performance of the aspartate aminotransferase-to-platelet ratio index for the staging of hepatitis C-related fibrosis: an updated meta-analysis. Hepatology. 53:726–736
70. Vallet-Pichard A, Mallet V, Nalpas B et al (2007) FIB-4: An inexpensive and accurate marker of fibrosis in HCV infection. Comparison with liver biopsy and fibrotest. *Hepatology.* 46:32–36
71. Harrison SA, Oliver D, Arnold HL et al (2008) Development and validation of a simple NAFLD clinical scoring system for identifying patients without advanced disease. Gut. 57:1441–1447
72. Angulo P, Hui JM, Marchesini G et al (2007) The NAFLD fibrosis score: a noninvasive system that identifies liver fibrosis in patients with NAFLD. Hepatology. 45:846–854
73. Cross TJ, Rizzi P, Berry PA et al (2009) King's score: an accurate marker of cirrhosis in chronic hepatitis C. *Eur J Gastroenterol Hepatol.* 21:730–738
74. Ohta T, Sakaguchi K, Fujiwara A et al (2006) Simple surrogate index of the fibrosis stage in chronic hepatitis C patients using platelet count and serum albumin level. *Acta Med Okayama.* 60:77–84
75. Cao W, Zhao C, Shen C et al (2013) Cytokeratin 18, alanine aminotransferase, platelets and triglycerides predict the presence of nonalcoholic steatohepatitis. PLoS One. 8:e82092

76. Alboraie M, Khairy M, Elsharkawy A et al (2014) Egy-Score as a noninvasive score for the assessment of hepatic fibrosis in chronic hepatitis C: a preliminary approach. Saudi J Gastroenterol. 20:170–174
77. Lichtinghagen R, Pietsch D, Bantel H et al (2013) The enhanced liver fibrosis (ELF) score: normal values, influence factors and proposed cut-off values. J Hepatol 59:236–242
78. Ratziu V, Massard J, Charlotte F et al (2006) Diagnostic value of biochemical markers (FibroTest-FibroSURE) for the prediction of liver fibrosis in patients with non-alcoholic fatty liver disease. BMC Gastroenterol. 6:6
79. Koda M, Matunaga Y, Kawakami M et al (2007) FibroIndex, a practical index for predicting significant fibrosis in patients with chronic hepatitis C. Hepatology. 45:297–306
80. Becker L, Salameh W, Sferruzza A et al (2009) Validation of hepascore, compared with simple indices of fibrosis, in patients with chronic hepatitis C virus infection in United States. Clin Gastroenterol Hepatol. 7:696–701
81. Forns X, Ampurdanès S, Llovet JM et al (2002) Identification of chronic hepatitis C patients without hepatic fibrosis by a simple predictive model. Hepatology. 36:986–992
82. Patel K, Gordon SC, Jacobson I et al (2004) Evaluation of a panel of non-invasive serum markers to differentiate mild from moderate-to-advanced liver fibrosis in chronic hepatitis C patients. J Hepatol. 41:935–942
83. Petta S, Wong VW, Camma C et al (2017) Serial combination of non-invasive tools improves the diagnostic accuracy of severe liver fibrosis in patients with NAFLD. Aliment Pharmacol Ther 46:617–627
84. Castera L, Vergniol J, Foucher J et al (2005) Prospective comparison of transient elastography, Fibrotest, APRI, and liver biopsy for the assessment of fibrosis in chronic hepatitis C. Gastroenterology. 128:343–350
85. Palmeri ML, Wang MH, Rouze NC et al (2011) Noninvasive evaluation of hepatic fibrosis using acoustic radiation force-based shear stiffness in patients with nonalcoholic fatty liver disease. J Hepatol. 55:666–672
86. Joo SK, Kim W, Kim D et al (2018) Steatosis severity affects the diagnostic performances of noninvasive fibrosis tests in nonalcoholic fatty liver disease. Liver Int 38:331–341
87. Frulio N, Trillaud H (2013) Ultrasound elastography in liver. Diagn Interv Imaging. 94:515–534
88. Lemoine M, Shimakawa Y, Njie R et al (2014) Food intake increases liver stiffness measurements and hampers reliable values in patients with chronic hepatitis B and healthy controls: the PROLIFICA experience in The Gambia. Aliment Pharmacol Ther. 39:188–196
89. Mederacke I, Wursthorn K, Kirschner J et al (2009) Food intake increases liver stiffness in patients with chronic or resolved hepatitis C virus infection. Liver Int. 29:1500–1506
90. Herrmann E, de Lédinghen V, Cassinotto C et al (2018) Assessment of biopsy-proven liver fibrosis by two-dimensional shear wave elastography: an individual patient data-based meta-analysis. Hepatology. 67:260–272
91. Takeuchi H, Sugimoto K, Oshiro H et al (2018) Liver fibrosis: noninvasive assessment using supersonic shear imaging and FIB4 index in patients with non-alcoholic fatty liver disease. J Med Ultrason 45:243–249
92. Wang QB, Zhu H, Liu HL et al (2012) Performance of magnetic resonance elastography and diffusion-weighted imaging for the staging of hepatic fibrosis: a meta-analysis. Hepatology. 56:239–247
93. Loomba R, Wolfson T, Ang B et al (2014) Magnetic resonance elastography predicts advanced fibrosis in patients with nonalcoholic fatty liver disease: a prospective study. Hepatology. 60:1920–1928
94. Mayo R, Crespo J, Martínez-Arranz I et al (2018) Metabolomic-based noninvasive serum test to diagnose nonalcoholic steatohepatitis: results from discovery and validation cohorts. Hepatol Commun. 2(7):807–820
95. Bell LN, Theodorakis JL, Vuppalanchi R et al (2010) Serum proteomics and biomarker discovery across the spectrum of nonalcoholic fatty liver disease. Hepatology. 51(1):111–120
96. Hou W, Janech MG, Sobolesky PM,et al. Proteomic screening of plasma identifies potential noninvasive biomarkers associated with significant/ advanced fibrosis in patients with nonalcoholic fatty liver disease. *Biosci Rep.* 2020; 40 (1): BSR20190395
97. Loomba R, Seguritan V, Li W, et al. Gut microbiome-based metagenomic signature for non-invasive detection of advanced fibrosis in human nonalcoholic fatty liver disease. Cell Metab. 2017; 25(5):1054-1062.e5.
98. National Institute for Health and Care Excellence (UK). Non alcoholic fatty liver disease: assessment and management. Available from: URL: http// www.niceorg.uk\guidance\ng49
99. Paul J, Venugopal RV, Peter L et al (2018) Effects of lifestyle modification on liver enzyme and Fibroscan in Indian patients with non-alcoholic fatty liver disease. Gastroenterol Rep (Oxf). 6:49–53
100. Saab S, Mallam D (2014) Cox 2nd GA, et al. Impact of coffee on liver diseases: a systematic review. Liver Int 34:495–504
101. Setiawan VW, Porcel J, Wei P et al (2017) Coffee drinking and alcoholic and nonalcoholic fatty liver diseases and viral hepatitis in the multiethnic cohort. Clin Gastroenterol Hepatol. 15(8):1305–1307
102. Salomone F, Galvano F, Li VG (2017) Molecular bases underlying the hepatoprotective effects of coffee. Nutrients. 9(1):85
103. Jegatheesan P, De Bandt JP (2017) Fructose and NAFLD: the multifaceted aspects of fructose metabolism. Nutrients. 9:230
104. Vos MB, Lavine JE (2013) Dietary fructose in nonalcoholic fatty liver disease. Hepatology 57:2525–2531
105. Liangpunsakul S, Chalasani N (2012) What should we recommend to our patients with NAFLD regarding alcohol use? Am J Gastroenterol 107:976–978
106. Wenxia Lu, Sainan Li, Jingjing Li, et al. Effects of omega-3 fatty acid in nonalcoholic fatty liver disease: a meta-analysis. Gastroenterol Res Pract 2016; 2016: 1459790.
107. Yan JH, Guan BJ, Gao HY et al (2018) Omega-3 polyunsaturated fatty acid supplementation and non-alcoholic fatty liver disease: a meta-analysis of randomized controlled trials. Medicine (Baltimore). 97(37):e12271
108. Marchesini G, Day CP, Dufour JF et al (2016) EASL-EASD-EASO clinical practice guidelines for the management of non-alcoholic fatty liver disease. J Hepatol. 64:1388–1402
109. Lewis JD, Habel LA, Quesenberry CP et al (2015) Pioglitazone use and risk of bladder cancer and other common cancers in persons with diabetes. JAMA 314:265–277
110. Sanyal AJ, Chalasani N, Kowdley KV et al (2010) Pioglitazone, vitamin E, or placebo for nonalcoholic steatohepatitis. N Engl J Med. 362:1675–1685
111. Chitturi S, Wong VW, Chan WK et al (2018) The Asia-Pacific Working Party on Non-alcoholic Fatty Liver Disease guidelines 2017-part 2: management and special groups. J Gastroenterol Hepatol 33:86–98
112. Kaul U, Parmar D, Manjunath K et al (2019) New dual peroxisome proliferator activated receptor agonist—Saroglitazar in diabetic dyslipidemia and non-alcoholic fatty liver disease: integrated analysis of the real world evidence. Cardiovasc Diabetol 18:80. https://doi.org/10.1186/s12933-019-0884-3
113. Joshi S, Ruby S, Saboo B, et al. Saroglitazar in non-alcoholic fatty liver disease. The American Association of Clinical Endocrinologists Annual Meeting Abstracts. Late breaking abstracts; 2016, p. 331.
114. Dadhich SK. Efficacy and safety of Saroglitazar in nonalcoholic fatty liver disease patients at 1 year: an investigator initiated study. American College of Gastroenterology Annual Scientific Meeting Abstracts; 2019, p. 1541.
115. Armstrong MJ, Gaunt P, Aithal GP et al (2016) Liraglutide safety and efficacy in patients with non-alcoholic steatohepatitis (LEAN): a multicentre, double blind, randomised, placebo-controlled phase 2 study. Lancet 387:679–690
116. Dufour JF, Oneta CM, Gonvers JJ et al (2006) Randomized placebo-controlled trial of ursodeoxycholic acid with vitamin E in nonalcoholic steatohepatitis. Clin Gastroenterol Hepatol 4:1537–1543
117. Leuschner UF, Lindenthal B, Herrmann G et al (2010) High-dose ursodeoxycholic acid therapy for nonalcoholic steatohepatitis: a double-blind, randomized, placebo-controlled trial. Hepatology 52:472–479
118. Parikh P, Ingle M, Patel J et al (2016) An open-label randomized control study to compare the efficacy of vitamin e versus ursodeoxycholic acid in nondiabetic and noncirrhotic Indian NAFLD patients. Saudi J Gastroenterol 22(3):192–197
119. Mappala H (2019) IDDF2019-ABS-0251 The efficacy of ursodeoxycholic acid in the treatment of non-alcoholic steatohepatitis: a 15-year systematic review. Gut 68:A152
120. Neuschwander-Tetri BA, Loomba R, Sanyal AJ et al (2015) Farnesoid X nuclear receptor ligand obeticholic acid for non-cirrhotic, non-alcoholic steatohepatitis (FLINT): a multicentre, randomised, placebo-controlled trial. Lancet 385:956–965
121. Hindson J (2020) Obeticholic acid for the treatment of NASH. Nat Rev Gastroenterol Hepatol. 17(2):66
122. Younossi ZM, Ratziu V, Loomba R et al (2019) Obeticholic acid for the treatment of non-alcoholic steatohepatitis: interim analysis from a multicentre, randomised, placebo-controlled phase 3 trial. Lancet. 394(10215):2184–2196

123. Raj H, Durgia H, Palui R et al (2019) SGLT-2 inhibitors in non-alcoholic fatty liver disease patients with type 2 diabetes mellitus: a systematic review. World J Diabetes 10:114–132
124. Ratziu V, Harrison SA, Francque S et al (2016) Elafibranor, an agonist of the peroxisome proliferator-activated receptor-α and -δ, induces resolution of nonalcoholic steatohepatitis without fibrosis worsening. Gastroenterology. 150(5):1147–1159
125. Westerouen Van Meeteren MJ, Drenth JPH, Tjwa ETTL (2020) Elafibranor: a potential drug for the treatment of nonalcoholic steatohepatitis (NASH). Expert Opin Investig Drugs. 29(2):117–123
126. Pawlak M, Lefebvre P, Staels B (2015) Molecular mechanism of PPARα action and its impact on lipid metabolism, inflammation and fibrosis in non-alcoholic fatty liver disease. J Hepatol. 62(3):720–733
127. Wettstein G, Luccarini JM, Poekes L et al (2017) The new-generation pan-peroxisome proliferator-activated receptor agonist IVA337 protects the liver from metabolic disorders and fibrosis. Hepatol Commun. 1(6):524–537
128. Friedman SL, Ratziu V, Harrison SA et al (2018) A randomized, placebo-controlled trial of cenicriviroc for treatment of nonalcoholic steatohepatitis with fibrosis. *Hepatology*. 67(5):1754–1767
129. Loomba R, Lawitz E, Mantry PS et al (2018) The ASK1 inhibitor selonsertib in patients with nonalcoholic steatohepatitis: a randomized, phase 2 trial. Hepatology. 67(2):549–559
130. Shiffman M, Freilich B, Vuppalanchi R et al (2019) Randomised clinical trial: emricasan versus placebo significantly decreases ALT and caspase 3/7 activation in subjects with non-alcoholic fatty liver disease. Aliment Pharmacol Ther. 49(1):64–73

13

Association of vitamin D supplementation with serum leptin and metabolic parameters in Egyptian patients with non-alcoholic steatohepatitis: a prospective study

Hany Haroun Kaisar* and Ahmed Samir Abo Halima

Abstract

Background: Nonalcoholic steatohepatitis (NASH) is the progressive form of NAFLD, a common cause of liver disease, with increased chance of progression to liver fibrosis, cirrhosis, and hepatocellular carcinoma. Circulating leptin is increased in patients with NASH. It is an independent positive predictor of the severity of hepatic steatosis. Vitamin D is a lipophilic molecule essential to maintain calcium and phosphate balance. Moreover, it has antifibrotic, antiproliferative, and anti-inflammatory effects on the liver. Vitamin D deficiency is a worldwide condition and very common in patients with NASH. Low serum vitamin D has been shown to predispose to intrahepatic lipid accumulation leading to NAFLD. The aim of this study was to investigate the association of vitamin D supplementation with serum leptin and metabolic parameters in Egyptian patients with non-alcoholic steatohepatitis

Results: Patients with NASH group had statistically significant higher values of diastolic blood pressure (94.3 ± 11.9 mmHg, $p < 0.0001$), glycated hemoglobin (8.0 ± 2.4%, $p < 0.0001$), fasting blood sugar (165.6 ± 62.0 mg/dL, $p < 0.0001$), fasting insulin level (24.2 ± 3.0 μU/ml, $p < 0.0001$), homeostatic model assessment of insulin resistance (HOMA-IR) (1.8 ± 0.7, $p < 0.0001$), alanine transferase (ALT) (78.2 ± 36.7 U/L, $p < 0.0001$), aspartate transferase (AST) (108.6 ± 85.6 U/L, $p < 0.0001$), NAFLD fibrosis score (− 0.78 ± 0.9, $p < 0.0001$), total cholesterol (233.0 ± 40.9 mg/dL, $p = 0.0011$), low-density lipoprotein (117.5 ± 41.6 mg/dL, $p = 0.0084$), and triglycerides (229.7 ± 62.1 mg/dL, $p < 0.0001$) than the control group. Moreover, they had lower serum vitamin D level (15.6 ± 6.6 ng/ml, $p = 0.0004$) and higher serum leptin level (35.9 ± 28.4 ng/ml, $p < 0.0001$) than the control group. Following vitamin D supplementation, there was a statistically significant reduction in HbA1c (6.8 ± 1.3%, $p = 0.0055$), fasting blood sugar (136.1 ± 32.7 mg/dL, $p = 0.0094$), fasting insulin level (22.9 ± 1.8 μU/ml, $p = 0.0236$), HOMA-IR (1.4 ± 0.4, $p = 0.0026$), ALT (55.3 ± 21.3 U/L, $p = 0.0010$), AST (73.1 ± 54.2 U/L, $p = 0.0297$), and triglycerides (203.6 ± 49.8 mg/dL, $p = 0.0415$) in patients with NASH. There was a statistically significant increase in serum vitamin D level (33.0 ± 7.6 ng/ml, $p < 0.0001$) and decrease in serum leptin level (23.5 ± 12.9 ng/ml, $p = 0.0140$) after treatment.

(Continued on next page)

* Correspondence: dr_hanyharoun@yahoo.com
Gastroenterology and Hepatology Department, Faculty of Medicine, Ain Shams University, Cairo 11211, Egypt

(Continued from previous page)

Conclusions: Vitamin D supplementation in patients with NASH in a dose of 4000 IU/day for 12 weeks improves severity of hepatic inflammation, decreases insulin resistance, improves glycemic control, corrects dyslipidemia, and protects against lipotoxicity by inhibition of serum leptin.

Keywords: Vitamin D, Nonalcoholic fatty liver disease, Nonalcoholic steatohepatitis, Leptin

Background

Nonalcoholic fatty liver disease (NAFLD) is considered as the most common cause of liver disease [1]. It is a condition histologically characterized by macrovesicular hepatic steatosis in individuals who do not consume alcohol in amounts generally considered to be harmful to the liver [2]. It is a broad term consisting of patients with simple steatosis or nonalcoholic fatty liver (NAFL) at one end of the spectrum, nonalcoholic steatohepatitis (NASH), NASH-related cirrhosis, and hepatocellular carcinoma (HCC) at the other end [3].

NAFLD is reported to be associated with other systemic diseases, such as cardiovascular diseases, insulin resistance (IR), obesity, dyslipidemia, and metabolic syndrome (MS) [4]. The prevalence of NAFLD is increasing and has been estimated to be between 10 and 30% worldwide [5].

Nonalcoholic steatohepatitis (NASH) is the progressive form of NAFLD characterized by lobular inflammation, hepatocyte degeneration, and ballooning, under the condition of macrovesicular hepatic steatosis. The danger of this specific form of NAFLD is expressed by its increased chance of progressing to liver fibrosis, cirrhosis, and hepatocellular carcinoma [6].

Leptin is a 167-amino acid protein produced by adipocytes in the hypothalamus [7]. Leptin is proportionally released to the amount of fat stored in the white adipose tissue and acts in hypothalamic suppression of food intake and increase in energy expenditure [8]. Circulating leptin is increased in both men and women with NASH. Serum leptin is an independent positive predictor of the severity of hepatic steatosis [9].

Vitamin D is a lipophilic molecule essential to maintain calcium and phosphate balance and osteometabolic system regulation [10]. Vitamin D also has antifibrotic, antiproliferative, and anti-inflammatory effects on the liver [11].

Vitamin D deficiency is also a worldwide condition and is present in approximately 30–60% of the general adult population [12]. Vitamin D-deficient individuals are more likely to develop alterations in glucose metabolism, such as impaired glucose tolerance, metabolic syndrome (MS), and type 2 diabetes mellitus (DM) [13]. Vitamin D levels have been reported to be inversely related with fasting glucose concentrations [14], adiposity [15], and blood pressure [16]. Low serum vitamin D has been shown to predispose to intrahepatic lipid accumulation leading to NAFLD as vitamin D is capable of reducing free fatty acid (FFA)-induced insulin resistance (IR) both in peripheral tissues and in hepatocytes [17].

Because NAFLD and vitamin D deficiency have similar risks for cardiovascular disease, insulin resistance, and metabolic syndrome in epidemiologic studies, there have been many reports debating a potential association between NAFLD and vitamin D deficiency [18].

Vitamin D substitution thus may represent a simple, cheap, and almost side effect-free approach to reduce the burden of end-stage liver failure and liver cancer in NASH as medical interventions with proven long-term efficacy are still lacking [19]. Vitamin D may influence hepatocytes and non-parenchymal hepatic cells (hepatic stellate cells, Kupffer cells) in NASH via metabolic, anti-inflammatory, and anti-fibrotic effects [20]. Several inflammatory cytokines, such as interleukin-6 (IL-6), tumor necrosis factor alpha (TNF-α), and IL-1β, and adipokines, such as adiponectin and leptin, may participate in these reactions [21].

The aim of this study was to investigate the association of vitamin D supplementation with serum leptin and metabolic parameters in Egyptian patients with nonalcoholic steatohepatitis.

Methods

This study was carried out in the Hepatology and Gastroenterology Department, Faculty of Medicine, Ain Shams University. The study included 40 patients with NASH referred to the hepatology clinic during the period between January 2019 and June 2019 in addition to 40 age- and sex-matched healthy individuals which were taken as the control group. All participants agreed to the study conditions and provided a written informed consent before enrollment in this study.

Inclusion criteria for patients with NASH included age more than 16 years, either total abstainers or consumption of less than 20 gm of alcohol per day, ultrasound showing features of steatosis, raised serum ALT level more than 40 IU/L for at least 6 months before enrollment in the study, negative viral markers (hepatitis B surface antigen and anti-hepatitis C virus), negative autoimmune markers (antinuclear antibody, anti-smooth muscle antibody, and antimitochondrial antibody), normal ceruloplasmin level, and normal iron workup (serum iron, total iron-binding capacity, ferritin, and transferrin saturation).

Exclusion criteria included pregnant females, patients with history of drug intake likely to cause NASH (e.g., corticosteroids, hormone replacement therapy, and non-steroidal anti-inflammatory drugs (NSAIDs)), patients with history of gastric bypass or extensive small bowel resection, and those with clinical, laboratory, and imaging features of acute hepatitis or liver cirrhosis. Moreover, patients with renal, respiratory, or cardiac failure and those who took vitamin D supplementation within 3 months prior to enrollment were excluded from the study.

All individuals participating in the study were subjected to complete medical history, full clinical examination, measurement of body weight (kg), height (m), BMI (kg/m^2), pelvi-abdominal U/S, complete blood count (CBC), liver function tests (AST, ALT, total bilirubin, alkaline phosphatase, gamma glutamyl transferase, albumin), hepatitis markers (HBsAg and HCVAb), fasting blood sugar (mg/dl), fasting insulin level (mU/L), serum glycated Hb (HbA1c) (%), serum creatinine (mg/dl), complete lipid profile (cholesterol (mg/dl), triglycerides (mg/dl), LDL (mg/dl), and HDL (mg/dl), and homeostasis model assessment of insulin resistance (HOMA-IR) was calculated using the formula (fasting plasma insulin (mU/L) × fasting plasma glucose (mmol/L)/22.5) [21]; NAFLD fibrosis score was calculated using the formula (– 1.675 + 0.037 × age (year) + 0.094 × BMI (kg/m^2) + 1.13 × impaired fasting glucose (IFG)/diabetes (yes = 1, no = 0) + 0.99 × AST/ALT ratio – 0.013 × platelet (× 10^9/L) – 0.66 × albumin (g/dL) [22], serum level of vitamin D (25-hydroxyvitamin D) (ng/mL), and serum level of leptin (ng/ml).

Vitamin D (25-hydroxyvitamin D) was measured by radioimmunoassay (vitamin D total, Roche Diagnostics, Mannheim, German) according to the manufacturer's instructions. An electrochemiluminescence binding assay was performed using Elecsys immunoassay analyzers, with measurement ranging from 3.00 to 70.0 ng/mL. Vitamin D status was defined based on the traditional classifications of "deficient" (< 20 ng/mL), "insufficient" (20–30 ng/mL), and "sufficient" (> 30 ng/mL) [23].

Quantitative determination of serum human leptin was performed using AssayMax Human Leptin ELISA Kit supplied by Assaypro LLC (Catalog No. EL2001-1). The AssayMax Human Leptin ELISA (Enzyme-Linked Immunosorbent Assay) kit was designed for detection of human leptin in plasma, serum, and cell culture samples. This assay employed a quantitative sandwich enzyme immunoassay technique. The reference value in normal weight/control subjects was 0.7–5.3 ng/ml in males and 3.3–18.3 ng/ml in females.

Patients with NASH were given vitamin D_3 (cholecalciferol) supplements. The supplementation procedure for vitamin D_3 was set at a 4000 IU per day with main meal for 12 weeks. To examine the possible toxicity and hypervitaminosis that might arise from taking vitamin D supplements, serum concentrations of calcium at study baseline and end will be quantified. All anthropometric measurements, imaging studies, and laboratory blood tests were repeated after the end of treatment.

Statistical analysis

This is a prospective cohort study, where the researchers conceive and design the study, recruit subjects, and collect background data on all subjects before enrollment in the study. Data collection in this study was done using paper questionnaire and checklists in addition to physical examinations and observations during interviews with the subjects.

Data were collected, revised, coded, and entered into the statistical package for social science (IBM SPSS, version 20, Chicago, USA). Data was described as mean ± standard deviation for quantitative variables and as number and percentage for qualitative variables. The comparison between two independent groups with quantitative data and parametric distribution was carried out by using the independent t test. The probability of error (p) was expressed as follows: p value more than 0.05: nonsignificant, p value less than or equal to 0.05: significant, and p value less than 0.01: highly significant.

Results

Forty patients with NASH were enrolled in this study in addition to forty age- and sex-matched healthy individuals which were taken as control. The NASH group included 21 (52.5%) men and 19 (47.5%) women while the control group included 24 (60%) men and 16 (40%) women. The mean age was 35.2 ± 7.0 years in the NASH group and 34.3 ± 8.2 years in the control group (p = 0.5899). The demographic and characteristic data are listed in Table 1. The mean weight and BMI were 106.3 ± 15.6 kg and 35.7 ± 5.7 kg/m^2 in the NASH group and 82.2 ± 8.2 kg and 27.5 ± 2.5 kg/m^2 in the control group respectively with a high statistically significant difference between both groups ($p < 0.0001$).

Subjects in the NASH group had higher levels than the control group as regards the following parameters: mean value in the NASH group/control group, diastolic blood pressure (94.3 ± 11.9/79.3 ± 11.2 mmHg), HbA1c (8.0 ± 2.4/5.2 ± 0.6%), fasting blood sugar (165.6 ± 62.0/101.7 ± 22.9 mg/dL), fasting insulin level (24.2 ± 3.0/17.0 ± 2.3 μU/ml), HOMA-IR (1.8 ± 0.7/0.8 ± 0.2), ALT (78.2 ± 36.7/29.9 ± 8.3 U/L), AST (108.6 ± 85.6/25.5 ± 7.5 U/L), NAFLD fibrosis score (– 0.78 ± 0.9/– 3.0 ± 1.6), total cholesterol (233.0 ± 40.9/201.9 ± 41.53 mg/dL), LDL

Table 1 Demographic, laboratory, and metabolic parameters of patients with the NASH and control groups

Characteristics	NASH	Control	*t* value	*p* value	Significance
Age (years)	**35.2 ± 7.0**	**34.3 ± 8.2**	**0.5412**	**0.5899**	**NS**
Male	**21 (52.5%)**	**24 (60%)**			
Female	**19 (47.5%)**	**16 (40%)**			
Weight (kg)	**106.3 ± 15.6**	**82.2 ± 8.2**	**8.6455**	**< 0.0001**	**HS**
Height (meter)	**1.7 ± 0.08**	**1.7 ± 0.1**	**0.0156**	**0.9876**	**NS**
BMI (kg/m^2)	**35.7 ± 5.7**	**27.5 ± 2.5**	**8.3947**	**< 0.0001**	**HS**
DBP (mmHg)	**94.3 ± 11.9**	**79.3 ± 11.2**	**5.8312**	**< 0.0001**	**HS**
Hepatomegaly	**20 (50%)**	**2 (5%)**			
HbA1c (%)	**8.0 ± 2.4**	**5.2 ± 0.6**	**7.2677**	**< 0.0001**	**HS**
Hemoglobin (gm/dL)	**13.5 ± 1.5**	**13.2 ± 1.3**	**0.8487**	**0.3986**	**NS**
Platelet ($\times 10^3/\mu L$)	**288.5 ± 114.9**	**322.1 ± 118.7**	**1.2836**	**0.2031**	**NS**
FBS (mg/dL)	**165.6 ± 62.0**	**101.7 ± 22.9**	**6.1141**	**< 0.0001**	**HS**
Fasting insulin (μU/ml)	**24.2 ± 3.0**	**17.0 ± 2.3**	**12.1379**	**< 0.0001**	**HS**
HOMA-IR	**1.8 ± 0.7**	**0.8 ± 0.2**	**8.8731**	**< 0.0001**	**HS**
Creatinine (mg/dL)	**0.9 ± 0.2**	**0.9 ± 0.3**	**2.6252**	**0.8252**	**NS**
ALT (U/L)	**78.2 ± 36.7**	**29.9 ± 8.3**	**8.1260**	**< 0.0001**	**HS**
AST (U/L)	**108.6 ± 85.6**	**25.5 ± 7.5**	**6.1183**	**< 0.0001**	**HS**
Albumin (gm/dL)	**3.8 ± 0.8**	**4.6 ± 0.6**	**4.7217**	**< 0.0001**	**HS**
NAFLD fibrosis score	**− 0.78 ± 0.9**	**− 3.0 ± 1.6**	**7.8602**	**< 0.0001**	**HS**
TCHOL (mg/dL)	**233.0 ± 40.9**	**201.9 ± 41.53**	**3.3796**	**0.0011**	**HS**
LDL (mg/dL)	**117.5 ± 41.6**	**95.35 ± 31.1**	**2.7022**	**0.0084**	**HS**
HDL (mg/dL)	**48.5 ± 7.59**	**64.58 ± 8.2**	**9.1398**	**< 0.0001**	**HS**
Triglycerides (mg/dL)	**229.7 ± 62.1**	**142.9 ± 36.3**	**7.6224**	**< 0.0001**	**HS**
ALP (mg/dL)	**70.4 ± 7.3**	**58.2 ± 6.9**	**7.6925**	**< 0.0001**	**HS**
GGT (U/L)	**43.3 ± 24.5**	**25.1 ± 7.1**	**4.5140**	**< 0.0001**	**HS**
Total bilirubin (mg/dL)	**1.1 ± 0.4**	**1.1 ± 1.1**	**0.2240**	**0.8234**	**NS**
Vitamin D (ng/ml)	**15.6 ± 6.6**	**21.0 ± 6.5**	**3.7323**	**0.0004**	**HS**
Leptin (ng/ml)	**35.9 ± 28.4**	**10.1 ± 1.8**	**5.7407**	**< 0.0001**	**HS**

(117.5 ± 41.6/95.35 ± 31.1 mg/dL), triglycerides (229.7 ± 62.1/142.9 ± 36.3 mg/dL), alkaline phosphates (70.4 ± 7.3/58.2 ± 6.9 mg/dL), and gamma glutamyl transferase (43.3 ± 24.5/25.1 ± 7.1 U/L) with significant statistical difference between both groups ($p < 0.0001$).

Twenty patients (50%) in the NASH group had hepatomegaly by abdominal ultrasonography in comparison to two subjects (5%) in the control group. There was no significant difference between the two groups regarding serum hemoglobin concentration, platelet count, serum creatinine, and total bilirubin.

Serum albumin level and HDL were significantly higher ($p < 0.0001$) in the control group (4.6 ± 0.6 gm/dL, 64.58 ± 8.2 mg/dL respectively) than in patients with NASH (3.8 ± 0.8 gm/dL, 48.5 ± 7.59 mg/dL respectively).

There was a statistically significant difference ($p < 0.0001$) between both groups as regards serum level of vitamin D and serum leptin. Patients with NASH had lower serum vitamin D level (15.6 ± 6.6 ng/ml) and higher serum leptin level (35.9 ± 28.4 ng/ml) than the control group where the mean values of vitamin D and serum leptin were 21.0 ± 6.5 ng/ml and 10.1 ± 1.8 ng/ml respectively.

All patients with NASH were given vitamin D_3 supplements as tablets. Each tablet contained 1000 IU vitamin D_3 (cholecalciferol). Every patient took 4 tablets (4000 IU) every day with main meal for 12 weeks. All demographic, laboratory, and clinical characteristics of the patients were measured again at the end of the 12th week of treatment and were represented in Table 2.

Following NASH treatment with vitamin D_3 supplements, there was a statistically significant ($p < 0.05$) reduction in HbA1c (6.8 ± 1.3%), fasting blood sugar (136.1 ± 32.7 mg/dL), fasting insulin level (22.9 ± 1.8 μU/ml), HOMA-IR (1.4 ± 0.4), ALT (55.3 ± 21.3 U/L), AST (73.1 ± 54.2 U/L), triglycerides (203.6 ± 49.8 mg/dL), alkaline

Table 2 Association of vitamin D supplementation with different demographic, laboratory, and metabolic parameters of patients with NASH

Characteristics	Before treatment	After treatment	*t* value	*p* value	Significance
Weight (kg)	106.3 ± 15.6	106.0 ± 15.9	0.0924	0.9266	NS
BMI (kg/m^2)	35.7 ± 5.7	35.6 ± 5.7	0.0901	0.9284	NS
DBP (mmHg)	94.3 ± 11.9	91.5 ± 11.5	1.0553	0.2946	NS
HbA1c (%)	8.0 ± 2.4	6.8 ± 1.3	2.8558	0.0055	S
Hemoglobin (gm/dL)	13.5 ± 1.5	13.3 ± 1.2	0.6176	0.5386	NS
Platelet (× 10^3/μL)	288.5 ± 114.9	285.2 ± 98.3	0.1412	0.8881	NS
FBS (mg/dL)	165.6 ± 62.0	136.1 ± 32.7	2.6637	0.0094	S
Fasting insulin (μU/ml)	24.2 ± 3.0	22.9 ± 1.8	2.3090	0.0236	S
HOMA-IR	1.8 ± 0.7	1.4 ± 0.4	3.1134	0.0026	S
Creatinine (mg/dL)	0.9 ± 0.2	0.9 ± 0.3	0.2439	0.8080	NS
ALT (U/L)	78.2 ± 36.7	55.3 ± 21.3	3.4135	0.0010	S
AST (U/L)	108.6 ± 85.6	73.1 ± 54.2	2.2143	0.0297	S
Albumin (gm/dL)	3.8 ± 0.8	4.2 ± 0.7	2.2273	0.0288	S
NAFLD fibrosis score	− 0.78 ± 0.9	− 0.9 ± 1.1	0.9934	0.3236	NS
TCHOL (mg/dL)	233.0 ± 40.9	226.5 ± 38.2	0.7431	0.4596	NS
LDL (mg/dL)	117.5 ± 41.6	129.8 ± 34.7	1.4286	0.1571	NS
HDL (mg/dL)	48.5 ± 7.59	48.1 ± 8.1	0.1858	0.8531	NS
Triglycerides (mg/dL)	229.7 ± 62.1	203.6 ± 49.8	2.0728	0.0415	S
ALP (mg/dL)	70.4 ± 7.3	63.7 ± 7.9	3.9422	0.0002	S
GGT (U/L)	43.3 ± 24.5	35.1 ± 8.7	2.0069	0.0482	S
Total bilirubin (mg/dL)	1.1 ± 0.4	1.1 ± 0.1	0.2267	0.8212	NS
Vitamin D (ng/ml)	15.6 ± 6.6	33.0 ± 7.6	11.0335	<0.0001	S
Leptin (ng/ml)	35.9 ± 28.4	23.5 ± 12.9	2.5129	0.0140	S

phosphatase (63.7 ± 7.9 mg/dL), and gamma glutamyl transferase (35.1 ± 8.7 U/L) and a statistically significant ($p < 0.05$) increase in serum albumin level (4.2 ± 0.7 gm/dL).

No significant changes were noted before and after vitamin D_3 treatment regarding mean body weight, BMI, diastolic blood pressure, hemoglobin concentration, platelet count, serum creatinine, NAFLD fibrosis score, serum cholesterol, LDL, HDL, and total bilirubin.

There was a statistically significant increase ($p < 0.0001$) in serum vitamin D_3 level after treatment (33.0 ± 7.6 ng/ml) than before treatment (15.6 ± 6.6 ng/ml). Moreover, serum leptin level decreased significantly ($p = 0.0140$) in patients with NASH following treatment with vitamin D_3 with mean value of 23.5 ± 12.9 ng/ml compared to 35.9 ± 28.4 ng/ml before treatment.

Discussion

Non-alcoholic fatty liver disease (NAFLD) comprises a whole spectrum of diseases, including simple steatosis and steatohepatitis (NASH) which can progress to liver fibrosis, cirrhosis, and hepatocellular carcinoma. NAFLD is highly associated with obesity, insulin resistance, and metabolic syndrome, and it is estimated to affect about 20–40% of the general population in developed countries [24].

Vitamin D has long been regarded as a regulatory factor for phospho-calcium metabolism and bone homeostasis. However, many studies have shown more properties, namely immunomodulatory role [25], involvement in cellular differentiation and proliferation [26], hormone secretion [27], and anti-inflammatory and antifibrotic effects [28]. All these roles support the importance of maintaining optimal vitamin D levels.

Vitamin D deficiency constitutes a largely unrecognized epidemic in many populations worldwide and has been reported in all age groups including healthy children, young adults, middle-aged, and elderly adults [29].

In this study, we measured different demographic, laboratory, and metabolic parameters in forty patients with NASH and compared them with those of age- and sex-matched forty healthy individuals as the control group. Then, vitamin D (4000 IU/day) was given to the NASH group for 12 weeks. All demographic, laboratory, and metabolic parameters including serum leptin level were repeated after the end of treatment. Then, we demonstrated the association of vitamin D supplementation with serum leptin and metabolic parameters in patients with NASH.

In this study, we found that patients with NASH had higher body weight and BMI than the control. Many former studies concluded that obesity is a condition most often associated with NASH as 69 to 100% of patients with NASH were also obese. Obesity is associated with increased FFA delivery to the liver, increased FFA synthesis within the liver, insufficient beta-oxidation of FFA, and insufficient very low-density lipoprotein synthesis or secretion [30].

This study concluded that insulin resistance and dyslipidemia were more common in NASH with higher levels of HbA1c, fasting blood glucose, fasting insulin level, HOMA-IR, cholesterol, LDL, and lower levels of HDL compared to the control. Insulin resistance is associated with various metabolic abnormalities especially hyperglycemia, hypertriglyceridemia, low HDL cholesterol, and high levels of LDL leading to the concept of "metabolic syndrome" [30]. When resistance to antilipolytic action of insulin is present, fatty acids are mobilized more rapidly from visceral (central) than from subcutaneous (peripheral) fat and drained directly to the liver via the portal vein. Excessive intracellular concentrations of fatty acids may be toxic and lead to oxidative stress and thus contribute to NASH [31].

In this study, patients with NASH have significantly low vitamin D levels. This agrees with previous studies that noted high prevalence of hypovitaminosis D in patients with NAFLD [19]. This may be explained by the increased amount of adipose tissue in which the vitamin D is distributed in obese patients with NASH; this will decrease the circulating serum of vitamin D level [32]. Another explanation could be related to sedentary lifestyle, poor micro-nutrient nutrition, and lack of exposure to sunlight [33]. Moreover, in view of the bile acid-dependent uptake of vitamin D, it is reasonable to expect an association between vitamin D status and both cholestatic and noncholestatic chronic liver diseases [19].

The study noted that serum leptin levels were raised in both men and women with NASH compared with age- and sex-matched controls. Several factors could contribute to increased serum leptin levels in NASH. Hyperleptinemia occurs in inflammatory disorders and has been attributed to cytokines such as tumor necrosis factor-α (TNF-α), which is also increased in NASH as TNF-α gene is overexpressed in adipose tissue of obese NASH subjects. Chronic hyperinsulinemia, which is especially relevant in the setting of NASH, is associated with persistent hyperleptinemia. Moreover, leptin also correlates with serum c-peptide. In patients with NASH, c-peptide is not significantly cleared by the liver [9].

Following vitamin D supplementation in a dose of 4000 IU/day for 12 weeks, there was significant improvement of NASH. There was significant decrease in ALT, AST, ALP, GGT, and NAFLD fibrosis score. Previous studies noticed significant improvement in serum levels of ALT in NASH patients who took standard medical treatment (SMT) together with vitamin D when compared with others who took SMT alone [20]. Vitamin D was effective in liver enzyme reduction in another study [34]. Vitamin D-mediated improvement in insulin secretion results in decreased adipose tissue inflammation with decreased hepatic inflammation and fibrosis via the regulation of the vitamin D receptor and several cytokines such as interleukin 6, TNF-α, and adiponectin [18]. New evidence revealed that vitamin D can prevent hepatic stellate cell (HSC) activation which increases cellular transformation and proliferation [35].

In this study, vitamin D treatment significantly decreased insulin resistance in NASH patients. Values of fasting blood sugar, fasting insulin level, and HOMA-IR were significantly decreased after treatment. Vitamin D, through its effect on peroxisome proliferator-activated receptor, can modulate FFA metabolism and reduce FFA-induced insulin resistance in bloodstream [34]. Other studies reported significant reduction in FBS, insulin, and HOMA-IR following vitamin D supplementation in NASH [36]. The decreased production of TNF-α and increasing adiponectin during therapy with vitamin D is expected to improve the underlying IR in patients with NASH [19].

Serum triglycerides (TGs) decreased after treatment with vitamin D while there were no significant change in levels of cholesterol, LDL, and HDL. Foroughi et al. [37] assessed vitamin D effect on TGs in patients with NASH. They stated that, after 10 weeks of vitamin D treatment (50,000 IU/week), a significant decrease in serum TGs was seen when compared with baseline values. Hariri and Zohdi [36] also found that vitamin D supplementation might improve lipid profile and inflammatory mediators (like C-reactive protein) in NASH patients when compared with placebo.

One of the main physiological roles of leptin is to prevent lipid accumulation in nonadipose sites, such as the myocardium, skeletal muscle, pancreas, and liver, a concept referred to as "lipotoxicity" [38]. In this study, treatment with vitamin D has led to significant decrease in serum leptin level. This agreed with previous studies which confirmed that vitamin D level was negatively correlated with leptin in patients with NASH [39]. Other studies also reported vitamin D-mediated inhibition of serum leptin [40].

Conclusion

Vitamin D deficiency is highly prevalent among NASH patients, and this deficiency is related to the degree of liver function and degree of fibrosis. Vitamin D supplementation in patients with NASH in a dose of 4000 IU/day for 12 weeks improves severity of hepatic inflammation, decreases insulin resistance, improves glycemic control, corrects dyslipidemia, and protects against lipotoxicity by inhibition of serum leptin.

Recommendation

Our findings regarding the relationship between vitamin D deficiency and NASH suggest that taking vitamin D supplements should be a therapeutic option for patients with NASH. Additional studies are recommended to determine the association of variable doses and duration of vitamin D treatment with histopathological, laboratory, and clinical aspects in patients with NASH.

Abbreviations

NAFLD: Non-alcoholic steatohepatitis; NASH: Non-alcoholic steatohepatitis; MS: Metabolic syndrome; BMI: Body mass index; DBP: Diastolic blood pressure; FBS: Fasting blood sugar; HOMA-IR: Homeostasis model assessment of insulin resistance; ALT: Alanine transferase; AST: Aspartate transferase; LDL: Low-density lipoprotein; HDL: High-density lipoprotein; TCHOL: Total cholesterol; ALP: Alkaline phosphatase; GGT: Gamma glutamyl transferase; TNF-α: Tumor necrosis factor-α; TGs: Triglycerides

Acknowledgements

The authors express their gratitude to all members of the Hepatology and Gastroenterology Department, Faculty of Medicine, Ain Shams University, for their valuable participation.

Authors' contributions

AS Abohalima has made substantial contribution to the conception and design in this study by collecting, revising, and coding the data. He shared in writing the manuscript. HH Kaisar has made substantial contribution to the analysis and interpretation in this study. He revised and drafted the work. He performed the statistical analysis of the data and shared in writing the manuscript. All authors have read and approved the submitted version of manuscript. Each author agreed to be personally accountable for his own contributions and ensured that questions related to the accuracy or integrity of any part of the work are appropriately investigated and resolved.

Competing interests

The authors declare that they have no competing interests in this section

References

1. Sattar N, Forrest E, Preiss D (2014) Non-alcoholic fatty liver disease. BMJ (Clin Res Ed) 349:g4596
2. Sanyal AJ (2002) AGA technical review on nonalcoholic fatty liver disease. Gastroenterology 123:1705–1725
3. Duseja A, Singh SP, Saraswat VA et al (2015) Non-alcoholic fatty liver disease and metabolic syndrome-position paper of the Indian National Association for the study of the liver, Endocrine Society of India, Indian College of Cardiology and Indian Society of gastroenterology. J Clin Exp Hepatol 5:51–68
4. Torres DM, Harrison SA (2008) Diagnosis and therapy of nonalcoholic steatohepatitis. Gastroenterology 134:1682–1698
5. Bellentani S (2017) The epidemiology of non-alcoholic fatty liver disease. Liver Int 37(Suppl 1):81–84
6. Chalasani N, Younossi Z, Lavine JE, Diehl AM, Brunt EM, Cusi K, Charlton M, Sanyal AJ (2012) The diagnosis and management of nonalcoholic fatty liver disease: practice guideline by the American Gastroenterological Association, American Association for the Study of Liver Diseases, and American College of Gastroenterology. Gastroenterology 142(7):1592–1609
7. Roubos EW, Dahmen M, Kozicz T et al (2012) Leptin and the hypothalamo-pituitary-adrenal stress axis. Gen Comp Endocrino 177(1):28 36
8. Belgardt BF, Brüning JC (2010) CNS leptin and insulin action in the control of energy homeostasis. Ann N Y Acad Sci 1212:97–113
9. Shivakumar Chitturi, Geoffrey Farrell, Linda Frost, Adamandia Kriketos, Rita Lin, Christopher Liddle, Dev Samarasinghe and Jacob George (2002) Serum leptin in NASH correlates with hepatic steatosis but not fibrosis: a manifestation of lipotoxicity? Hepatology; August Vol. 36, No. 2:403-408
10. Bruyere O, Malaise O, Neuprez A et al (2007) Prevalence of vitamin D inadequacy in European postmenopausal women. Curr Med Res Opin 23: 1939–1944
11. Abramovitch S, Dahan-Bachar L, Sharvit E, Weisman Y, Ben Tov A, Brazowski E et al (2011) Vitamin D inhibits proliferation and profibrotic marker expression in hepatic stellate cells and decreases thioacetamide-induced liver fibrosis in rats. Gut 60:1728–1737
12. Gagnon C, Lu ZX, Magliano DJ et al (2012) Low serum 25-hydroxyvitamin D is associated with increased risk of the development of the metabolic syndrome at five years: results from a national, population-based prospective study (the Australian diabetes, obesity and lifestyle study: AusDiab). J Clin Endocrinol Metab 97:1953–1961
13. Pittas AG, Lau J, Hu FB et al. (2007) The role of vitamin D and calcium in type 2 diabetes. A systematic review and meta-analysis. J Clin Endocrinol Metab.; 92: 2017–2029.
14. Scragg R, Sowers M, Bell C (2004) Serum 25-hydroxyvitamin D, diabetes, and ethnicity in the third National Health and nutrition examination survey. Diabetes Care 27:2813–2818
15. Parikh SJ, Edelman M, Uwaifo GI, Freedman RJ, Semega-Janneh M, Reynolds J, Yanovski JA (2004) The relationship between obesity and serum 1,25-dihydroxy vitamin D concentrations in healthy adults. J Clin Endocrinol Metab 89:1196–1199
16. Snijder MB, van Dam RM, Visser M, Deeg DJ, Dekker JM, Bouter LM, Seidell JC, Lips P (2005) Adiposity in relation to vitamin D status and parathyroid hormone levels: a population-based study in older men and women. J Clin Endocrinol Metab 90:4119–4123
17. Zhou QG, Hou FF, Guo ZJ et al (2008) 1,25-Dihydroxyvitamin D improved the free fatty-acid-induced insulin resistance in cultured C2C12 cells. Diabetes Metab Res Rev 24:459–464
18. Eliades M, Spyrou E (2015) Vitamin D: a new player in non-alcoholic fatty liver disease? World J Gastroenterol 21(6):1718–1727
19. Sakpal M, Satsangi S, Mehta M, Duseja A, Bhadada S, Das A, Dhiman RK, Chawla YK. (2017) Vitamin D supplementation in patients with nonalcoholic fatty liver disease: a randomized controlled trial. J Gastroenterol Hepatol, 1; 62–67.
20. Kwok RM, Torres DM, Harrison SA (2013) Vitamin D and nonalcoholic fatty liver disease (NAFLD): is it more than just an association? Hepatology 58: 1166–1174
21. Matthews DR, Hosker JP, Rudenski AS et al (1985) Homeostasis model assessment: insulin resistance and beta-cell function from fasting plasma glucose and insulin concentrations in man. Diabetologia 28: 412–419
22. Angulo P, Hui JM, Marchesini G et al (2007) The NAFLD fibrosis score: a noninvasive system that identifies liver fibrosis in patients with NAFLD. Hepatology 45:846–854
23. Holick MF (2009) Vitamin D status: measurement, interpretation, and clinical application. Ann Epidemiol 19:73–78
24. Fabbrini E, Sullivan S, Klein S (2010) Obesity and nonalcoholic fatty liver disease: biochemical, metabolic and clinical implications. Hepatology 51(2): 679–689
25. Chen S, Sims GP, Chen XX, Gu YY, Chen S, Lipsky PE (2007) Modulatory effects of 1,25 dihydroxyvitamin D3 on human B cell differentiation. J Immunol 179(3):1634–1647
26. Bikle B (2009) Nonclassic actions of vitamin D. J Clin Endocrinol Metab 94(1): 26–34
27. Li YC, King J, Wei M, Chen ZF, Liu SQ, Cao LP (2002) 1,25-Dihydroxyvitamin D (3) is a negative endocrine regulator of the renin-angiotensin system. J Clin Invest 110(2):229–238
28. Beilfuss A, Sowa JP, Sydor S, Beste M, Bechmann LP, Schlattjan M, Syn WK, Wedemeyer I, Mathé Z, Jochum C, Gerken G, Gieseler RK, Canbay A (2015) Vitamin D counteracts fibrogenic TGF-β signalling in human hepatic stellate cells both receptor dependently and independently. Gut 64(5):791–799
29. Gordon CM, DePeter KC, Feldman HA et al (2004) Prevalence of vitamin D deficiency among healthy adolescents. Arch Pediatr Adolesc Med 158:531–537

30. Howard BV. (1999) Insulin resistance and lipid metabolism. Am J Cardiol, 84 (Suppl 1A), 28 J-32 J.
31. Sheth SG, Gordon FD, Chopra S (1997) Nonalcoholic steatohepatitis. Ann Intern Med 126:137–145
32. Wortsman J, Matsuoka LY, Chen TC, Lu Z, Holick MF (2000) Decreased bioavailability of vitamin D in obesity. Am J Clin Nutr 72(3):690–693
33. Bradlee ML, Singer MR, Qureshi MM, Moore LL (2010) Food group intake and central obesity among children and adolescents in the third National Health and nutrition examination survey (NHANES III). Public Health Nutr 13(6):797–805
34. Hariri M, Zohdi S (2019) Effect of vitamin D on non-alcoholic fatty liver disease: a systematic review of randomized controlled clinical trials. Int J Prev Med 10:14
35. Seydel S, Beilfuss A, Kahraman A, Aksoy K, Gerken G, Akkiz H et al (2011) Vitamin D ameliorates stress ligand expression elicited by free fatty acids in the hepatic stellate cell line LX-2. Turk J Gastroenterol 22:400–407
36. Lorvand Amiri H, Agah S, Tolouei Azar J, Hosseini S, Shidfar F, Mousavi SN et al (2017) Effect of daily calcitriol supplementation with and without calcium on disease regression in non-alcoholic fatty liver patients following an energy-restricted diet: randomized, controlled, double-blind trial. Clin Nutr 36:1490–1497
37. Foroughi M, Maghsoudi Z, Ghiasvand R, Iraj B, Askari G (2014) Effect of vitamin D supplementation on C-reactive protein in patients with nonalcoholic fatty liver. Int J Prev Med 5:969–975
38. Unger RH, Orci L (2001) Diseases of liporegulation: new perspective on obesity and related disorders. FASEB J 15:312–321
39. Chen L-W, Chien C-H, Kuo S-F, Yu C-Y, Lin C-L, Chien R-N (2019) Low vitamin D level was associated with metabolic syndrome and high leptin level in subjects with nonalcoholic fatty liver disease: a community-based study. BMC Gastroenterol 19:126. https://doi.org/https://doi.org/10.1186/s12876-019-1040-y
40. Hajimohammadi M, Shab-Bidar S, Neyestani TR (2017) Vitamin D and serum leptin: a systematic review and meta-analysis of observational studies and randomized controlled trials. Eur J Clin Nutr 71:1144–1153

14

A study of the different parameters in acute and chronic Budd–Chiari syndrome

Ramin Niknam[1], Nemattellah Hajizadegan[1], Vahid Mohammadkarimi[2*†] and Laleh Mahmoudi[3*†]

Abstract

Background: Budd–Chiari syndrome (BCS) is a rare and potentially life-threatening vascular disease of the liver. There are a few studies on the differences between acute and chronic BCS in clinical and laboratory characteristics, as well as the outcomes, so we designed this research to study the different parameters in acute and chronic BCS. Diagnosis of BCS was made using Doppler ultrasound, magnetic resonance imaging, and venography. Patients with BCS were then divided into chronic and acute groups based on both imaging characteristics and disease duration. Finally, the outcomes, clinical features, and laboratory parameters of acute and chronic BCS were compared.

Results: In total, 60 patients were included in this study, of whom 28.3% and 71.7% had acute and chronic BCS, respectively. According to clinical features, spontaneous bacterial peritonitis (PR 1.289; 95% CI 1.115–1.489; P = 0.001) and jaundice (PR 1.308; 95% CI 1.148–1.490; $P < 0.001$) were significantly associated with chronic than acute BCS. According to laboratory parameters, the levels of international normalized ratio (INR) (PR 0.953; 95% CI 0.918–0.989; P = 0.012), blood urea nitrogen (BUN) (PR 0.996; 95% CI 0.993–1.000; P = 0.039), and model for end-stage liver disease (MELD) score (PR 1.024; 95% CI 1.012–1.037; $P < 0.001$) in chronic group were significantly higher than in the acute BCS. The hospital length of stay (LOS) and mortality rate between the two groups did not differ significantly.

Conclusions: This study showed that the spontaneous bacterial peritonitis, jaundice, increased levels of MELD score, INR, and BUN were significantly associated with the chronic group compared with the acute group. The hospital LOS and mortality rate between the two groups did not differ significantly. Further research is recommended to clarify this issue.

Keywords: Budd–Chiari syndrome, Liver, Acute, Chronic, Outcome

Background

Budd–Chiari syndrome (BCS) is a rare and potentially life-threatening disorder caused by a partial or complete occlusion from small hepatic veins till inferior vena cava including the main hepatic veins [1–3]. The true incidence of BCS is unknown due to its rarity, and various results have been reported in different regions [3, 4].

Based on the onset of the disease in most studies, BCS is classified as acute (less than 6 months) and chronic (more than 6 months), and these two types of BCS differ in clinical manifestations, treatment, and prognosis [3, 5, 6].

Although some studies suggest that clinical presentations have little relationship with the actual duration of BCS [7], acute BCS is usually associated with severe symptoms, poor prognosis, and high mortality, while chronic BCS in most patients has an insidious onset and present with cirrhosis and surface varicose veins. Therefore, accurate diagnosis is essential for a rational treatment, to improve symptoms and increase survival [5].

* Correspondence: Vahid.mohammadkarimi@gmail.com; Mahmoudi_l@sums.ac.ir
†Vahid Mohammadkarimi and Laleh Mahmoudi contributed equally to this work.
[2]Department of Internal Medicine, School of Medicine, Shiraz University of Medical Sciences, Shiraz, Iran
[3]Department of Clinical Pharmacy, School of Pharmacy, Shiraz University of Medical Sciences, Shiraz, Iran

The signs and symptoms of BCS vary, so this diagnosis should be considered in any patient with acute or chronic liver disease [2, 7]. Most physicians differentiate between the acute and chronic forms of the disease based solely on the patient's history, which makes it difficult to diagnose BCS with insidious presentation. Therefore, imaging techniques such as Doppler ultrasound, magnetic resonance imaging (MRI), and computed tomography are necessary to diagnose BCS, as well as to differentiate acute from chronic disease [5]. Hepatic venography is recommended if the clinical suspicion of BCS is high (the presence of hepatomegaly, abdominal pain, and ascites with unknown cause), and there are no typical findings in other imaging [8].

There is controversy about the association of clinical and laboratory characteristics with the actual duration of BCS. On the other hand, there are few reports comparing clinical features, laboratory parameters, and outcomes between acute and chronic BCS [1, 5, 7]. Therefore, we conducted this study with the aim of comparing outcomes, clinical features, and laboratory parameters in different types of BCS in Namazi Hospital, as the main referral center for patients with liver disease in southern Iran.

Methods

Participants and groups

A cross-sectional study was performed at a referral hospital affiliated with Shiraz University of Medical Sciences between 2016 and 2020. All participants who were referred to our hospital for diagnosis and treatment for BCS from other centers were included in the study. Exclusion criteria as conditions that could act as confounders were heart failure, non-cooperative patients, sinusoidal obstruction syndrome, liver transplantation, and hepatic cancer. All eligible patients were followed for types and clinical and laboratory parameters of BCS.

Final diagnosis of BCS as well as follow-up of patients was performed by a hepatologist. Necessary variables including age, sex, ethnicity, individual habits, etiology, clinical features, associated disorders, and laboratory data were recorded in the checklist. BCS participants were divided into acute and chronic groups according to the criteria identified below. Finally, clinical and laboratory parameters between acute and chronic BCS were compared.

Diagnosis of BCS and its types

All patients with suspected BCS were examined using Doppler ultrasound and MRI. The diagnosis of BCS was based on the presence of thrombosis in the hepatic veins or inferior vena cava, decreased or reversed flow in these veins, and dampening of hepatic vein spectral waveform. If the diagnosis of BCS could not be confirmed by previous two methods, direct venography was used for further examination. Patients with BCS were then divided into chronic and acute groups based on both imaging characteristics and disease duration. Chronic BCS was defined as a disease duration more than 6 months [5, 6] and replacement of the hepatic vein and/or inferior vena cava by collateral veins in Doppler ultrasound or the presence of MRI findings indicating chronic BCS including collateral veins, regenerative nodules, decreased T1- and T2-weighted signal intensity on unenhanced MRI, and delayed enhancement on contrast-enhanced imaging because of replacement of parenchymal edema by fibrosis [8]. Acute BCS was defined as a disease onset of less than 6 months without evidence of chronicity in Doppler ultrasound and MRI.

The differentiation between hepatocellular carcinoma and regenerative nodules was based on imaging characteristics and alpha-fetoprotein levels. If the diagnosis was still unclear, a biopsy of the liver lesion was performed. Thrombophilia testing was performed to evaluate the underlying hypercoagulable states in all patients with BCS.

Ethical approval/statement

This research was carried out taking into account the ethics Declaration of the Helsinki research and was approved by the ethics committee of Shiraz University of Medical Sciences (IR.SUMS.MED.REC.1397.442). Written consent was obtained from all patients.

Measurement of laboratory parameters

Blood samples were taken to evaluate complete blood count, liver biochemical tests, partial thromboplastin time (PTT), international normalized ratio (INR), blood urea nitrogen (BUN), creatinine, and blood sugar for all participants. Jaundice was defined as the total serum bilirubin level greater than 2.5 mg/dL. Paracentesis was performed to assess the albumin, protein, culture, cell counts, and differentiation for all patients with ascites. All laboratory parameters were tested under international standards, and blood samples were transported to the laboratory in less than an hour. Finally, serum-ascites albumin gradient (SAAG) and model for end-stage liver disease (MELD) score was also calculated based on the results of lab data for all participants.

Statistical analysis

The data was stored in a SPSS software, version 25.0, Chicago, USA. Qualitative data analysis was performed using chi-square test. Quantitative data was expressed as the mean and standard deviation, and the differences between the groups were examined using two independent *t* tests and Mann-Whitney test, where appropriate. Robust Poisson regression models were used to estimate prevalence ratio (PR) and 95% confidence interval (CI) to evaluate the association of various independent clinical and laboratory variables on the types of BCS. The Kaplan–Meier method and log rank test was used for comparing hospital length of stay (LOS) between groups, defining in-hospital mortality as the main event. P value lower than 0.05 was considered as significant difference.

Results

In total, 60 patients were included in this study, of whom 17 (28.3%) had acute BCS and 43 (71.7%) participants were considered as the chronic BCS group. The median/mean age (SD) was 37.5/37.68 (12.78) years ranging from 19 to 90 years. Twenty-one (35.0%) and 39 (65.0%) patients were male and female, respectively. Diagnosis was made in 58 patients based on Doppler ultrasound and MRI, while 2 patients underwent direct venography due to uncertain results in imaging studies. The most common predisposing factor of BCS was myeloproliferative neoplasms (8.3%). Overall, 22 (36.7 %) patients had Fars ethnicity and 19 (31.7 %) were smokers. The demographic and clinical characteristics of the participants are shown in Table 1.

Although most of the patients were male, there was no significant difference compared to women in terms of acute or chronic BCS (P = 0.24). According to clinical features, jaundice in chronic BCS group was significantly higher than acute group (P < 0.001) but there was no significant difference in other variables between two groups. The comparison of clinical and demographic characteristics between acute and chronic BCS is shown in Table 2.

According to laboratory parameters, levels of PTT, INR, bilirubin, and end-stage liver disease (MELD) score in chronic BCS were significantly higher than acute group. There were no significant differences between the two groups in other laboratory variables such as hemoglobin, platelet, alanine transaminase (ALT), aspartate transaminase (AST), albumin, protein, and ascitic fluid parameters. The comparison of laboratory parameters between acute and chronic BCS is shown in Table 3.

Robust Poisson regression models was used for estimating the PRs and 95% CIs to evaluate the association of various clinical and laboratory variables on the types of BCS. Spontaneous bacterial peritonitis (PR 1.289; 95% CI 1.115–1.489; P = 0.001) and jaundice (PR 1.308; 95% CI 1.148–1.490; P < 0.001) were significantly associated with chronic than acute BCS. However, other variables including gender, age, encephalopathy, gastrointestinal (GI) bleeding, and renal failure were not significantly associated with acute compared to chronic BCS group (Table 4).

According to laboratory parameters, the levels of INR (PR 0.953; 95% CI 0.918–0.989; P = 0.012), BUN (PR 0.996; 95% CI 0.993–1.000; P = 0.039), and MELD score (PR 1.024; 95% CI 1.012–1.037; P < 0.001) in chronic group were significantly higher than in the acute BCS. However, the levels of other variables including platelet, PTT, total bilirubin, and ascitic fluid parameters did not differ significantly between the two groups (Table 5).

The median/mean (SD) hospital LOS in patients with acute BCS was 12/13.29 (10.042) days and in chronic BCS patients was 9/10.40 (6.97) days. The Kaplan–Meier method and log rank test for comparing hospital LOS between acute and chronic BCS patients showed that there was no significant difference between the two groups (P = 0.34). Hospital LOS curves for patients with acute and chronic BCS are shown in Fig. 1. The in-hospital mortality rate was 1 (5.9%) and 5 (11.6%) in

Table 1 Demographic and clinical characteristics of participants with Budd–Chiari syndrome (n = 60)

Gender	
Male	21 (35.0%)
Female	39 (65.0%)
Age (years); mean ± SD	37.68 ± 12.78
Ethnicity	
Fars	22 (36.7 %)
Turke	15 (25.0%)
Arabs	5 (8.3%)
Lurs	5 (8.3%)
Kurds	4 (6.7%)
Baloch	4 (6.7%)
Mazandarani	3 (5.0%)
Turkomen	2 (3.3%)
Past medical history	
Myeloproliferative neoplasms	5 (8.3%)
Paroxysmal nocturnal hemoglobinuria	3 (5.0%)
Myelodysplastic syndromes	2 (3.3%)
Antiphospholipid syndrome	1 (1.7%)
Protein C deficiency	1 (1.7%)
Lymphoma	1 (1.7%)
Positive human immunodeficiency virus	1 (1.7%)
Systemic lupus erythematosus	3 (5.0%)
Pseudotumor cerebri	1 (1.7%)
Diabetes mellitus	3 (5.0%)
Cigarette smoking	19 (31.7 %)
Alcohol use	12 20.0 (%)
Abdominal pain	46 (76.7%)
Jaundice	29 (48.3%)
Ascites	60 (100.0%)
Spontaneous bacterial peritonitis [1]	5 (8.3%)
Gastrointestinal bleeding [1]	16 (26.7%)
Encephalopathy	14 (23.3%)
Renal failure	12 (20.0%)
Hospital length of stay (days); mean ± SD	11.22 ± 7.98
Mortality	6 (10.0%)

[1]Spontaneous bacterial peritonitis was defined as ascitic fluid polymorphonuclear leukocyte count ≥ 250 cells/mm^3 and positive ascitic fluid culture; gastrointestinal bleeding including hematemesis and melena

Table 2 Comparison of clinical and demographic characteristics between acute (*n* = 17) and chronic (*n* = 43) Budd–Chiari syndrome (BCS)

Variables	Acute BCS; *N* (%)	Chronic BCS; *N* (%)	*P* value
Gender[2]			0.241
Male	4 (23.5%)	17 (39.5%)	
Female	13 (76.5%)	26 (60.5%)	
Age (years); mean ± SD	34.47 ± 11.07	38.95 ± 13.30	0.224
Ethnicity[1]			0.649
Fars	7 (41.2%)	15 (34.9%)	
Others	10 (58.8%)	28 (65.1%)	
Abdominal pain[1]	13 (76.5%)	33 (76.7%)	0.982
Jaundice[1]	2 (11.8%)	27 (62.8%)	< 0.001
Dyspnea[1]	4 (23.5%)	15 (34.9%)	0.394
Peripheral edema[1]	8 (47.1%)	25 (58.1%)	0.437
Fever[1]	4 (23.5%)	14 (32.6%)	0.492
Vomiting[1]	13 (76.5%)	25 (58.1%)	0.184
Weight loss[1]	13 (76.5%)	27 (62.8%)	0.311
Encephalopathy[1]	2 (11.8%)	12 (27.9%)	0.183
Gastrointestinal bleeding	2 (11.8%)	14 (32.6%)	0.101
Spontaneous bacterial peritonitis[1]	0 (0.0%)	5 (11.6%)	0.142
Renal failure[1]	1 (5.9%)	11 (25.6%)	0.086
Cigarette smoking[1]	3 (17.6%)	16 (37.2%)	0.142
Alcohol use[1]	1 (5.9%)	11 (25.6%)	0.081

[1]Chi-square test
[2]*T* test

patients with acute and chronic BCS, respectively, but there was no significant difference between the two groups (P = 0.45). There was no significant association between the predisposing causes of BCS and the increase in in-hospital mortality. The mean (SD) age of patients who died in hospital was 35.50 (6.25) years, and there was no significant association between patients' age and increased mortality (P = 0.66).

Discussion

BCS is a rare vascular disease of the liver with heterogeneous clinical manifestations caused by obstruction of hepatic venous outflow. According to the etiology of the disease, BCS is classified as primary and secondary. Primary BCS is caused by acquired conditions such as myeloproliferative neoplasms, hereditary conditions such as Factor V Leiden, and systemic prothrombotic conditions. Secondary BCS is caused by vascular compression due to pyogenic infectious process or benign and malignant tumors [1, 2]. Regardless of the cause of the venous outflow obstruction, increased hepatic sinusoidal pressure and portal hypertension occur rapidly, leading to ischemic damage to the hepatocytes, followed by nodular regeneration, fibrosis, and eventually cirrhosis. In addition, large regenerative nodules may in turn lead to compression of intrahepatic veins [1, 4].

This study is the first report to compare the clinical features, laboratory parameters, and outcomes between acute and chronic BCS from Iran. This cross-sectional study showed that spontaneous bacterial peritonitis and jaundice were significantly associated with the chronic group compared with the acute group. The study also showed that levels of MELD score, INR, and BUN in chronic BCS was significantly higher than in the acute group. There was no significant difference between the outcomes of the two groups in terms of hospital LOS and mortality. In our patients the most common predisposing factor for BCS were myeloproliferative neoplasms, paroxysmal nocturnal hemoglobinuria, and systemic lupus erythematosus (Table 1)

The definitions of acute and chronic of BCS are not clearly defined [9]; however, most studies have classified the BCS with an onset of less than 6 months as acute and more than 6 months as chronic [3, 5, 6]. When BCS is suspected, color Doppler ultrasound is typically the first imaging procedure with high sensitivity and specificity [8]. Doppler ultrasound, MRI, and computed tomography are usually sufficient to diagnose BCS. Liver biopsy is only useful if the thrombosis is limited to the small intrahepatic veins and the large vessels appear

Table 3 Comparison of laboratory parameters between acute (*n* = 17) and chronic (*n* = 43) Budd–Chiari syndrome (BCS)

Variables	Acute BCS; *N* (%)	Chronic BCS; *N* (%)	*P* value	Normal range
White blood cells; μl[1]	8386.47 ± 3412.33	8837.21 ± 5014.17	0.902	4000–10,000
Hemoglobin; g/dL[2]	11.51 ± 1.98	11.43 ± 2.31	0.901	12–16
Platelet; μl[1]	257,058.82 ± 228,189.47	155,441.86 ± 121,008.32	0.075	140,000–400,000
PTT; seconds[1]	37.34 ± 4.44	45.73 ± 17.63	0.016	25–35
INR* [1]	1.77 ± 0.71	3.04 ± 2.16	0.003	< 1.1
Aspartate transaminase; IU/L[1]	123.06 ± 152.68	140.09 ± 205.22	0.844	< 31
Alanine transaminase; IU/L[1]	189.82 ± 271.73	133.56 ± 207.81	0.634	< 31
Alkaline phosphatase; IU/L[2]	320.94 ± 191.68	307.65 ± 155.08	0.781	64–306
Serum albumin; g/dL[2]	3.48 ± 0.66	3.30 ± 0.68	0.356	3.5–5.4
Serum protein; g/dL[2]	6.26 ± 1.05	6.16 ± 1.64	0.811	6.0–8.3
Total bilirubin; mg/dL[1]	2.04 ± 2.55	4.20 ± 3.59	0.020	0.1–1.2
Direct bilirubin; mg/dL[1]	0.81 ± 1.13	1.94 ± 1.69	0.023	< 0.2
Blood urea nitrogen; mg/dL[1]	18.77 ± 21.68	28.44 ± 26.51	0.071	7–20
Creatinine; mg/dL[1]	0.99 ± 0.37	1.49 ± 1.70	0.645	0.8–1.2
Blood sugar; mg/dL[1]	98.77 ± 50.55	104.30 ± 49.95	0.475	70–99
Ascitic fluid cell counts; μL[1]	587.24 ± 933.40	2527.72 ± 7496.39	0.123	-
Ascitic fluid albumin; g/dL[1]	1.45 ± 0.50	1.26 ± 0.75	0.230	-
Ascitic fluid protein; g/dL[1]	2.02 ± 0.69	2.00 ± 1.22	0.480	-
SAAG[2]	2.03 ± 0.50	2.04 ± 0.71	0.754	-
SAAG[3]			0.551	-
Low	0 (0.0%)	3 (7.0%)		
High	17 (100.0%)	40 (93.0%)		
MELD score[1]	14.65 ± 7.42	24.00 ± 10.17	< 0.001	-

PTT partial thromboplastin time, *INR* international normalized ratio, *SAAG* serum-ascites albumin gradient, *MELD* model for end-stage liver disease
[1]Mann–Whitney test
[2]*T* test
[3]Chi-square test

normal on imaging [2, 7]. In our study, most patients were in the chronic BCS group.

The clinical manifestations of BCS are heterogeneous and depend on the extent and speed of the obstruction of the hepatic venous outflow and the presence of collateral venous ducts. All of our participants were symptomatic, although the literature reported that up to 20% of patients with BCS were asymptomatic [1]. This difference may be due to the fact that all of our participants were referred from other centers for diagnostic and therapeutic procedures and were hospitalized, so we did not evaluate outpatients. Although the classic triad of abdominal pain, ascites, and hepatomegaly is common in BCS patients, other clinical features, including fever, pedal edema, truncal hepatic veins, GI bleeding, and hepatic encephalopathy, may be seen in this disease [1].

In a study by Darwish Murad et al. [10], they found that 61% and 83% of patients with BCS had ascites and abdominal pain, while esophageal bleeding and hepatic encephalopathy have been reported in approximately 5% and 9% of their patients, respectively. The frequency of all of these manifestations was higher in our results. 76.7% of our patients had abdominal pain, while GI bleeding and hepatic encephalopathy in our participants was about 15%, but there was no significant difference in terms of these manifestations between acute and chronic BCS. Another complication of liver failure is spontaneous bacterial peritonitis, which was significantly higher in our study in the chronic group than in the acute group.

In a study conducted by Mahmoud et al. [11] on BCS patients, the frequency of abdominal pain (84%) and hepatic encephalopathy (36%) was higher than our results, while the frequency of peripheral edema (4%), GI bleeding (9%), jaundice 4 (9%), and vomiting (27%) was less than our study. According to clinical manifestations, in our research, the presence of jaundice in chronic BCS was significantly higher than acute group, but there was no significant difference in other clinical features including peripheral edema, and fever between two groups (Tables 2 and 4).

Serum aminotransferases, alkaline phosphatase, serum albumin, serum bilirubin, and prothrombin may be normal or high in patients with BCS [12]. In our

Table 4 Robust Poisson regression models estimating prevalence ratio (PR) and 95% confidence interval (CI) to evaluate the association of various independent variables on the types of Budd–Chiari syndrome

Variable	Crude model		Adjusted model	
	PR (95% CI)	*P* value	PR (95% CI)	*P* value
Gender		0.209		0.739
Female	0.921 (0.810–1.047)		1.022 (0.897–1.165)	
Male	1.0		1.0	
Age	1.003 (0.999–1.008)	0.144	1.001 (0.996–1.005)	0.706
Jaundice		< 0.001		< 0.001
Yes	1.274 (1.123–1.444)		1.308 (1.148–1.490)	
No	1.0		1.0	
Vomiting	ss	0.154		0.094
Yes	0.912 (0.803–1.035)		0.904 (0.803–1.018)	
No	1.0		1.0	
Encephalopathy		0.111		0.569
Yes	1.109 (0.977–1.261)		1.039 (0.911–1.184)	
No	1.0		1.0	
Gastrointestinal bleeding		0.047		0.114
Yes	1.130 (1.002–1.275)		1.087 (0.980–1.206)	
No	1.0		1.0	
Renal failure		0.017		0.826
Yes	1.150 (1.026–1.289)		1.014 (0.893–1.152)	
No	1.0		1.0	
Spontaneous bacterial peritonitis		< 0.001		0.001
Yes	1.183 (1.100–1.271)		1.289 (1.115–1.489)	
No	1.0		1.0	
Cigarette smoking		0.099		0.911
Yes	1.111 (0.980–1.258)		0.992 (0.865–1.138)	
No	1.0		1.0	
Alcohol use		0.017		0.208
Yes	1.150 (1.026–1.289)		1.075 (0.961–1.204)	
No	1.0		1.0	

Table 5 Robust Poisson regression models estimating prevalence ratio (PR) and 95% confidence interval (CI) to evaluate the association of various laboratory parameters on the types of Budd–Chiari syndrome

Variable	Crude model		Adjusted model	
	PR (95% CI)	*P* value	PR (95% CI)	*P* value
PTT	1.004 (1.001–1.006)	0.003	1.002 (1.000–1.005)	0.086
INR	1.037 (1.013–1.062)	0.002	0.953 (0.918–0.989)	0.012
Platelet	1.000 (1.000–1.000)	0.009	1.000 (1.000–1.000)	0.083
Total bilirubin	1.021 (1.005–1.038)	0.012	1.001 (0.980–1.022)	0.961
Blood urea nitrogen	1.002 (0.999–1.004)	0.139	0.996 (0.993–1.000)	0.039
Ascitic fluid cell counts	1.000 (1.000–1.000)	0.005	1.000 (1.000–1.000)	0.326
Ascitic fluid albumin	0.951 (0.868–1.042)	0.281	0.978 (0.894–1.071)	0.638
MELD score	1.010 (1.005–1.015)	< 0.001	1.024 (1.012–1.037)	< 0.001

PTT partial thromboplastin time, *INR* international normalized ratio, *MELD* model for end-stage liver disease

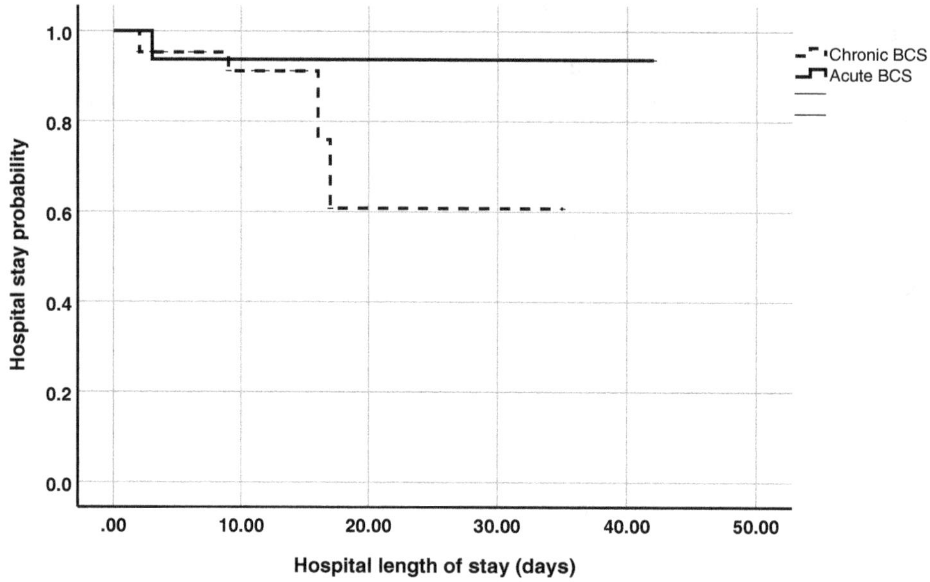

Fig. 1 Kaplan–Meier graph showing hospital length of stay curves for patients with acute and chronic Budd–Chiari syndrome (BCS)

participants, although the mean ALT, AST, bilirubin, INR, and PTT were high in both acute and chronic groups, the differences between the two groups were significant only in bilirubin, INR, and PTT. In a study by Rautou et al. [13], in 96 BCS patients, they concluded that high levels of ALT reflected acute and severe but potentially reversible ischemic liver cell necrosis. Another study of 45 BCS patients who were admitted to four medical centers concluded that serum ALT appeared to be a prognostic indicator [14]. Serum creatinine levels can also be high, usually due to pre-renal dysfunction [12], and may be associated with patient death [15]. The levels of BUN and creatinine in the chronic group of our patients were higher than acute, which was significant in terms of BUN.

The classic composition of ascitic fluid in BCS is high SAAG (> 1.1 g/dL) [1, 12]. All patients with acute BCS in our study had high SAAG ascites, but 7% of patients in the chronic group had low SAAG ascites (Table 3); the reason for this difference was unclear and requires further research with higher sample size. Although standard laboratory analyzes are of little help in diagnosing BCS, they are useful in predicting the severity of the disease, the likelihood of death, and the possible response to treatment. One of the common prognostic indices in BCS is the MELD score [1, 7]. MELD score and INR in chronic BCS group of our patients were significantly higher than the acute group (Table 5).

An important limitation in our research was that only symptomatic hospitalized participants were studied, so the results of this study may not be generalizable to asymptomatic patients. Another limitation of our study was that it was conducted in a single center, but the main strength of our research was the optimal evaluation of clinical features as well as the detailed assessment of laboratory parameters in acute and chronic BCS patients.

Conclusions

The present study found that the spontaneous bacterial peritonitis, jaundice, increased levels of MELD score, INR, and BUN were significantly associated with the chronic group compared with the acute group. The hospital LOS and mortality rate between the two groups did not differ significantly. Further research is recommended to clarify this issue.

Supplementary information

Supplementary information accompanies this paper at https://doi.org/10.1186/s43066-020-00058-4.

Additional file 1. STROBE checklist .

Abbreviations

BCS: Budd–Chiari syndrome; MRI: Magnetic resonance imaging; PTT: Partial thromboplastin time; INR: International normalized ratio; BUN: Blood urea nitrogen; SAAG: Serum-ascites albumin gradient; MELD: Model for end-stage liver disease; PR: Prevalence ratio; CI: Confidence interval; LOS: Hospital length of stay; ALT: Alanine transaminase; AST: Aspartate transaminase; GI: Gastrointestinal

Acknowledgements

This study was a part of a MD thesis written by Nemattellah Hajizadegan and was supported by the research Council of Shiraz University of Medical Sciences, Shiraz, Iran (1396-01-01-15890).

Authors' contributions

RN generates the research idea. VM study design. LM study design and data collection. RN and NH perform the clinical examination. NH performs the laboratory analysis. All authors shared in analyzing and interpreting the patient data and in writing the manuscript. All authors read and approved the final manuscript.

Competing interests
The authors declare that they have no competing interests.

Author details
[1]Department of Internal Medicine, School of Medicine, Gastroenterohepatology Research Center, Shiraz University of Medical Sciences, Shiraz, Iran. [2]Department of Internal Medicine, School of Medicine, Shiraz University of Medical Sciences, Shiraz, Iran. [3]Department of Clinical Pharmacy, School of Pharmacy, Shiraz University of Medical Sciences, Shiraz, Iran.

References

1. Martens P, Nevens F (2015) Budd-Chiari syndrome. United European Gastroenterol J. 3(6):489–500
2. Van Wettere M, Bruno O, Rautou PE, Vilgrain V, Ronot M (2018) Diagnosis of Budd-Chiari syndrome. Abdom Radiol (NY). 43(8):1896–1907
3. Zanetto A, Pellone M, Senzolo M (2019) Milestones in the discovery of Budd-Chiari syndrome. Liver Int. 39(7):1180–1185
4. Grus T, Lambert L, Grusova G, Banerjee R, Burgetova A (2017) Budd-Chiari syndrome. Prague Med Rep. 118(2-3):69–80
5. Cheng D, Xu H, Hua R, Xu K, Lv W, Lu X et al (2015) Comparative study of MRI manifestations of acute and chronic Budd-Chiari syndrome. Abdom Imaging. 40(1):76–84
6. Singh V, Sinha SK, Nain CK, Bambery P, Kaur U, Verma S et al (2000) Budd-Chiari syndrome: our experience of 71 patients. J Gastroenterol Hepatol. 15(5):550–554
7. Valla DC (2018) Budd-Chiari syndrome/hepatic venous outflow tract obstruction. Hepatol Int. 12(Suppl 1):168–180
8. Copelan A, Remer EM, Sands M, Nghiem H, Kapoor B (2015) Diagnosis and management of Budd Chiari syndrome: an update. Cardiovasc Intervent Radiol. 38(1):1–12
9. Shin N, Kim YH, Xu H, Shi HB, Zhang QQ, Colon Pons JP et al (2016) Redefining Budd-Chiari syndrome: A systematic review. World J Hepatol. 8(16):691–702
10. Darwish Murad S, Plessier A, Hernandez-Guerra M, Fabris F, Eapen CE, Bahr MJ et al (2009) Etiology, management, and outcome of the Budd-Chiari syndrome. Ann Intern Med. 151(3):167–175
11. Mahmoud AE, Mendoza A, Meshikhes AN, Olliff S, West R, Neuberger J et al (1996) Clinical spectrum, investigations and treatment of Budd-Chiari syndrome. QJM. 89(1):37–43
12. DeLeve LD, Valla DC, Garcia-Tsao G (2009) American Association for the Study Liver D. Vascular disorders of the liver. Hepatology. 49(5):1729–1764
13. Rautou PE, Moucari R, Cazals-Hatem D, Escolano S, Denie C, Douarin L et al (2009) Levels and initial course of serum alanine aminotransferase can predict outcome of patients with Budd-Chiari syndrome. Clin Gastroenterol Hepatol. 7(11):1230–1235
14. Tang TJ, Batts KP, de Groen PC, van Hoek B, Haagsma EB, Hop WC et al (2001) The prognostic value of histology in the assessment of patients with Budd-Chiari syndrome. J Hepatol. 35(3):338–343
15. Parekh J, Matei VM, Canas-Coto A, Friedman D, Lee WM (2017) Acute Liver Failure Study G. Budd-chiari syndrome causing acute liver failure: A multicenter case series. Liver Transpl. 23(2):135–142

15

Effect of eradication of HCV infection by direct-acting antivirals in diabetic HCV-infected patients as regards glycemic control

Mohamed Mohei El Badry[1*], Doaa Abdelhady Ali[1], Noha Hamdy Eltaweel[2] and Marwa A. Abdel-Wahed[3]

Abstract

Background: A burden of data suggests that insulin signaling could be impaired with hepatitis C virus infection, and this boost the onset of type 2 diabetes mellitus beyond and in addition to the histological effect on the associated liver disease. We aimed to evaluate the hemoglobin A1c (HbA1c) levels before and after therapy with direct-acting antivirals (DAAs) in HCV-diabetic patients who achieved sustained virological response (SVR) at Aswan Fever Hospital. This prospective study was conducted at the Viral Hepatitis Treatment Center, Aswan Fever Hospital, Aswan, Egypt, between November 2017 and May 2018. A total of 85 randomly selected diabetic patients (type 2 diabetes mellitus) with chronic HCV infection were received sofosbuvir and daclatasvir as a dual therapy for 3 months, then followed up for week 12 after the end of DAA therapy, Changes in the levels of hemoglobin A1c (HbA1c) were measured at baseline then 12 weeks after the end of treatment with DAAs.

Results: Thirty-two patients (37.6%) showed a significant glycemic improvement after receiving DAAs therapy; in the form of > 1% reduction in HbA1c level (p value < 0.001). Their baseline mean HbA1c level was 7.98 ± 0.62% which was significantly improved 12 weeks after the end of therapy (SVR) to reach a level of 6.88 ± 0.81%. Meanwhile, 53 patients (62.4%) had a baseline mean HbA1c of 8.24 ± 0.64% and a post-treatment mean HbA1c level of 8.34 ± 0.61% (p value = 0.083).

Conclusion: DAAs-based eradication of HCV is associated with improved glycemic control in 37.6% of patients with diabetes as evidenced by a significant reduction of mean HbA1c.

Keywords: Direct-acting antiviral drugs (DAAs), HCV, Glycated hemoglobin (HA1C), Glycemic control, Eradication, Diabetic

Background

Hepatitis C virus (HCV) affects over 185 million people, with an estimated 2.8% increase globally over the last decade. It has been estimated that HCV is the leading cause of cirrhosis and hepatocellular carcinoma (HCC) cases worldwide. Global- and region-specific estimates of HCV prevalence vary greatly [1, 2], but the highest prevalence has been reported in China, Pakistan, Nigeria, Egypt, India, and Russia which together accounted for more than half of the total infections [3].

In Egypt, HCV was estimated to affect 14.7% of the population; over 90% of the infections have been reported to be HCV genotype 4. The spread of chronic HCV infection in Egypt is thought to be largely due to needle re-use during mass-treatment programs for schistosomiasis during the late 1950s through the early 1980s. Unfortunately, transmission continues to occur,

* Correspondence: melbadry2002@yahoo.com
[1]Department of Tropical Medicine and Gastroenterology, Faculty of Medicine, Aswan University, Aswan, Egypt

primarily through iatrogenic sources, such as blood transfusions, injections, and dental care [4].

It is widely recognized that there is a link between infection with HCV and type 2 diabetes mellitus (T2DM). Patients chronically infected with HCV are 4 times more likely to have T2DM than HCV negative subjects. Several studies focused on the treatment of HCV with pegylated interferon (peg)/ribavirin (RBV) based therapy prior to the widespread use of the new direct-acting antiviral drugs (DAAs) [5].

With recent advances, many DAAs developed and led to a more promising future for HCV infected patients. Excellent advantages were related to their high potency, pangenotypic coverage and intermediate to high barrier to resistance. They paved the way to the possible application of oral interferon-free regimens. In addition, these regimens can be taken once daily and may result in global HCV eradication in the near future [6].

The effect of sustained virological response (SVR) on various clinical outcomes provides another line of evidence linking HCV infection with Insulin resistance (IR). Sustained virological response (SVR) is associated with a reduction in HCC incidence, liver-related mortality, and overall mortality. A number of clinical trials demonstrate that SVR was associated also with improved IR. For instance, a longitudinal study of the Hepatitis C Antiviral Long-Term Treatment against Cirrhosis Trial found that SVR was associated with an improvement in IR [7]. Another study based on the Milan Safety Tolerability study cohort found a reduction of de novo IR development in SVR patients compared to non-SVR patients although the mean baseline and post-treatment Homeostatic Model Assessment for Insulin Resistance (HOMA) values were similar in SVR patients [8]. Gilad et al. (2019) reported that HCV eradication leads to a decrease in HbA1c ≥ 0.5% with no increase in diabetes medications or a decrease in diabetes medications with a stable HbA1c. Thus, the association between HCV eradication and glycemic improvement has been widely postulated. However, a little is known about the exact percent of glycemic improvement within SVR patients. Therefore, the aim of this study is to evaluate the HbA1c levels before and after therapy with DAAs in HCV-diabetic patients who achieved SVR [9].

Methods

This prospective observational study was done in the Viral Hepatitis Treatment Center, Aswan Fever Hospital, Egypt, which is one of the centers affiliated to the Egyptian National Committee for Control of Viral Hepatitis (NCCVH) in the period between November 2017 and May 2018. Preliminary, 100 randomly selected diabetic patients with chronic HCV infection who intended to receive DAAs were participated, then followed up for week 12 after the end of DAAs therapy, only 85 patients continued till the end of the study. The remaining fifteen patients were excluded due to loss of follow-up, also those who demonstrated a viremic relapse 4 weeks after the end of therapy and remained HCV-RNA positive at week 12 were excluded.

The study was performed according to the ethical guidelines of the 1975 Declaration of Helsinki after approval from the Institutional Review Board (IRB) for human subject research at the National Hepatology and Tropical Medicine Research Institute. Written informed consents were obtained from all enrolled participants before enrolment to the study. Diabetes was defined according to American Diabetes Association (ADA) guidelines and confirmed by a hemoglobin Alc > 6.5% [10]. The SVR was defined as undetectable HCV-RNA at week 12 after the end of therapy. The stated glycemic improvement in our study was defined as a ≥ 1% reduction of baseline HbA1c levels. Other previous studies involving DAAs therapy reported a decline of HbA1C by 0.5–1.95% [9, 11].

Patients were included in the study according to the standardized protocol for HCV management issued by NCCVH. Key exclusion criteria were Child–Turcotte–Pugh (CTP) class C, hemoglobin level < 10 g/dL, platelet count < 50,000/mm3, hepatocellular carcinoma (HCC) except 6 months following a successful intervention and cure with no proof of recurrence by dynamic imaging (CT, MRI), extra-hepatic malignancy except after 2 years of cure, co-infection with hepatitis B or HIV, and hypersensitivity to any of study medications. All patients included in this study were subjected to full history taking and thorough clinical examination. Baseline demographics (age, gender, and treatment medications) were recorded. Baseline laboratory investigations were done, including complete blood count (CBC), prothrombin time (PT), international normalized ratio (INR), hemoglobin A1c (HbA1c), renal function tests (BUN, creatinine), hepatitis B virus surface antigen (Hbs Ag), alpha fetoprotein (AFP), and liver function tests including AST and ALT. Patients were followed up for 12 weeks after the end of DAAs therapy and post-treatment laboratory values were obtained at the time of SVR response (HCV-RNA clearance 12 weeks after the end of therapy).The analysis of CBC was done using Coulter LH 750 Cell Counter, measurement of PT was performed using Stago Compact Autoanalyzer using Neoplastine CI Plus supplied by Diagnostica Stago and serum chemistry was performed using Beckman Coulter AU480 Autoanalyzer, HCV (RNA) PCR using the COBAS® TaqMan® HCV Test v2.0. The HbA1c measurement is based on a turbidimetric inhibition immunoassay (TINIA) principle and was performed using Roche Diagnostics Cobas c 311 Autoanalyzer.

Statistical analysis

Statistical analysis was done using IBM SPSS software version 20. The values for the biochemical markers were expressed as mean and standard deviation in case of parametric data, and as median and interquartile ranges in case of skewed data, while categorical variables were summarized using frequency measures. Independent t test was used in the comparison between two groups with quantitative data and parametric distribution and Mann-Whitney test was used in the comparison between two groups with quantitative data and non-parametric distribution. Chi-square test was used in the comparison between two groups with qualitative data and Fisher exact test was used instead of the chi-square test when the expected count in any cell found to be less than 5. Univariate analysis was performed using paired t test for continuous variables. In all statistical analyses, $p < 0.05$ was considered significant.

Results

This study included 85 adult diabetic patients with chronic HCV infection, 5 patients (5.8%) of them were cirrhotic (child A) and 14 patients (16.4%) were hypertensive; by history and clinical examinations, there were no any associated diabetic microvascular or macrovascular complications. All included patients were HCV genotype 4. The mean (SD) diabetic duration of the enrolled patients was 11 (5.3). The baseline demographic and clinical characteristics of all included patients are summarized in Table 1. Table 2 demonstrates the statistical comparison of the post-treatment parameters in glycemic improved patients versus glycemic non-improved patients.

Statistical comparison between pre-treatment and post-treatment parameters in both glycemic improved and glycemic non-improved patients are shown in Tables 3 and 4, respectively. At the end of therapy, there was a significant decrease in hemoglobin, bilirubin, AST, ALT levels, AFP, and FIB-4 scores, in both studied groups (p value < 0.001) (Table 4).

At the end of treatment, 32 patients (37.6%) showed a significant improvement in the form of > 1% reduction in HbA1c level (p value < 0.001). Their baseline mean HbA1c level was 7.98 ± 0.62% which was significantly improved at the end of therapy to reach a level of 6.88 ± 0.81%. Meanwhile, 53 patients (62.4%) had a baseline mean HbA1c of 8.24 ± 0.64% and a post-treatment mean HbA1c level of 8.34 ± 0.61% (p value = 0.083).

Discussion

Chronic HCV infection is a major health-related burden in Egypt which affects 14.7% of the Egyptian population. Moreover, the incidence rate of HCV infection was reported to range between 2 and 6 per 1000 every year; this leads to an estimated 170,000 new cases every year to add to the 11.5 million patients suffering from the disease. Chronic infection with HCV is the leading cause of end-stage liver disease, HCC, and liver-related death in Egypt [12]. However, with a recent introduction of genotype 4 effective DAAs to the treatment protocol, there was a revolutionary reduction HCV epidemic in Egypt; DAAs combinations were reported to show high rates of SVR and pan-genotypic clinical efficacy in HCV genotypes 1–6 [13].

On the other hand, the current body of evidence shows a higher prevalence of T2DM among patients with chronic HCV infection, it was proposed that HCV proteins increase serine and threonine phosphorylation of insulin receptor substrate-1, which contributes to insulin resistance. In addition, HCV proteins enhance the release of proinflammatory cytokines such as interleukin-6 and tumor necrosis factor-α, which then upregulate gluconeogenesis and enhance lipid accumulation in the liver [14].

Therefore, it is presumed that effective HCV management would result in improved glycemic control in diabetic patients. A growing body of evidence has shown a promising role of effective HCV eradication on glycemic control of diabetic patients; previous reports showed that the change in HbA1c was greater in those who achieved SVR (0.98%) with DAAs than in those who sustained treatment failure. Also, the use of anti-diabetic medications decreased more in patients who achieved SVR than in those who failed to achieve SVR [15].

This was further confirmed by recent studies focusing on the association of SVR achievement and the glycemic improvement in HCV patients who received DAAs regimen [15, 16]. Meanwhile, we conducted our study only on patients who achieved SVR, in order to verify whether this suggested improvement is occurring to all patients who achieved SVR with DAAs or not.

The drop in average HbA1c level after treatment was greater in 37.6% of our included patients, from 7.98 to 6.88% (yielding a mean HA1C difference more than 1%), than in those for whom glycemic control failed (from 8.24 to 8.34%). Moreover, our results revealed that those who achieved a significant glycemic improvement were less likely to have hepatic fibrosis as presented by the FIB-4 score. In agreement with our findings, Abdel Alem and his colleagues reviewed the clinical records of 65 diabetic HCV patients; there were statistically significant declines in fasting plasma glucose and HbA1c values at SVR24. Notably, whatever the degree of hepatic fibrosis, the level of fasting plasma glucose and HbA1c decreased at SVR24 in comparison to the baseline level. The improvement rate of HbA1c was as high as 78% of the included patients [17].

Table 1 Baseline demographic and clinical characteristics of all included patients

	Glycemic non-improved Patients (no = 53)	Glycemic improved Patients (no = 32)	*P* value
Male, *n* (%)	21(39.6%)	12(37.5%)	0.846
Age (year)[a]	55.26 ± 9.24	57.50 ± 7.37	0.248
Insulin therapy, *n* (%)	23(43.4%)	13(40.6%)	0.538
Oral hypoglycemic therapy, *n* (%)	30(56.6%)	19(59.4%)	0.538
Family history of DM, *n* (%)	29(54.7%)	15(46.9%)	0.483
Hemoglobin (g/dL)[a]	12.98 ± 1.34	13.07 ± 1.05	0.764
Leukocytes (× 103/μL cells)[a]	6.53 ± 1.67	6.53 ± 1.91	0.998
Platelets (× 103/μL cells)[a]	223.57 ± 50.09	206.56 ± 53.82	0.144
Albumin (g/dL)[a]	4.25 ± 0.42	4.30 ± 0.40	0.622
Bilirubin, total (mg/dL)[a]	0.81 ± 0.15	0.78 ± 0.22	0.436
INR[a]	1.29 ± 1.36	1.41 ± 1.75	0.722
AST (IU/L)[a]	50.65 ± 24.36	51.59 ± 28.20	0.871
ALT (IU/L)[a]	55.71 ± 27.48	64.13 ± 35.90	0.227
Creatinine (mg/dL)[a]	1.02 ± 0.86	0.87 ± 0.15	0.304
AFP (ng/mL)[a]	7.08 ± 5.01	7.41 ± 6.24	0.789
HCV RNA viral load (log10 IU/mL)[a]	6.77 ± 6.661	6.77 ± 6.640	0.847
HbA1c (%)[a]	8.17 ± 0.58	7.91 ± 0.69	0.062
FIB-4[b] score[a]	1.89 ± 0.85	1.75 ± 0.76	0.442

[a]Mean ± SD. Glycemic improved group: ≥ 1% reduction of baseline HbA1c levels at SVR. Non-glycemic improved group: < 1% reduction of baseline HbA1c levels at SVR

AFP Alpha-fetoprotein, *ALT* Alanine transaminase, *AST* Aspartate transaminase, [b]FIB-4 score = [age 3AST]/[platelets 3 ALT1/2], *INR* international normalized ratio, *HbA1c* glycated hemoglobin

Table 2 Statistical comparison of the post-treatment parameters in glycemic improved patients versus glycemic non-improved patients

	Glycemic non-improved Patients (no = 53)	Glycemic improved Patients (no = 32)	*P* value
Hemoglobin (g/dL)[a]	12.25 ± 1.44	12.57 ± 1.23	0.289
Leukocytes (× 103/μL cells)[a]	6.98 ± 1.72	6.58 ± 2.03	0.337
Platelets (× 103/μL cells)[a]	228.9 ± 51.77	217.31 ± 47.82	0.307
Albumin (g/dL)[a]	4.28 ± 0.39	4.31 ± 0.37	0.664
Bilirubin, total (mg/dL)[a]	0.67 ± 0.16	0.67 ± 0.19	0.848
INR[a]	1.07 ± 0.06	1.07 ± 0.09	0.992
AST (IU/L)[a]	22.38 ± 7.83	24.53 ± 8.27	0.232
ALT (IU/L)[a]	23.87 ± 9.43	24.22 ± 7.98	0.861
Creatinine (mg/dL)[a]	0.93 ± 0.18	0.88 ± 0.15	0.181
HbA1c (%)[a]	7.91 ± 0.79	6.50 ± 0.72	< 0.001
AFP (ng/mL)[a]	6.43 ± 4.09	6.56 ± 5.94	0.906
FIB-4[b] score[a]	1.38 ± 0.47	1.17 ± 0.44	0.039

[a]Mean ± SD. Glycemic improved group: ≥ 1% reduction of baseline HbA1c levels at SVR. Non-glycemic improved group: < 1% reduction of baseline HbA1c levels at SVR

AFP Alpha-fetoprotein, *ALT* Alanine transaminase, *AST* Aspartate transaminase, [b]FIB-4 score = [age 3AST]/[platelets 3 ALT1/2], *INR* international normalized ratio, *HbA1c* glycated hemoglobin

Table 3 Statistical comparison between pre-treatment and post-treatment parameters in glycemic improved patients

	Pre-treatment (no = 32)	Post-treatment (no = 32)	*P* value
Hemoglobin (g/dL)[a]	13.07 ± 1.05	12.57 ± 1.23	0.002
Leukocytes (× 103/μL cells)[a]	6.53 ± 1.91	6.58 ± 2.03	0.876
Platelets (× 103/μL cells)[a]	206.56 ± 53.82	217.31 ± 47.82	0.130
Albumin (g/dL)[a]	4.30 ± 0.40	4.31 ± 0.37	0.501
Bilirubin, total (mg/dL)[a]	0.78 ± 0.22	0.67 ± 0.19	0.009
INR[a]	1.41 ± 1.75	1.07 ± 0.09	0.290
AST (IU/L)[a]	51.59 ± 28.20	24.53 ± 8.27	0.001
ALT (IU/L)[a]	64.13 ± 35.90	24.22 ± 7.98	0.001
Creatinine (mg/dL)[a]	0.87 ± 0.15	0.88 ± 0.15	0.525
HbA1c (%)[a]	7.91 ± 0.69	6.50 ± 0.72	0.001
AFP (ng/mL)[a]	7.41 ± 6.24	6.56 ± 5.94	0.032
FIB-4[b] score[a]	1.75 ± 0.76	1.17 ± 0.44	0.001

[a]Mean ± SD. Glycemic improved group: ≥ 1% reduction of baseline HbA1c levels at SVR. Non-glycemic improved group: < 1% reduction of baseline HbA1c levels at SVR

AFP Alpha-fetoprotein, *ALT* Alanine transaminase, *AST* Aspartate transaminase, [b]FIB-4 score = [age 3AST]/[platelets 3 ALT1/2], *INR* international normalized ratio, *HbA1c* glycated hemoglobin

Another report from Egypt by Dawood and his colleagues who included 460 T2DM patients with chronic HCV genotype 4 infection in order to evaluate the role of DAAs therapy on glycemic status. Their results showed that almost 77% of the patients achieved the improved glycemic control status after HCV-eradication by DAAs; moreover, the HbA1c and fasting blood glucose levels changed significantly 6 months following treatment [18].

In concordance with our findings, Pavone and his colleagues reported a statistically significant reduction in HbA1c, with a reduction of the mean value of 1.95%, during the DAAs treatment [11]. The impact of HCV eradication on the glycemic control was also evaluated by Gilad and his colleagues who studied the clinical characteristics of 122 diabetic patients with chronic HCV infection; the authors reported that HbA1c at the nearest time point before treatment was 8.4% ± 1.9%, compared with 7.8% ± 1.7% after treatment, a mean difference of 0.6% [9].

As regards to our patients who did not achieve the expected glycemic improvement at the end of therapy, this may be explained by two factors as proposed by Hashim et al. (2018); first, the etiology of T2DM in HCV-infected individuals has been postulated to result from either hepatogenous T2DM or classical T2DM due to

Table 4 Statistical comparison between pre-treatment and post-treatment parameters in glycemic non-improved patients

	Pre-treatment (no = 53)	Post-treatment (no = 53)	*P* value
Hemoglobin (g/dL)[a]	12.98 ± 1.34	12.25 ± 1.44	0.001
Leukocytes (× 103/μL cells)[a]	6.53 ± 1.67	6.98 ± 1.72	0.038
Platelets (× 103/μL cells)[a]	223.57 ± 50.09	228.91 ± 51.77	0.150
Albumin (g/dL)[a]	4.25 ± 0.42	4.28 ± 0.39	0.249
Bilirubin, total (mg/dL)[a]	0.81 ± 0.15	0.67 ± 0.16	0.001
INR[a]	1.29 ± 1.36	1.07 ± 0.06	0.253
AST (IU/L)[a]	50.65 ± 24.36	22.38 ± 7.83	0.001
ALT (IU/L)[a]	55.71 ± 27.48	23.87 ± 9.43	0.001
Creatinine (mg/dL)[a]	1.02 ± 0.86	0.93 ± 0.18	0.404
HbA1c (%)[a]	8.17 ± 0.58	7.91 ± 0.79	0.001
AFP (ng/mL)[a]	7.08 ± 5.01	6.43 ± 4.09	0.012
FIB-4[b] score[a]	1.89 ± 0.85	1.38 ± 0.47	0.001

[a]Mean ± SD. Glycemic improved group: ≥ 1% reduction of baseline HbA1c levels at SVR. Non-glycemic improved group: < 1% reduction of baseline HbA1c levels at SVR

AFP Alpha-fetoprotein, *ALT* Alanine transaminase, *AST* Aspartate transaminase, [b]FIB-4 score = [age 3AST]/[platelets 3 ALT1/2], *INR* international normalized ratio, *HbA1c* glycated hemoglobin

virally mediated IR. Second explanation, HCV infection may affect glucose level by an autoimmune mechanism on β cells and is not related to IR [19].

However, it should be noted that there were limitations in the present study; the sample size and the duration of follow-up, it is well established that the micro-vascular complications of diabetes, including nephropathy, neuropathy, and retinopathy, improve with lowered HbA1c level. Therefore, early treatment of HCV could potentially slow the onset and progression of micro-vascular complications of diabetes. Given the study period, we were unable to evaluate whether improved glycemic control was durable beyond 3 months. Therefore, larger studies with a longer duration of follow-up are recommended to validate these findings.

Conclusion

In conclusion, our study reported that HCV eradication with DAAs leads to a significant reduction in HbA1c level (HbA1C improvement of more than 1%) in 37.6% of patients with diabetes. Meanwhile, 62.4% patients showed a reduction in HbA1c level less than 1% at 12 weeks after the end of therapy. These findings raise the question to whether the HCV eradication may also impact the future morbidity due to T2DM and slowing the onset and progression of micro-vascular complications of diabetes, as well as the degree of improvement of hepatic fibrosis induced by chronic HCV. For this reason, close follow-up post-HCV treatment is needed, and large prospective studies are recommended to validate these results.

Abbreviations

AFP: Alpha fetoprotein; CTP: Child–Turcotte–Pugh; CBC: Complete blood count; DAAs: Direct-acting antivirals; Hba1c: Hemoglobin A1c; Hbs Ag: Hepatitis B virus surface antigen; HCV: Hepatitis C virus; HCC: Hepatocellular carcinoma; HOMA: Homeostatic model assessment; IRB: Institutional Review Board; IR: Insulin resistance; INR: International normalized ratio; NCCVH: National Committee for Control of Viral Hepatitis; Peg: Pegylated interferon; RBV: Ribavirin; PT: Prothrombin time; SVR: Sustained virological response; T2DM: Type 2 diabetes mellitus

Acknowledgements

I wish to express my great appreciation to all those who assisted us to complete this work in the Tropical Medicine Department, Aswan University Hospital.

Authors' contributions

MME contributed in conception of the study design, clinical supervision and acceptance of the final form of the manuscript. DAA contributed in clinical examinations and collection of data. NHE contributed in statistical analysis and writing of the manuscript. MAA contributed in the laboratory investigations' design, supervision, and writing of the manuscript. All authors read and approved the final manuscript.

Competing interests

The authors have no conflict of interest to declare.

Author details

[1]Department of Tropical Medicine and Gastroenterology, Faculty of Medicine, Aswan University, Aswan, Egypt. [2]Department of Moleculer genetics, National Research Center, Cairo, Egypt. [3]Department of Clinical Pathology, Faculty of Medicine, Ain Shams University, Cairo, Egypt.

References

1. Mohd Hanafiah K, Groeger J, Flaxman AD, Wiersma ST (2013) Global epidemiology of hepatitis C virus infection: new estimates of agespecific antibody to HCV seroprevalence. Hepatology (Baltimore, Md) 57(4):1333–1342
2. Petruzziello A, Marigliano S, Loquercio G, Cozzolino A, Cacciapuoti C (2016) Global epidemiology of hepatitis C virus infection: an up-date of the distribution and circulation of hepatitis C virus genotypes. World J Gastroenterol 22(34):7824–7840
3. Gower E, Estes C, Blach S, Razavi-Shearer K, Razavi H (2014) Global epidemiology and genotype distribution of the hepatitis C virus infection. J Hepatol 61(1 Suppl):S45–S57
4. El-Ghitany E (2019) Hepatitis C virus infection in Egypt: current situation and future perspective. J High Inst Public Health 49(1):1–9. https://doi.org/10.21608/jhiph.2019.29460
5. Hum J, Jou JH (2018) The link between hepatitis C virus and diabetes mellitus: improvement in insulin resistance after eradication of hepatitis C virus. Clin Liver Dis (Hoboken) 11(3):73–76
6. Gaetano JN (2014) Benefit-risk assessment of new and emerging treatments for hepatitis C: focus on simeprevir and sofosbuvir. Drug Healthc Patient Saf 6:37–45
7. Delgado-Borrego A, Jordan SH, Negre B, Healey D, Lin W, Kamegaya Y (2010) Reduction of insulin resistance with effective clearance of hepatitis C infection: results from the HALT-C trial. Clin Gastroenterol Hepatol 8(5):458–462
8. Aghemo A, Prati GM, Rumi MG, Soffredini R, D'Ambrosio R, Orsi E, De Nicola S, Degasperi E, Grancini V, Colombo M (2012) Sustained virological response prevents the development of insulin resistance in patients with chronic hepatitis C. Hepatology 56(5):1681–1687
9. Gilad A, Fricker ZP, Hsieh A, Thomas DD, Zahorian T, Nunes DP (2019) Sustained improvement in type 2 diabetes mellitus is common after treatment of hepatitis C virus with direct-acting antiviral therapy. J Clin Gastroenterol 53(8):616–620
10. American Diabetes Association (2020) Standards of medical care in diabetes—2020. Diabetes Care 43(8):1981–1981. https://doi.org/10.2337/dc20-ad08c
11. Pavone P, Tieghi T, d'Ettorre G, Lichtner M, Marocco R, Mezzaroma I, Vullo V (2016) Rapid decline of fasting glucose in HCV diabetic patients treated with direct-acting antiviral agents. Clin Microbiol Infect 22:462.e1–462.e3
12. Elgharably A, Gomaa AI, Crossey MM, Norsworthy PJ, Waked I, Taylor-Robinson SD (2016) Hepatitis C in Egypt - past, present, and future. Int J Gen Med 10:1–6
13. Omran D, Alboraie M, Zayed RA, Wifi MN, Naguib M, Eltabbakh M, Abdellah M, Sherief AF, Maklad S, Eldemellawy HH, Saad OK, Khamiss DM, El Kassas M (2018) Towards hepatitis C virus elimination: Egyptian experience, achievements and limitations. World J Gastroenterol 24(38):4330–4340
14. Parvaiz F, Manzoor S, Iqbal J, Sarkar-Dutta M, Imran M, Waris G (2015) Hepatitis C virus NS5A promotes insulin resistance through IRS-1 serine phosphorylation and increased gluconeogenesis. World J Gastroenterol 21(43):12361–12369
15. Hum J, Jou JH, Green PK, Berry K, Lundblad J, Hettinger BD, Ioannou GN (2017) Improvement in glycemic control of type 2 diabetes after successful treatment of hepatitis C virus. Diabetes Care 40:1173–1180
16. Ciancio A, Bosio R, Bo S, Pellegrini M, Sacco M, Vogliotti E, Fassio G, AGF BMD, Gallo M, Giordanino C, Terzi di Bergamo L, Ribaldone D, Bugianesi E, Smedile A, Rizzetto M, Saracco GM (2018) Significant improvement of glycemic control in diabetic patients with HCV infection responding to direct-acting antiviral agents. J Med Virol 90:320–327
17. Abdel Alem S, Elsharkawy A, Fouad R, Adel E, Abdellatif Z, Musa S, Nagy A, Hussein MS, Yosry A, Esmat GJ (2017) Improvement of glycemic state among responders to Sofosbuvir-based treatment regimens: single center experience. J Med Virol 89(12):2181–2187
18. Dawood AA, Nooh MZ, Elgamal AA (2017) Factors associated with improved glycemic control by direct-acting antiviral agent treatment in Egyptian type 2 diabetes mellitus patients with chronic hepatitis C genotype 4. Diabetes Metab J 41:316–321

16

Apparent diffusion coefficient for differentiating between benign and malignant hepatic focal lesions

Sherif Abugamra[1], Aya Yassin[1], Asmaa Saber Mostafa Abdel-Rehim[2] and Dina Sayed Sheha[2*]

Abstract

Background: The aim of this study was to prospectively evaluate the role of diffusion weight MRI (DWI) in the characterization of hepatic focal lesions by using apparent diffusion coefficient (ADC). Thirty patients (18 women, 12 men; mean age 48.5 years) with hepatic focal lesions were included in this study. Patients underwent DW MR imaging with the SPLICE sequence. ADC of each focal lesion carcinoma was calculated from DW MR Images obtained with low and high *b* values. ADCs were compared among pathological types of focal lesions.

Results: Among the 30 patients included in the study, 46 focal lesions were detected. Twenty-four lesions were metastatic lesions from primary cancer, 7 lesions were hepatocellular carcinoma (HCC), 9 lesions were hemangiomas, and 6 lesions were simple cysts. There was highly significant difference between the mean ADC of the malignant lesions (metastasis and HCC) and the mean ADC of benign lesions (hemangiomas and cysts). The ADC of malignant lesion was much less than that of benign lesion. The mean ADC of malignant lesions ($n = 31$) was $0.73 \pm 0.19 \times 10^{-3}$ mm^2/s, and the mean ADC of benign lesions ($n = 15$) was $1.94 \pm 0.68 \times 10^{-3}$ mm^2/s (p value < 0.001). There was no significant difference between the cysts and hemangiomas. There was no statistically significant difference between the metastases and hepatocellular carcinoma.

Conclusion: ADCs values were able to differentiate benign from malignant lesions. ADC should be considered in the work up of patients with hepatic focal lesions.

Keywords: Liver, Diffusion, Hepatic focal lesions, Hepatocellular carcinoma

Background

Liver masses have currently been recognized and gained great attention. Most of these masses are known to be benign. Also, many cancer patients may coincidently have benign liver focal lesions that are confused for metastasis or primary liver malignancy [1]. The precise characterization of hepatic focal lesions is crucial for the diagnosis and management of patients [2], and accurate evaluation is essential to avoid unnecessary and incorrect intervention or treatment [1]. Common benign tumors include hemangiomas, fatty infiltration, adenoma, and cysts. As regards malignant liver tumors, metastases are considered 20 times more common than primary hepatocellular carcinoma [3].

Egypt is known for its high prevalence of hepatitis C virus [4], and therefore, close follow-up is essential to identify and detect the cases with hepatocellular carcinoma (HCC), which represents the fourth most common cancer in Egypt [5]. The serum biomarker, alpha-fetoprotein (AFP), is most commonly used in early diagnosis of HCC [6], However, some studies showed that AFP levels appeared to be normal in 40% of cases with HCC especially in their early stages [7, 8]. Other studies demonstrated high levels of AFP in cirrhotic patients and patients with chronic hepatitis [9, 10]. Usually confirmation of diagnosis of HCC is done by routine biopsy. Unfortunately, biopsy exposes

* Correspondence: shehadina@yahoo.com
[2]Department of Internal Medicine, Allergy and Clinical Immunology Unit, Ain Shams University, Khalifa El-Maamon St., Abbasiya sq, Cairo 11566, Egypt

the patient to undesirable risks and may delay diagnosis and treatment [11].

In the past few years, diagnosis of HCC through radiology has gained great support and attention. The international guidelines, European Association for the Study of the Liver (EASL) and American Association of the Study of Liver Disease (AASLD), accept and approve the use of radiology for diagnosis of HCC provided that it meets high-quality and defined imaging criteria [11].

The current imaging procedures to diagnose focal lesions are ultrasonography and computed tomography. Magnetic resonance imaging (MRI) is reserved to characterize lesions when not specified by other modalities. The inherent advantages of high contrast resolution, lack of ionizing radiation, as well as usage of advanced sequences and MR techniques renders it a favored modality [12].

The hepatic focal lesions are diagnosed based on their morphology and intensity on different sequences and their contrast behavior. There is still further accuracy needed for further differentiation between benign and malignant lesions [13].

Diffusion MRI has been used recently as a tool for further characterization of the hepatic focal lesions. This is available through measurement of apparent diffusion coefficient (ADC). Several studies have reported that ADC can contribute to the differentiation between benign and malignant lesions. The concomitant use with contrast enhancement criteria increases the accuracy of detection and characterization [14].

Therefore, the aim of the current work was to study a group of patients with hepatic focal lesions using the diffusion sequence as well as calculating the ADC value to differentiate between benign and malignant lesions.

Methods

Thirty patients with focal hepatic lesions were included in this study. The study was performed between June 2017 and January 2018. Patients with liver disease or known focal liver lesions who attended the Internal Medicine outpatient clinic or the emergency room at Ain Shams University Hospital were admitted and referred to the MRI unit of Ain Shams University Hospital for completion of the study. Informed verbal consent was taken from the patients and the local ethical committee approved the study. Patients were diagnosed according to AASLD practice guidelines [15]. Biopsy was done for some cases (to confirm whether HCC or metastases) and imaging, including MRI with diffusion-weighted imaging (DWI), was done for participants.

MRI examination

Conventional MRI, post-Gd-DTPA dynamic and diffusion MR imaging were performed. First blind characterization and detection of focal lesions was performed, and then the diffusion images with ADC values were reviewed. All imaging results were verified against a standard of reference, which is a pathological verification. MR imaging was performed on high-field system (1.5 Tesla) magnet units (Philips Intera) using a phased array coil to cover the whole liver.

MR protocol used

Pre-contrast imaging included

Steps of pre-contrast imaging:

1. Axial T1-weighted imaging (T1WI)
2. Coronal T2-weighted imaging
3. Axial T2 SPAIR
4. Axial T1 in and out of phase
5. Axial heavy T2-weighted imaging

- T1-weighted (T1W) images: repetition time (TR) = 10 ms, echo time (TE) = 4.58 ms, matrix 179/320, slice thickness 7–8 mm, slice gap 1–2 mm, and FOV 355 mm.
- T2-weighted (T2W) images (single shot free breathing): TR ≥ 445 ms, TE = 26–28 ms, matrix 180–200 × 240 with a field of view: 365, slice thickness 7–8 mm, slice gap 1–2 mm.

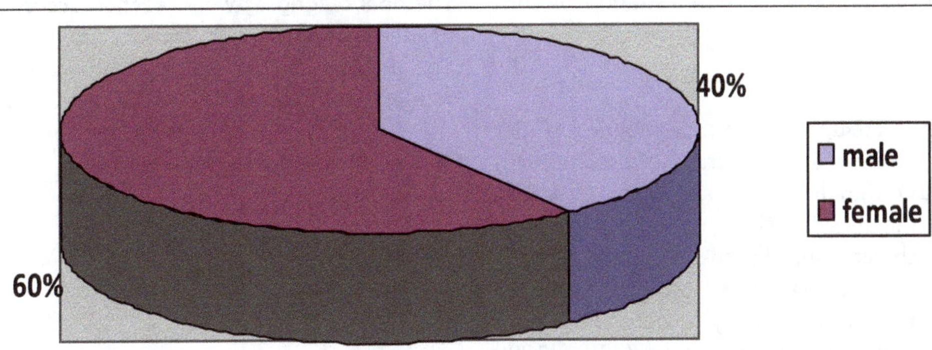

Fig. 1 Gender distribution of patients

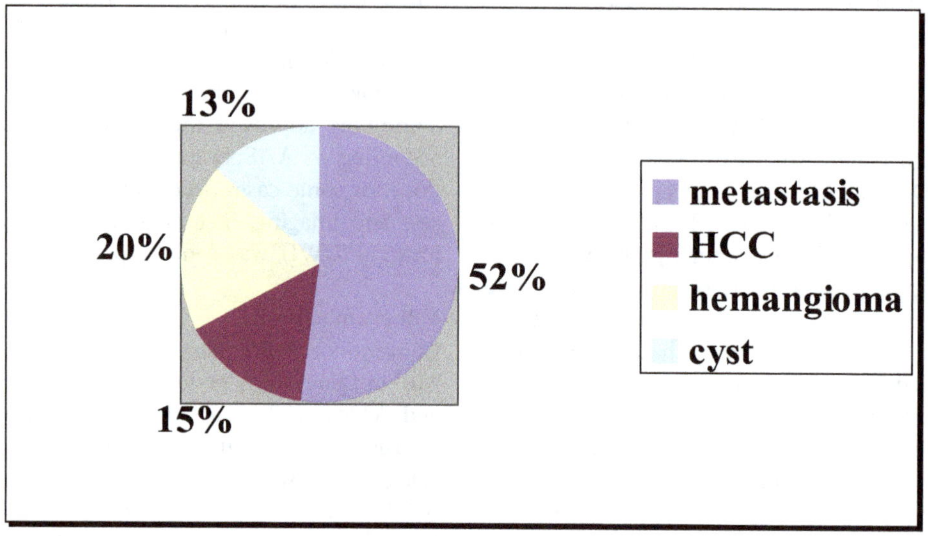

Fig. 2 Percentage of the lesions according to the pathological types

- T2 SPAIR (Spectral Attenuated Inversion Recovery) fat suppression sequence: TR ≥ 400 ms, TE = 80 ms, matrix 204 × 384 with a field of view: 365 slice thickness 7–8 mm, slice gap 1–2 mm.
- In phase and out phase gradient echo sequence (Dual/FFE): TR = 75–100 ms, TE = 4.6 ms for in phase and 2.3 ms for out phase, matrix 143 × 240 with a field of view: 345 slice thickness 7–8 mm, slice gap 0 mm.
- Heavy T2-weighted images: TR = 520 ms, TE = 200 ms, matrix 235/384 with a field of view: 375 slice thickness 7–8 mm, slice gap 1–2 mm.

Dynamic study

Dynamic study was performed after bolus injection of 0.1 mmol/kg body weight of Gd-DTPA at a rate of 2 ml/s, flushed with 20 ml of sterile 0.9% saline solution from the antecubital vein. The injection of contrast media and saline solution was performed manually. Dynamic imaging using T1 THRIVE (high resolution isotropic volume Examination) technique was performed in triphasic way [arterial phase (16–20 s), porto-venous phase (45–60 s), and delayed equilibrium phase (3–5 min) after administration of contrast media.

Diffusion study

Respiratory-triggered fat-suppressed single-shot echoplanar DW imaging was performed in the transverse plane with tri-directional diffusion gradients by using *b* values 0, 500, and 1000 s/mm^2 to increase sensitivity to cellular packing. Parallel imaging with generalized auto-calibrating partially parallel acquisition (GRAPPA) with an acceleration factor of two was applied to improve image quality. The other parameters were as follows: repetition time (TR) ≥ 1880 ms, echo time (TE) = 70 ms, number of excitations (NEX) = 3, matrix 256 × 256 with a field of view as small as possible with 52% rectangular field of view, slice thickness 7–8 mm, slice gap 1–2 mm, scan time 3–4 min.

Imaging evaluation

The morphological features of each lesion were recorded included size, shape, margin, signal characteristics, pattern of enhancement in the dynamic imaging, and as number and site of the detected focal lesions. Then provisional diagnosis was reported. A 10-year experienced radiologist (AY) reviewed the diffusion images with ADC values for final radiological characterization and detection of focal lesions.

ADC calculation

The mean ADC of each focal lesion detected was measured by drawing a region of interest over the lesion. The ADC was measured twice and the two measurements were averaged. To ensure that the same areas were measured, regions of interest were copied and pasted from DW images to ADC maps.

The final diagnoses were reached according to standard of reference (SOR)

For lesion characterization, all imaging results were refined against a predefined SOR. A range of procedures

Table 1 Number of lesions according to the size

Size of lesions (cm)	Number of lesions
0.5–1	8
1.1–2	9
2.1–5	21
5.1–10	6
> 10	2

Table 2 ADC of metastatic lesions and HCC

Sup-groups		ADC				T test	
		Min.	Max.	Mean	±SD	T	p value
Metastasis	24	0.20	0.90	0.70	0.18	− 1.427	0.164
HCC	7	0.50	1.10	0.81	0.21		

was identified as valid "gold standards" for the characterization of lesions. The pathological results of the lesions were reviewed after blinded radiological diagnosis.

Statistical analysis

Data were analyzed using IBM© SPSS© Statistics version 23 (IBM© Corp., Armonk, NY) and MedCalc© version 18.2.1 (MedCalc© Software bvba, Ostend, Belgium).

Quantitative data were expressed as mean ± standard deviation (SD). Qualitative data were expressed as frequency and percentage. Comparative analysis was done using Student's t test and chi-square tests for quantitative and qualitative data, respectively. Correlations were done using Spearman's correlation coefficient. Probability (p value) was considered significant if it is < 0.05, highly significant if $p < 0.01$ and insignificant if $p > 0.05$.

Results

Thirty patients were enrolled in this study. The age ranged between 18 years and 73 years with mean age of 48.5 ± 18.37 years (Fig. 1).

There were 46 focal hepatic lesions in our patients. Twenty-four lesions (52%) were metastatic lesions from primary cancer, 7 lesions (15%) were HCC, 9 lesions (20%) were hemangiomas, and 6 lesions (13%) were simple cystic (Fig. 2).

As regards the size of the lesions, 8 lesions were measured as 0.5–1 cm, 9 lesions were measured as 1.1–2 cm, 21 lesions were measured as 2.1–5 cm, 6 lesions were measured as 5.1–10 cm, and only 2 lesions were measured as more than 10 cm (Table 1).

All cystic lesions showed facilitated diffusion, where they showed reduction of signal intensity on increasing the b values, and those which did not show reduction of signal showed high signal on ADC map, which also reflects facilitated diffusion. On the other hand, all solid lesions showed restricted diffusion evidenced by increased signal on increasing the b values and low signal on ADC maps.

ADC values

ADC values were obtained for all 46 focal hepatic lesions detected at consensus reading. The mean ADC value of the 24 metastatic lesions was 0.7 ± 0.18 × 10^{-3} mm^2/s. The mean ADC value of the 7 cirrhotic lesions in HCC patients was 0.81 ± 0.21 × 10^{-3} mm^2/s. The difference between the mean ADC of the two subtypes of malignant lesions was statistically insignificant (p value 0.16, NS) (Table 2) (Figs. 3, 4 and 5).

As regards the ADC of benign lesions (hemangioma and cystic lesions), the mean ADC of hemangioma was

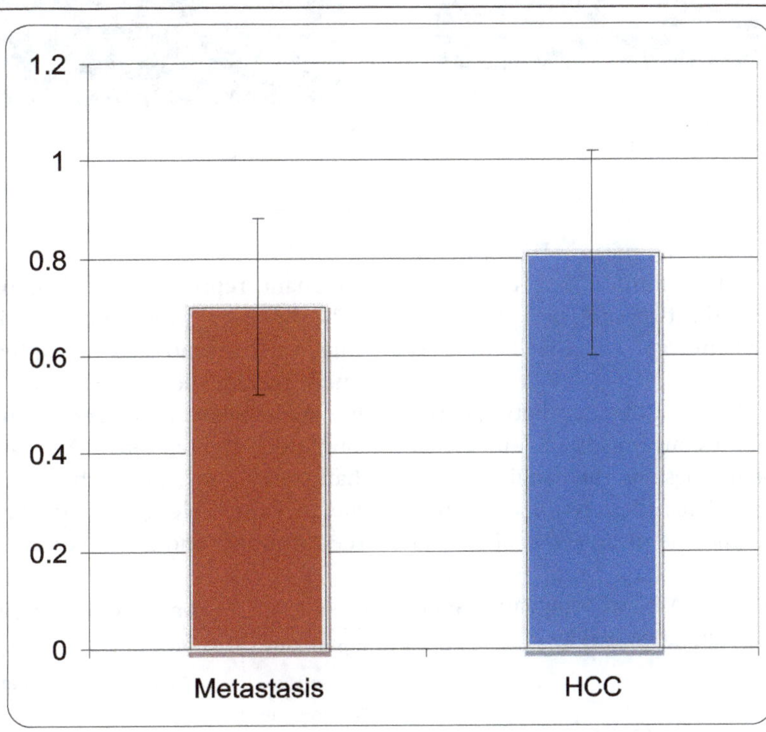

Fig. 3 ADC of metastatic lesions and HCC

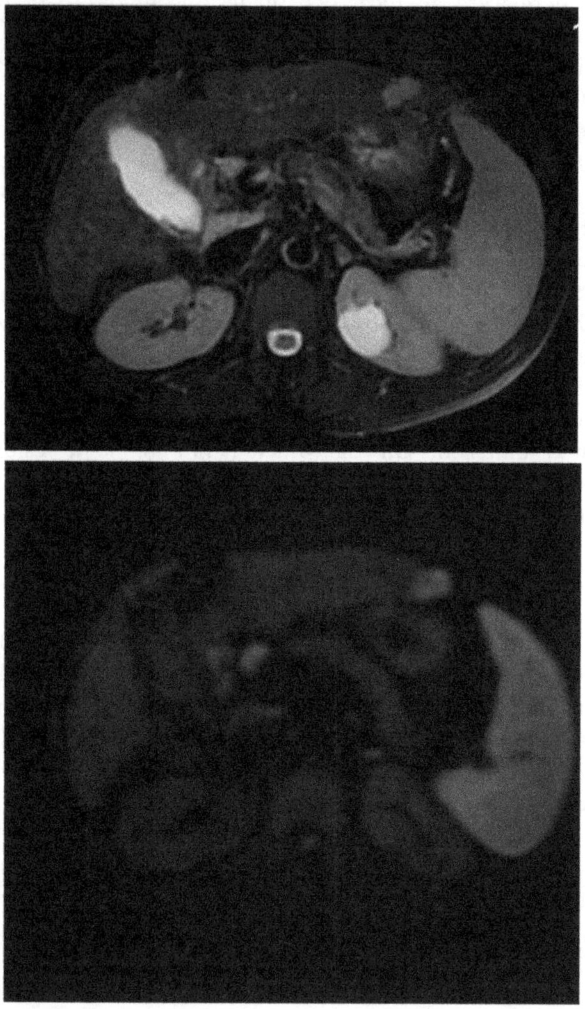

Fig. 4 a A 54-year-old male with liver cirrhosis and elevated Alfa feto protein proved to be hepatocellular carcinoma. Axial T2 fat sat shows a hyperintense focal lesion (arrowed). **b** Axial DWI, *b* value = 600 showing restricted diffusion within the lesion

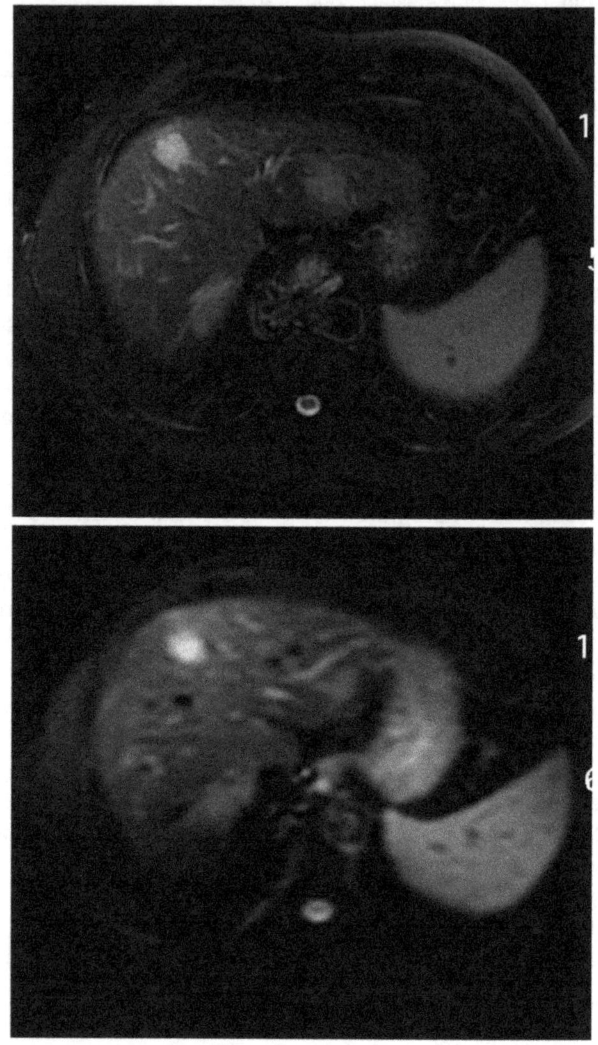

Fig. 5 a A 64-year-old male with history of pancreatic carcinoma. Axial T2 WI fat sat shows hyperintense focal lesion (arrowed). **b** Axial DWI *b* value = 600 showing restricted diffusion

$1.72 \pm 0.55 \times 10^{-3}$ mm^2/s, and the mean ADC of cystic lesions was $2.27 \pm 0.78 \times 10^{-3}$ mm^2/s. The difference between the mean ADC of the two subtypes of benign lesions was statistically insignificant (*p* value 0.13, NS) (Table 3) (Fig. 5).

There was a highly significant difference between the mean ADC of the malignant lesions (metastasis and HCC) and the mean ADC of benign lesions (hemangioma and cyst). The mean ADC of malignant lesions (n = 31) was $0.73 \pm 0.19 \times 10^{-3}$ mm^2/s and the mean ADC of benign lesions (n = 15) was $1.94 \pm 0.68 \times 10^{-3}$ mm^2/s (*p* value < 0.001, S) (Table 4, Fig. 6). The ADC of malignant lesions was much less than that of benign lesions (Fig. 7).

Discussion

Focal lesions of the liver are a commonly encountered incidental finding. Focal lesions could be benign or malignant, representing a diagnostic dilemma, especially with the high prevalence of viral hepatitis in Egypt. Thus, early diagnosis is warranted to ensure optimal and timely management of hepatic focal lesions. Currently, the guidelines are dependent on ultrasonography and computed tomography; MR is reserved for further characterization since it has higher contrast resolution, safe in vulnerable groups of patients due to radiation-free technique and a safe contrast agent [16].

Table 3 ADC of hemangioma and cyst

Sup-groups		ADC				*T* test	
		Min.	Max.	Mean	±SD	*T*	*p* value
Hemangioma	9	1.30	3.00	1.72	0.55	− 1.593	0.135
CYST	6	1.50	3.20	2.27	0.78		

Table 4 ADC of malignant and benign lesions

Groups	ADC			*T* test	
	N	Mean	±SD	*T*	*p* value
Malignant	31	0.73	0.19	− 9.279	< 0.001
Benign	15	1.94	0.68		

Diffusion imaging carries the advantage of using non-contrast agent, in addition to being dependent on tissue cellularity, organization, and integrity of cell membranes. These factors render it useful for detecting malignant lesions and differentiating tumorous from non-tumorous tissues [17].

In the current study, we aimed to demonstrate the use of diffusion MRI in differentiating benign from malignant liver lesions using the current sequence and comparing it to previously published literature. We used 3 *b* values 0, 200, and 800 as used in several studies including Demir et al. in 2007, Koike et al. in 2009, and Hosny et al. in 2010 [18–20].

In our study, the lesions were detected on DWI. Interestingly, the smallest detected lesion was 0.5 cm, thus demonstrating its capability of detecting small lesions. While cysts and hemangiomas showed facilitated diffusion, solid neoplastic lesions showed restricted diffusion. This came in agreement with *Taouli and Koh* who reported that cellular hepatic lesions such as tumors demonstrated restricted diffusion at *b* values higher than 500 s/mm^2 [17]. This could be explained by the fact that DWI depends on several factors including tissue cellularity. Since the main target of DWI is extracellular diffusion, high cellular tissue leads to a short diffusion path, resulting in low ADC values as seen in solid malignant lesions. On the other hand, low cellular lesions with less structural barriers as seen in cysts enhance longer diffusion path [21–23].

The absolute ADC values of different types of lesions were variable due to differences in techniques applied by *b* values, different breath measurement techniques, and mathematical logarithms. Petra and Eric stated similar findings in 2010 [24]. The authors compared their findings with previous studies that used different DWI techniques, and reported that some publications preferred using breath-hold, or in other words respiratory triggered DWI, rather than using the conventional T2-weighed MRI, while others favored both modalities in conjunction to obtain better results especially in atypical lesions, in order to avoid artifacts that might occur with measuring techniques of DWI.

The ADC measurement of benign and malignant lesions was significantly different with *p* value < 0.0001, which comes in agreement with a previous study by Onur et al. 2012. The authors found the mean ADC values differentiating benign and malignant lesions were statistically significant [25]. According to another study,

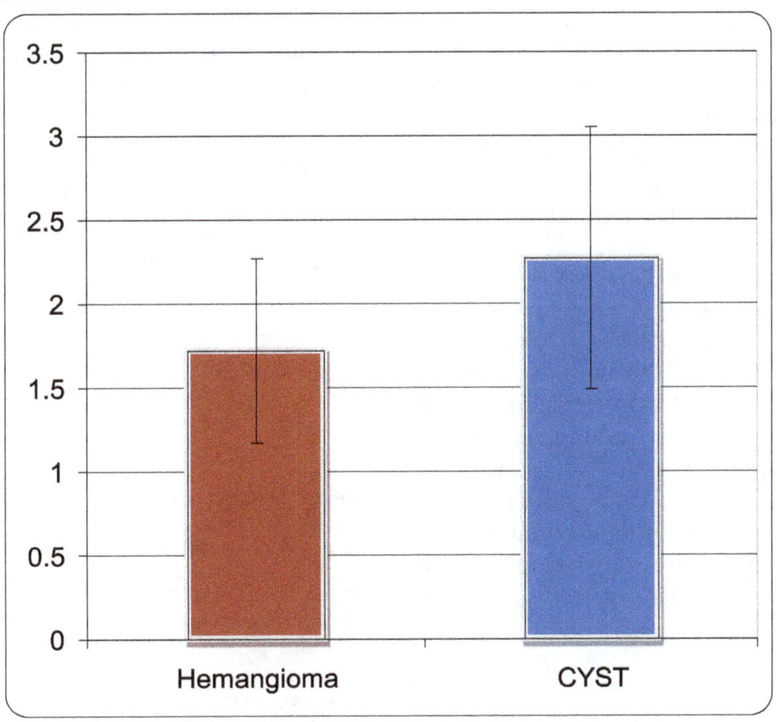

Fig. 6 ADC of hemangioma and cyst

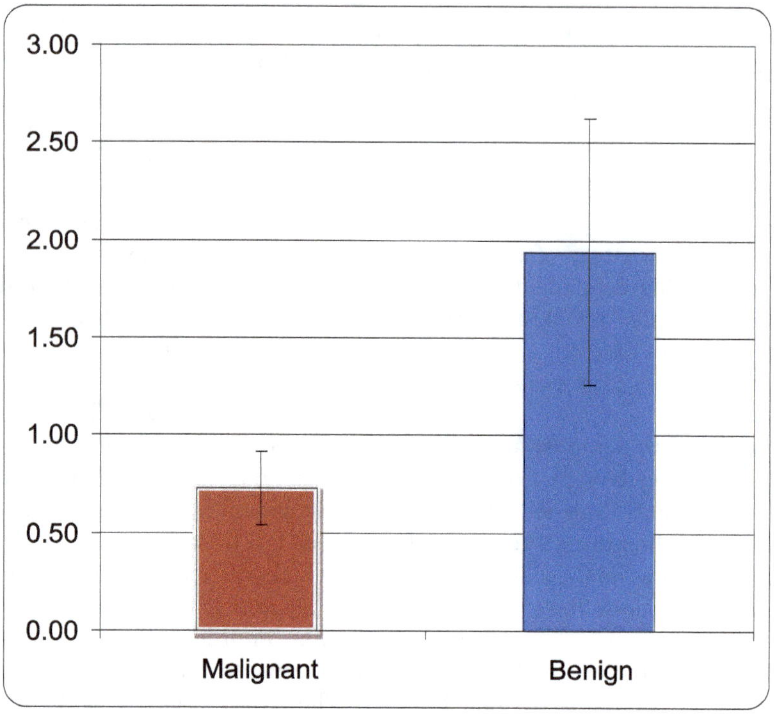

Fig. 7 ADC of malignant and benign lesions

although the authors recommended that the value of DWI should be highly considered, and showed the importance of ADC in focal lesions, they advised it careful interpretation since overlaps may occur between focal lesions as hemangiomas and metastases [26].

Some studies have indicated that AFP has substantially limited diagnostic accuracy in detecting small HCC [27]. As mentioned previously, AFP may be normal. We hence speculate that combination of AFP and ADC together could be useful in predicting malignancy. Unfortunately, they cannot differentiate primary from secondary malignancy.

Our study has some limitations. First, the DW data set was only respiratory triggered which has some limitations including cardiac motion artifacts and noise contamination that may distort ADC values. Second, the small number of patients included, especially in the subgroups of benign and malignant groups respectively. Additionally, benign lesions were limited to hemangiomas and cysts, while adenomas, focal nodular hyperplasia, and abscesses were not studied. Future multi-center studies with a larger sample size and including more pathologies of benign liver focal lesions are warranted to confirm our findings.

Conclusion

In conclusion, the DWI with ADC calculation could be used to differentiate between benign and malignant liver focal lesions. We recommend incurring such calculation in institutions across Egypt for accurate characterization of liver focal lesions. However, it is still not of clear value in identifying individual lesions; thus, we recommend further larger scale, multi-center studies to detect further modalities to identify individual lesions and differentiate between benign and malignant liver focal lesions.

Abbreviations

ADC: Apparent diffusion coefficient; AFP: Alpha-fetoprotein; AASLD: American Association of the study of liver disease; DWI: Diffusion-weighted imaging; TE: Echo time; EASL: European association for the study of the liver; GRAPPA: Generalized auto-calibrating partially parallel acquisition; HCC: Hepatocellular carcinoma; MRI: Magnetic resonance imaging; NEX: Number of excitations; TR: Repetition time; SD: Standard deviation; SPSS: Statistical Program for Social Science; T1W: T1 weighted

Acknowledgements

We would like to acknowledge the contributions of the Public Health and community department for helping in the biostatistical analysis.

Authors' contributions

SA made substantial contributions to the design of the work. AY made substantial contributions to the conception of the idea and substantial revision of the work. AS made substantial contributions to acquisition and analysis of data. DS contributed to revising the work and interpretation, acquisition, and analysis of data. All authors have read and approved the final manuscript.

Competing interests

The authors declare that they have no competing interests.

Author details
[1]Department of Radiodiagnosis, Ain Shams University, Khalifa El-Maamon St., Abbasiya sq, Cairo 11566, Egypt. [2]Department of Internal Medicine, Allergy and Clinical Immunology Unit, Ain Shams University, Khalifa El-Maamon St., Abbasiya sq, Cairo 11566, Egypt.

References

1. Heiken JP (2007) Distinguishing benign from malignant liver tumours. Cancer Imaging. 7:S1–S14
2. Heslin MJ, Medina-Franco H, Parker M et al (2001) Colorectal hepatic metastases: resection, local ablation, and hepatic artery infusion pump are associated with prolonged survival. Arch Surg. 136(3):318–323
3. Xia Q, Feng Y, Wu C et al (2015) Differentiation between malignant and benign solitary lesions in the liver with FDG PET/CT: accuracy of age-related diagnostic standard. Journal of Cancer. 6:40–47
4. Doss W, Hermez J, Atta H, Jabbour J (2018) Towards a hepatitis-free Egypt: is this achievable? East Mediterr Health J. 24(7):609–610. https://doi.org/10.26719/2018.24.7.609
5. Akinyemiju T, Abera S, Ahmed M, Alam N, Alemayohu MA, Allen C et al (2017) The burden of primary liver cancer and underlying etiologies from 1990 to 2015 at the global, regional, and national level. JAMA Oncol. 3: 1683–1691
6. Song PP, Feng X, Zhang K et al (2013) Perspectives on using des-ycarboxyprothrombin (DCP) as a serum biomarker: facilitating early detection of hepatocellular carcinoma in China. Hepatobiliary Surg Nutr. 2: 227–231
7. Daniele B, Bencivenga A, Megna AS et al (2004) Alpha-fetoprotein and ultrasonography screening for hepatocellular carcinoma. Gastroenterology. 127(Suppl 1):S108–S112
8. Marrero JA (2005) Screening tests for hepatocellular carcinoma. Clin Liver Dis. 9(235-251):vi
9. Di Bisceglie AM, Hoofnagle JH (1989) Elevations in serum alpha-fetoprotein levels in patients with chronic hepatitis B. Cancer. 64:2117–2120
10. Colli A, Fraquelli M, Casazza G et al (2006) Accuracy of ultrasonography, spiral CT, magnetic resonance, and alpha fetoprotein in diagnosing hepatocellular carcinoma: A systematic review. Am J Gastroenterol. 101: 513–523
11. Heuman DM, Gilles HS, Solomon C et al (2012) Should a radiological diagnosis of hepatocellular carcinoma be routinely confirmed by a biopsy? No. Eur J Intern Med. 23(1):37–39
12. Chandarana H, Block TK, Rosenkrantz AB et al (2011) Free-breathing radial 3D fat-suppressed T1-weighted gradient echo sequence: a viable alternative for contrast-enhanced liver imaging in patients unable to suspend respiration. Invest Radiol. 46(10):648–653
13. Vergara ML, Fernández M, Pereira R (2010) Diffusion-weighted MRI characterization of solid liver lesions. Revista Chilena De Radiología. 16(1):510
14. Parikh T, Drew SJ, Lee VS et al (2008) Focal liver lesion detection and characterization with diffusion-weighted MR imaging: comparison with standard breath-hold T2-weighted imaging. Radiology. 246(3):812–822
15. Bruix J, Sherman M (2011) Management of hepatocellular carcinoma: An Update. AASLD Practice Guideline. Hepatology 53(3):1020–1022
16. Iwasaki Y, Arai K, Katayanagi S et al (2004) Biomarkers for neoplasmas in digestive organs. Gan To Kagaku Ryoho. 31(7):1015–1020
17. Taouli B, Koh DM (2010) Diffusion-weighted MR imaging of the liver. Radiology 254(1):47–66
18. Demir OI, Obuz F, Sagul O et al (2007) Contribution of diffusion-weighted MRI to the differential diagnosis of hepatic masses. Diagn Interv Radiol. 13(2):81–86
19. Koike N, Cho O, Nasu K et al (2009) Role of diffusion-weighted magnetic resonance imaging in the differential diagnosis of focal hepatic lesions. World J Gastroenterol. 15(46):5805–5581
20. Hosny IA (2010) Diffusion MRI of focal liver lesions. Pakistan journal of Radiology 20:01–07
21. Charles-Edwards EM, deSouza NM (2006) Diffusion-weighted magnetic resonance imaging and its application to cancer. Cancer Imaging 6:135–143
22. Thoeny HC, De Keyzer F (2007) Extracranial applications of diffusion-weighted magnetic resonance imaging. Eur Radiol 17:1385–1393
23. Kwee TC, Takahara T, Ochiai R et al (2008) Diffusion-weighted whole-body imaging with background body signal suppression (DWIBS): features and potential applications in oncology. Eur Radiol 18:1937–1952
24. Petra GK, Eric J (2010) Diffusion-weighted Imaging in the liver. World journal of gastroenterology 16:1567–1576
25. Onur MR, Çiçekçi M, Kayalı A et al (2012) The role of ADC measurement in differential diagnosis of focal hepatic lesions. Eur J Radiol. 81(3):e171–e176
26. Bruegel M, Holzapfel K, Gaa J et al (2008) Characterization of focal liver lesions by ADC measurements using a respiratory triggered diffusion-weighted single-shot echo-planar MR imaging technique. Eur Radiol. 18(3): 477–485
27. Tateishi R, Yoshida H, Matsuyama Y et al (2008) Diagnostic accuracy of tumor markers for hepatocellular carcinoma: A systematic review. Hepatol Int. 2:17–30

17

Natural history of hepatic hemangiomas as a guide for surgical indication

Mohamed M. Mogahed[1], Ashraf Anas Zytoon[2*], Bassem Essa[3], Wessam Abdellatif[4], Nashwa Ghanem[5] and Bahaa ElWakeel[1]

Abstract

Background: Generally, hemangiomas are asymptomatic and most lesions are incidentally diagnosed on abdominal ultrasonography. The indications for surgery are still debated mainly due to limited data about the natural history of hepatic hemangiomas. The aim of this study is to investigate the natural history of hepatic hemangiomas, the effects of age and sex on their growth, and their tendency to increase in size or causing symptoms or complications as a guide for surgical indication. In this current study, combined retrospective and prospective analysis was conducted on 186 Egyptian adult patients having 244 hepatic hemangiomas who attended to the outpatient clinics. Follow-up was performed to observe the accurate site, size, number, rate of growth of the lesions, and their tendency to cause symptoms or complications.

Results: Ninety-one percent of patients were asymptomatic and 9% were symptomatic. During follow-up, 48% of patients showed an increase in tumor diameter, 22% decreased, and 30% were stable. The growth rate at 18–45-year group showed an increasing trend that was higher in females; it was 3.3 ± 2 mm/year for males and 3.9 ± 1.8 mm/year for females. At ˃ 45 year group, the female patients showed a decreasing trend (− 2.1 ± 1.1 mm/year) while in males showed an increasing trend that was slower than in 18–45-year group (2.6 ± 1.7 mm/year).

Conclusion: Growth pattern of liver hemangiomas is affected by age and sex. The majority of hemangiomas are asymptomatic and complications are rare. Hemangioma size alone is not an indication for surgery in asymptomatic patients. Surgical indications are limited to patients with severe symptoms, complications, or suspicious lesions. Most hemangiomas can be managed conservatively even giant hemangiomas.

Keywords: Hepatic hemangiomas, Natural history, Surgical indication

Background

Hepatic hemangioma is the most common benign tumor of the liver [1], with an incidence reach up to 7.3% on autopsy [2] and up to 20% in the general population [3]. This tumor is typically observed in females with female to male ratio that may reach 5:1 at age of 50 years [4]. Hepatic hemangiomas are usually asymptomatic and diagnosed incidentally on abdominal ultrasonography [5]. MRI has high sensitivity and specificity for diagnosis of small and atypical hepatic hemangiomas [5]. The indications for surgery are still not clearly defined up till now. The main reason is the limited and inconsistent data available on the natural history of hepatic hemangiomas and on their tendency to increase in size or causing complications [6]. Ultrasonography is the first diagnostic and most available imaging test. US shows the hemangioma as well-defined, occasionally lobulated, homogeneously hyperechoic with posterior acoustic enhancement, and frequently located close to a hepatic or a portal vein with sensitivity of 96.9% and specificity of 60.3% [7]. Color-Doppler US does not improve accuracy in diagnosis, and it only shows blood flow in liver hemangioma with an intralesional arterio-portal shunt [8, 9]. Liver hemangiomas appears by CT as well-demarcated hypo-dense masses that is showing

* Correspondence: ashradio@gmail.com
[2]Radiodiagnosis Department, Faculty of Medicine, Menoufia University, Menoufia, Egypt

arterial peripheral nodular enhancement followed by progressive centripetal homogeneous filling toward the center at delayed images in triphasic post contrast study; however, small lesions of liver hemangiomas appears with cystic areas, fibrosis, or thrombosis may show atypical patterns [10]. CT has a sensitivity of 98.3% and a specificity of 55% [7]. Dynamic MRI is the best diagnostic imaging for liver hemangioma with sensitivity of 100% and specificity of 85.7% [7]. MRI shows a smooth, well-defined, homogenous lesion, hypointense on T1 and hyperintense on T2-weighted images. Some malignant hepatic lesions may show a similar hyperintensity on T2; to differentiate liver hemangioma from solid neoplastic liver lesions, the echo time is increased which causes signal from malignant lesions to decrease and signal from liver hemangioma to increase. With gadolinium administration, hemangioma shows a peripheral enhancement on arterial phase and contrast retention on delayed phases; this allows differentiation from hypervascular tumors that have a contrast washout on delayed phase [11].

This study aimed to investigate the natural history of hepatic hemangiomas and the effects of age and sex on their growth as a guide for surgical indications.

Methods

Study population

This combined retrospective and prospective study from April 2014 to March 2020 on 186 adult patients (54 males and 132 females) with 244 hepatic hemangioma lesions. The median age of patients was 45 years and the range was 18–68 years.

Patient inclusion criteria

Adult patients (age is more than 18 years) having hepatic hemangioma.

Patient exclusion criteria

Patients younger than 18 years, females receiving oral contraceptive pills, and patients who had received treatment for the hemangiomas were excluded.

Follow-up was performed to observe the accurate site, size, number, rate of growth of the lesions, and their tendency to cause symptoms or complications. Diagnosis of hemangiomas was done by typical ultrasonographic findings and patients with atypical manifestations underwent enhanced computed tomography or magnetic resonance imaging.

Patients were divided into two age groups: 18–45 years and > 45 years. Data regarding sex, age, tumor diameter, and follow-up period were recorded. The maximum diameter was used to assess the tumor size. The change of tumor growth was expressed in mm/year. Ultrasound examinations for all patients were done every 6 months for at least 2 times after the initial diagnosis.

Follow-up period of 12 to 24 months was performed in the outpatient clinics, with repeated US and blood examinations (complete blood count, prothrombin time and liver function tests) every 6 months. Giant hemangiomas were defined in the current study as hemangiomas with a diameter > 10 cm [7].

Written consent form was filled by every patient after detailed explanation of the study and the plane of management.

The study was approved by the Ethics Review Committee of our institute.

Study design

Combined retrospective and prospective study was conducted on 186 adult patients (more than 18 years) having 244 hepatic hemangiomas who attended to the outpatient clinics, 54 males and 132 females. Follow-up was performed to observe the accurate site, size, number, rate of growth of the lesions, and their tendency to cause symptoms or complications.

Imaging proctocol

Ultrasound examination was performed by ultrasound scanner (EPIQ 7 Machine-Philips ultrasound). Ultrasonography of the whole liver parenchyma was done with several imaging access, and many application techniques were used during examination (subcostal diagonal, subcostal longitudinal, sagittal and transverse, right intercostal lateral plans). The selection of planes depends on the accessibility of the lesion by the ultrasound beam intra-abdominally away from ribs and gas containing viscera.

CT examination was performed by CT scanner (Aquilion PRIM-Canon Medical). Triphasic CT scanning of the liver where performed at 120 kvp and 200–250 mAs. Patients were fasting for 5 h before procedure then were given non-ionic I/V contrast of 1.5 ml/kg with dose ranging from 80 to 100 ml. Patient preparation also included administration of 1000 ml of water 30–60 min prior to the examination as oral contrast. First, we scan all the liver before I/V contrast injection (non-contrast images) then after injection of intravenous contrast material, liver was scanned in the arterial phase for 15–35 s, the portal was scanned for 60–70 s, venous phase for 70–90 s, and delayed scanning after 5–10 min).

MRI examination was performed by MRI scanner (Ingenia Philips Medical Systems). Technique of MRI requires numerous sequences and imaging at multiple times after the administration of contrast at different axial and coronal plans. T2-weighted sequence: T2 HASTE and T2 fat-saturated, non-contrast T1-weighted sequences: T1 in-phase and out-of-phase, T1 fat-saturated, diffusion-weighted imaging (DWI): fat-saturated single-shot diffusion-weighted EPI, post-contrast dynamic sequences T1 2D or 3D gradient-echo sequences: arterial phase: 20–

30 s, portal venous phase: 60–70 s, equilibrium phase: 5–10 min, with and without fat sat.

We used the longitudinal, sagittal, and transverse plans for measuring the size of lesions by ultrasonography. By CT and MRI, we estimated the volume of the lesion from the axial and coronal images by measuring the antero-posterior, transverse, and longitudinal diameters.

Statistical analysis

Statistical analysis was performed using SPSS, Version 23 (SPSS Inc., Chicago, IL). Chi-square test was used to compare between the groups with respect to categorical data. Comparisons between two groups for normally distributed numeric variables were done using Student's *t* test while for non-normally distributed numeric variables, comparisons were done by Mann–Whitney *U* test. Numerical variables were presented as mean ± SD. Descriptive statistics were reported as frequencies and percent.

Results

Of the 186 patients (54 males and 132 females; male/female ratio was 1:2.4) having 244 lesions, 137 had single lesion and 49 had more than 1 lesion. The smallest hemangioma was 1 cm, and the largest was 19 cm in diameter with median 4.7 cm.

During the median 16 (range 12–30) months follow-up, 89 patients (48%) showed an increase in tumor diameter, 41 (22%) tumor diameters decreased, and 56 (30%) tumor diameters were stable. Patient data are summarized in Table 1

Table 1 Data of hepatic hemangioma patients included in the study

Total number of patients	186
Males	54
Females	132
Age (median, range) years	45, (18–68)
Total number of hemangioma lesions	244
Number of patients with single lesion	137
Number of patients with multiple lesions	49
Hemangioma diameter (median, range) cm	4.7 (1–21)
Hemangioma location (total = 244 lesion)	
Right lobe	178 (73%)
Left lobe	66 (27%)
Surface hemangioma	212 (87%)
Intraparenchymatous hemangioma	32 (13%)
Hemangioma growth pattern (number, %)	
Increased in diameter	89 (48%)
Decreased	41 (22%)
Stable	56 (30%)
Clinical presentation (number, %)	
Asymptomatic	169 (91%)
Symptomatic	17 (9%)
Patients with hemangioma diameter ≥ 10 cm	35 (19%)
Growth rate at (18–45-year group) mm/year, (mean ± SD)	
Males	3.3 ± 2
Females	3.9 ± 1.8
Growth rate at (˃ 45-year group) mm/year	
Males	2.6 ± 1.7
Females	− 2.1 ± 1.1

Data are presented as number and % unless otherwise indicated

The current study showed that hemangioma more frequently affects the right lobe than the left lobe as 178 (73%) of hemangiomas were in the right lobe and 66 (27%) were in the left lobe.

Typical appearance of hemangioma by ultrasound was detected in 151 patient that all of them presented by a well-defined, lobulated and homogeneously hyperechoic lesions that is showing posterior acoustic enhancement, some of them located close to a hepatic or a portal vein. 35 patients presented by atypical findings, some lesions showed homogenous hypoechoic texture and other lesions showed peripheral high echogenicity and hypoechoic center, according to these atypical findings we decided to do further imaging modalities to confirm diagnosis (Fig. 1).

Twenty patient did triphasic CT and lesions gives typical features that is seen hypo-attenuating to hepatic parenchyma at non contrast images, then gives discontinuous, nodular, peripheral enhancement at the arterial phase followed by progressive peripheral enhancement with centripetal fill-in at portal and venous phases, finally at delayed phase lesions showed irregular fill-in and therefore become iso- or hyper-attenuating to hepatic parenchyma (Fig. 2). Fifteen patients did dynamic MRI and all lesions gives the typical features of hemangioma by MRI, all lesions was relatively hypointense to liver parenchyma at T2 images, hyperintense to liver parenchyma at T2 images, at dynamic sequences all lesions showed peripheral nodular discontinuous enhancement that is progresses centripetally toward the center at portal images, then retained contrast on delayed images, all was hyperintense on diffusion-weighted imaging due to slow blood flow, and hyperintense or mixed (hyper and hypointense regions) on ADC map (Fig. 3).

The majority of patients with liver hemangiomas were asymptomatic, 169 patients (91%), and most of the lesions were diagnosed during physical examination and investigations for other gastrointestinal diseases and abdominal discomfort. Seventeen patient were symptomatic (9%), 6 of those 17 patients had severe symptoms in the form of abdominal pain, distension and discomfort while 11 of them had mild symptoms. The six patients with severe symptoms were fully investigated to exclude other gastrointestinal causes of their symptoms. 19% of patients (35/186) had hemangioma 10 cm diameter or more, all symptomatic patients were in this group (17/35 = 48.5%), while (18/35 = 51.5%) were asymptomatic in spite of the large diameter of hemangioma (Fig. 4).

Nineteen percent of patients (35/186) had hemangioma 10 cm diameter or more; all symptomatic patients were in this group (17/35 = 48.5%), while (18/35 = 51.5%) were asymptomatic in spite of the large diameter of hemangioma.

At the time of diagnosis, serum laboratory tests were within normal levels in 90.3% (168/186) of patients. Eighteen patients had slight elevation in liver transaminases, alkaline phosphatase, or bilirubin.

Growth pattern of hepatic hemangiomas

The median age of patients was 45 years and the range was 18–68 years. Patients were subdivided according to their age into two groups (18–45 and more than 45 years) to describe the effect of age and sex on hemangioma growth pattern.

The growth rate at 18–45-year group showed an increasing trend that was higher in females than in males. It was 3.3 ± 2 mm/year for males and 3.9 ± 1.8 mm/year for females in this group.

The growth rate at (> 45-year group) the female patients showed a decreasing trend (− 2.1 ± 1.1 mm/year) with regression of hemangioma size most obvious between the ages of 55–68 years while in males, it showed an increasing trend that was slower than in 18–45-year group with 2.6 ± 1.7 mm/year.

As regards the 17 symptomatic patients, 11 patients with mild symptoms continued follow-up and responded to medical treatment of other associated gastrointestinal disorders and reassurance. Six patients with severe symptoms, 2 patients refused the operation and continued follow-up, 4 patients underwent surgery, 2 underwent enucleation, and 2 underwent liver resection with no postoperative complications or mortality. One asymptomatic case was suspicious and malignancy could not be excluded by imaging; the patient underwent surgery and proved to be negative for malignancy. Data of patients underwent surgery are summarized in Table 2.

Surgically treated lesions were huge, occupying nearly most of the right or left lobe and not only segment and were mainly peripheral.

No spontaneous or traumatic intraperitoneal hemorrhage occurred in the current study, and no recorded Kasabach–Merritt syndrome as it is a rare condition recorded only in children and our cases were adults.

Discussion

In the current study during follow-up, 48% of patients showed an increase in tumor diameters, 22% tumor diameters decreased, and 30% tumor diameters were stable. This is comparable to results of Ankang Wang et al.'s study who reported 40.3% of patients showed increased diameter, 40.6% decreased, and 19.1% stable. While in Jing L et al.'s study, 61.0% patients had hemangiomas that increased in size; 23.7% had stable lesions, and 8.5% decreased in size [12, 13].

Studies have reported that hepatic hemangioma is more likely to occur in female patients, and long exposure to estrogen promotes the growth of hepatic hemangioma [14]. In this study, male:female ratio was 1: 2.4. Age is an important factor affecting the growth rate of hepatic hemangiomas [15]. In the current study, the growth before the age of 45 years showed an increasing trend that was higher in females than in males and after the age of 45 years the female patients showed a decreasing trend with regression of hemangioma size most obvious between the ages of 55 and 68 years while in males showed an increasing trend that was slower than in 18–45-year group.

The role of female gender in hemangioma growth has been discussed in a long-term follow-up study of Ankang Wang which revealed that there were significant differences in hemangioma growth between males and females [12].

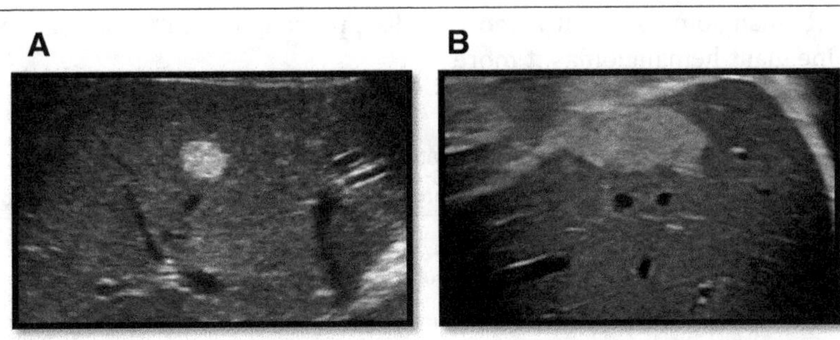

Fig. 1 Hemangioma as seen by ultrasonography. **a** Right lobe segment V well-defined hyper-echoic lesion close to hepatic vein. **b** Left lobe subcapsular segment II hyperechoic lesion

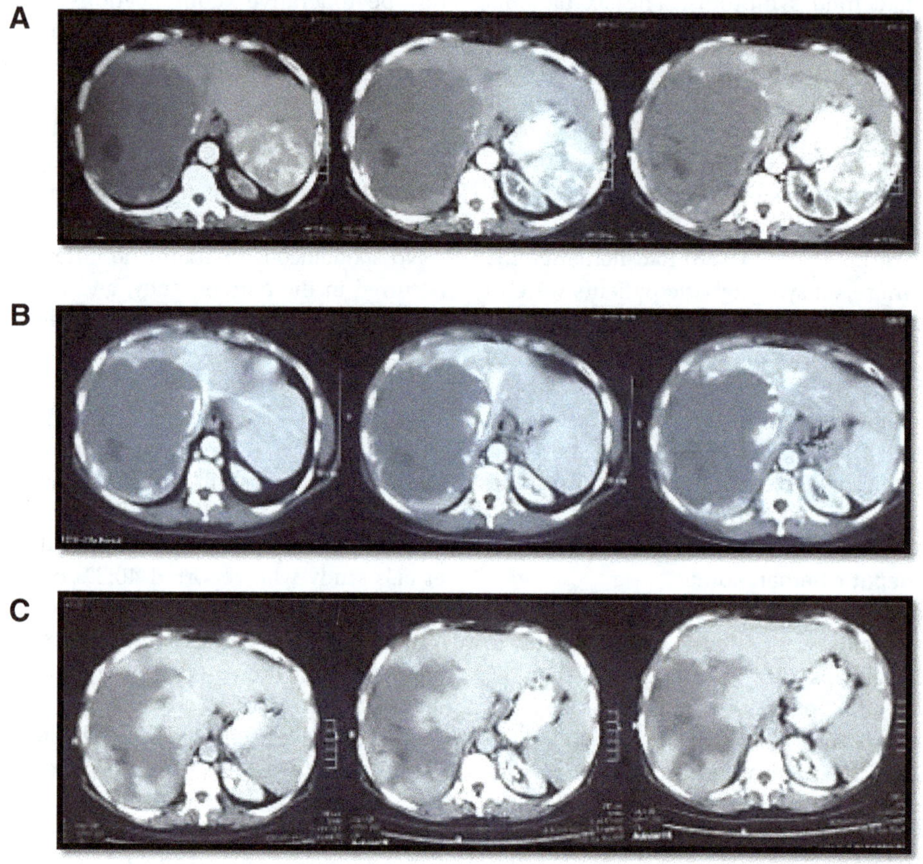

Fig. 2 Large right hepatic lobe hemangioma as seen by triphasic CT. **a** Arterial phase showing faint peripheral enhancement of the lesion. **b** Porto-venous phase showing more pronounced peripheral nodular enhancement by the lesion. **c** Delayed images showing progressive contrast enhancement toward the center of the lesion

Abdominal pain and discomfort caused by distension of the liver capsule are the most common presentations of symptomatic hepatic hemangioma. In the current study, 91% of patients with liver hemangiomas were asymptomatic and 9% were symptomatic with no mortality or complications during the follow-up period. This is comparable to results of Jing L et al.'s study who reported that 21 of 220 patients (9.5%) were symptomatic while in Ankang Wang's study, the symptomatic patient were about 6% [12, 13].

Some authors define the hemangioma as giant if more than 5 cm, and others define giant hemangiomas if more than 10 cm [16, 17]. Nineteen percent of the current study patients (35/186) had hemangioma diameter of ˃ 10 cm; 51.5% were asymptomatic in spite of the large diameter of hemangioma and need no treatment but only observation, while 48.5% were symptomatic. This goes with Boukerrouche A's study who concluded that size of the tumor alone is not indication for surgery [18].

Exclusion of other causes of abdominal pain in patient with liver hemangioma is mandatory. As in many recorded studies like in Farges and colleagues' study, pain disappeared in 54% of patients after treatment of

Table 2 Data of the five patients who underwent surgery for hepatic hemangioma

n	Age (years)	Gender	Tumor (cm)	Surgical indication	Surgical approach	Site	Relief of symptom	Complications
1	57	Female	12.7	Abdominal pain	Enucleation	Right lobe	Yes	No
2	53	Male	11.3	Abdominal pain	Enucleation	Right lobe	Yes	No
3	44	Female	13.1	Abdominal discomfort	Laparoscopic resection	Left lobe	Yes	No
4	49	Female	19	Abdominal pain	Open resection	Left lobe	Yes	No
5	58	Male	10.5	Atypical lesion	Open resection	Right lobe	Yes	No

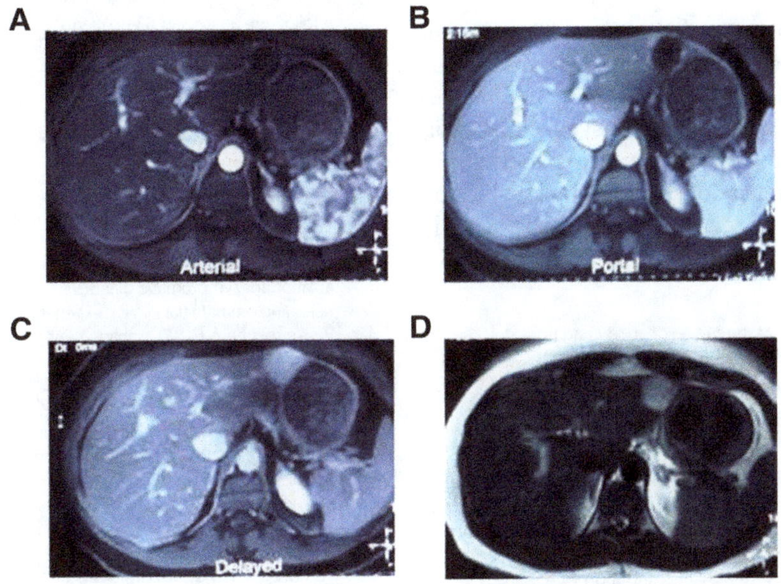

Fig. 3 Axial dynamic MRI sequences of the liver for left lobe 3 cm sub-capsular hemangioma. **a** Axial T1 arterial phase showing faint peripheral enhancement. **b** Progressive enhancement at axial T1 portal phase. **c** Axial T1 delayed phase showing homogenous enhancement of the lesion. **d** The lesion showing bright signal at axial T2 images

associated disorders and in 4/11 patients, pain persisted even after tumor resection [19].

Many patients after incidental diagnosis of liver hemangioma get anxiety. Anxiety alone should never be considered as indication for surgery [20]. Malignant transformation is practically inexistent and the patients have to be reassured. Patients operated for hemangioma because of anxiety continued to have anxiety after surgery [21].

Spontaneous hemorrhage and Kasabach-Merritt syndrome are rare [22, 23]. In the current study, there was no spontaneous or traumatic intraperitoneal hemorrhage occurred, no recorded Kasabach–Merritt syndrome as it is recorded in children and our cases were adult. This is comparable to results of Jing L et al.'s study with no reported cases, while Akang Wang's study reported only one case of 590 hepatic hemangioma patients diagnosed as spontaneous internal hemorrhage at surgery [12, 13].

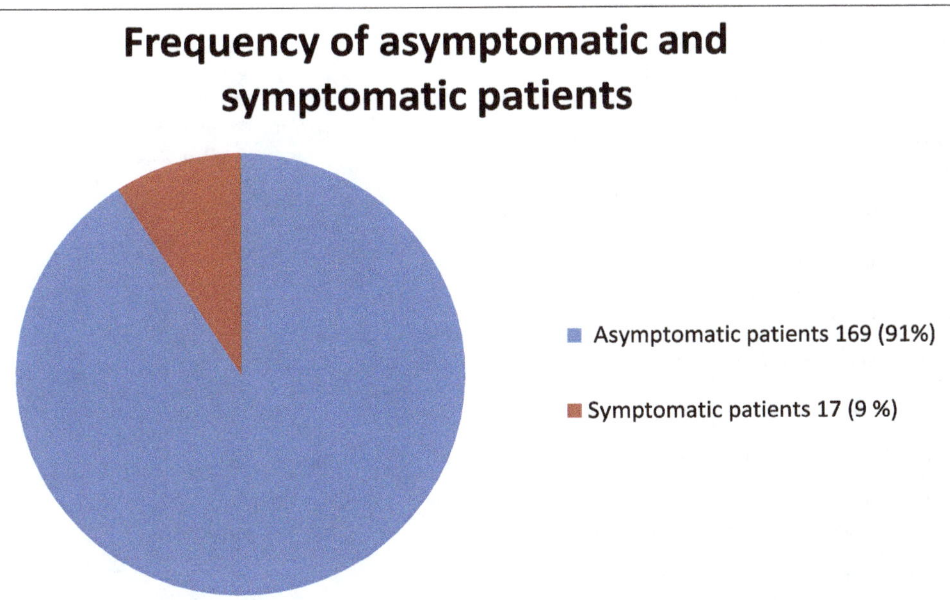

Fig. 4. Frequency of asymptomatic and symptomatic hemangioma patients

Conclusion

Growth pattern of hemangiomas is affected by age and sex. The majority of hepatic hemangiomas are asymptomatic and complications are rare. Hemangioma size alone is not indication for surgery in asymptomatic patients. Surgical indications are limited to patients with severe symptoms, complications, or suspicious lesion. Most hemangiomas, even giant hemangiomas, can be managed conservatively.

Abbreviations
CT: Computed tomography; MRI: Magnetic resonance imaging

Acknowledgements
N/A

Authors' contributions
M. M. M., A. A. Z., B. E., W. AL., N. G., and B. EW. made substantial contribution to the conception of the study; substantial contribution to the design of the study; substantial contribution to the acquisition and analysis of the data; substantial contribution to the interpretation of data; substantial contribution to the creation of the final work; substantial contribution to the study revision; and substantial contribution to the accuracy or integrity of the submitted manuscript. All authors have read and approved the manuscript.

Competing interests
The authors declare that they have no competing interests.

Author details
[1]Departments of Surgery, NHTMRI, Cairo, Egypt. [2]Radiodiagnosis Department, Faculty of Medicine, Menoufia University, Menoufia, Egypt. [3]Tropical Medicine Department, NHTMRI, Cairo, Egypt. [4]Radiology Department, NHTMRI, Cairo, Egypt. [5]Internal Medicine Department, Faculty of Medicine, Cairo University, Cairo, Egypt.

References
1. Yin X, Huang X, Li Q et al (2018) Hepatic hemangiomas alter morphometry and impair hemodynamics of the abdominal aorta and primary branches from computer simulations. Front Physiol 9:334
2. Herman P, Costa ML, Machado MA et al (2005) Management of hepatic hemangiomas: a 14-year experience. J Gastrointest Surg 9:853–859
3. Bahirwani R, Reddy KR (2008) The evaluation of solitary liver masses. Aliment Pharmacol Ther. 28:953–965
4. Duxbury MS, Garden OJ (2010) Giant haemangioma of the liver: observation or resection? DigSurg 27:7–11
5. Caseiro-Alves F, Brito J, Araujo AE et al (2007) Liver haemangioma: common and uncommon findings and how to improve the differential diagnosis. Eur Radiol 17:1544–1554
6. Giuliante F, Ardito F, Vellone M et al (2011) Reappraisal of surgical indications and approach for liver hemangioma: single center experience on 74 patients. Am J Surg 201:741–748
7. Toro A, Mahfouz AE, Ardiri A et al (2014) What is changing in indications and treatment of hepatic hemangiomas. A review. Ann Hepatol. 13:327–339
8. Perkins AB, Imam K, Smith WJ, Cronan JJ (2000) Color and power Doppler sonography of liver hemangiomas: a dream unfulfilled ? J Clin Ultrasound. 28:159–165
9. Lim KJ, Kim KW, Jeong WK et al (2012) Colour Doppler sonography of hepatic haemangiomas with arterioportal shunts. Br J Radiol 85:142–146
10. Yamashita Y, Ogata I, Urata J, Takahashi M (1997) Cavernous hemangioma of the liver: pathologic correlation with dynamic CT findings. Radiology 203: 121–125
11. McFarland EG, Mayo-Smith WW, Saini S, Hahn PF, Goldberg MA, Lee MJ (1994) Hepatic hemangiomas and malignant tumors: improved differentiation with heavily T2-weighted conventional spin-echo MR imaging. Radiology 193:43–47
12. Wang A, Deng J, Qian B et al (2019) Natural history of hepatic hemangioma: a follow-up analysis of 534 patients. Frontiers in Life Science 12:27–32
13. Jing L, Liang H, Caifeng L et al (2016) New recognition of the natural history and growth pattern of hepatic hemangioma in adults. Hepatol Res 46:727–733
14. Van Malenstein H, Maleux G, Monbaliu D et al (2011) Giant liver hemangioma: the role of female sex hormones and treatment. Eur J Gastroenterol Hepatol 23:438–443
15. Liu X, Yang Z, Tan H, Xu L, Liu L, Huang J, Si S, Sun Y, Zhou W (2018) Patient age affects the growth of liver haemangioma. HPB 20:64–68
16. Grieco MB, Miscall BG (1978) Giant hemangiomas of the liver. Surg Gynecol Obstet 147:783–787
17. Van Tilborg AA, Nielsen K, Scheffer HJ et al (2013) Bipolar radiofrequency ablation for symptomatic giant (> 10 cm) hepatic cavernous haemangiomas: initial clinical experience. Clin Radiol 68:e9–e14
18. Boukerrouche A (2017) Management of giant liver hemangioma. J Gastroenterol Dig Dis. 2:12–16
19. Farges O, Daradkeh S, Bismuth H (1995) Cavernous hemangiomas of the liver: are there any indications for resection ? World J Surg 19:19–24
20. Di Carlo I, Toro A (2013) Discomfort and anxiety should never be considered surgical indications for hemangioma of the liver. World J Surg 37:2723–2724
21. Di Carlo I, Sofia M, Toro A (2005) Does the psychological request of the patient justify the surgery for hepatic hemangioma? Hepatogastroenterology 52:657–661
22. Vernuccio F, Ronot M, Burgio MD et al (2018) Uncommon evolutions and complications of common benign liver lesions. Abdom Radiol 43:2075–2096
23. Kamyab AA, Rezaei-Kalantari K (2019) Hepatic hemangioma in a cluster of Iranian population. J Med Ultrasound 27:97–100

18

Sofosbuvir and daclatasvir are safe and effective in treatment of recurrent hepatitis C virus in Egyptian patients underwent living donor liver transplantation

Osama Aboelfotoh Aly[1], Wael Ahmed Yousry[1], Nahla Mohamed Teama[2*], Eman Mohammed Shona[1] and Ahmed Mohamed ElGhandour[1]

Abstract

Background: Liver transplant population has been considered as a special population in the treatment of hepatitis C virus infection, not only because of lower sustained virological response (SVR) rates in comparison with pretransplant setting, but also for other aspects (i.e., immunosuppressive therapy, renal function, drug–drug interactions). We aimed to evaluate the efficacy and safety of the combined treatment with sofosbuvir and daclatasvir with or without ribavirin in liver transplant recipients with recurrent hepatitis C following transplantation and screening for the development of hepatocellular carcinoma during treatment, after the end of treatment, or during follow-up. This multicenteric prospective study was conducted in Egypt. This study included 40 patients who underwent living donor liver transplantation that started treatment at least 3 months following transplantation. All participants received 400 mg sofosbuvir once daily plus daclatasvir 60 mg daily ± ribavirin. Treatment lasted for up to 24 weeks, and participants were followed up as outpatients monthly for 12 and 24 weeks and 36 weeks post-treatment to determine sustained virological response (SVR12 and SVR24), considered to be a cure and detection of any changes in tumor markers or radiological imaging during follow-up.

Results: In the current study, 40 patients (100%) have good response to treatment during treatment and during follow-up (SVR 12 was 100%). No abnormal side effects to treatment were detected; also, no drug–drug interactions were noted during the treatment.

Conclusions: Treatment of HCV after living donor liver transplantation with combined sofosbuvir and daclatasvir is safe and well-tolerated and provides high rates of SVR.

Keywords: Hepatitis C virus infection, Sofosbuvir, Daclatasvir, Living donor liver transplantation

Background

End-stage liver disease (ESLD) caused by hepatitis C virus (HCV) infection is the main indication of liver transplantation (LT) in most transplant programs [1].

Most patients will go on to develop viral recurrence, and it has been widely appreciated that the clinical course of HCV in LT recipients is accelerated in comparison with chronic hepatitis C in the non-transplant population, such that 8 to 44% of the patients will go on to develop cirrhosis within 5 to 10 years after transplantation [2].

Clinical decompensation in a significant proportion of HCV recipients who have developed cirrhosis of the allograft, with 40% developing clinical decompensation at 1 year, and up to 60% will suffer a decompensation episode 3 years after the diagnosis of cirrhosis. This unfortunately significantly affects patient survival, with an estimated survival rate of less than 10% at 3 years [3].

* Correspondence: nahlateama@med.asu.edu.eg
[2]Division of Nephrology, Department of Internal Medicine, Faculty of Medicine, Ain Shams University, Ramsis street 38, Abbasia, Cairo 11566, Egypt

Treatment of hepatitis C in the post-liver transplantation patient is a rapidly evolving field. When treating hepatitis C in this setting, the main goals of therapy include (a) cure of HCV chronic infection in the allograft post-transplant; (b) minimize the risk of developing HCV-associated complications in the allograft, such as fibrosing cholestatic hepatitis and allograft failure; and (c) prevent the development of hepatic fibrosis and thus preserve the function of the transplanted liver [4].

Treatment with pegylated interferon (PEG-IFN) and ribavirin (RBV) had been the standard of care for HCV patients for a decade, until the development of several direct-acting antivirals (DAAs) [5].

The association of sofosbuvir and daclatasvir has been shown to have very high antiviral efficacy when administered with or without ribavirin to previously naïve or non-responder patients with chronic HCV infection. Combination with daclatasvir in a LT recipient with severe recurrent cholestatic hepatitis C has been reported, showing a favorable outcome and the lack of drug interactions with calcineurin inhibitors (CNI) [6].

Owing to the low incidence of HCC among SVR patients, the study of factors associated with liver cancer development in this population is rather problematic. So far, no single clinical or histological predictor of HCC development has been identified in SVR patients, reinforcing therefore the concept that HCC risk in HCV patients may be multifactorial [7].

The aim of this study was to evaluate the virological response, clinical efficacy, and safety of the combined sofosbuvir and daclatasvir in living donor liver transplant recipients with recurrent hepatitis C following transplantation and screening for the development of hepatocellular carcinoma during treatment, after the end of treatment, or during follow-up.

Methods

This was a multicenteric prospective study conducted in Egypt. This study included 40 patients who underwent living donor liver transplantation who started treatment at least 3 months following transplantation provided that no abnormality was detected in liver functions related to immunosuppression and no prior history of treatment of hepatitis C infection. All patients were fully investigated for complete blood picture, liver function tests, coagulation profile, sodium, potassium, kidney function tests, HCV antibodies and quantitative HCV RNA by PCR, HBV markers, tumor markers including alpha fetoprotein (AFP), and abdominal ultrasonography.

Eligible patients had no evidence of advanced fibrosis (METAVIR score ≤ F2) on fibroscan performed not more than 6 months before screening.

All participants received 400 mg sofosbuvir once daily plus daclatasvir 60 mg daily ± ribavirin. Treatment lasted for up to 24 weeks, and participants were followed up as outpatients monthly for 12 and 24 weeks and 36 weeks post-treatment to determine sustained virological response (SVR12 and SVR24); also, patients were followed up for any changes in tumor markers or radiological imaging during follow-up.

A stable tacrolimus-based or cyclosporine-based immunosuppressive regimen was required, and glucocorticoids were permitted at a dose of 5 mg per day.

Statistical analysis

All collected data were analyzed and correlated. Statistical analysis was performed using the Statistical Package for Social Sciences (SPSS) version 24. Basic descriptive statistics including means and standard deviations were performed. A comparison of qualitative data between groups was performed using the chi-square test. Independent test or Mann–Whitney *U* test was used to compare quantitative data between groups with parametric distribution or non-parametric distribution, respectively. The continuous variables across time were compared using the paired *t* test or Wilcoxon signed-rank test. Differences were considered statistically significant if the p value was less than 0.05.

Results

This prospective multicenteric study included 40 patients, 37 males (92.5%) and 3 females (7.5%); their mean age was 55.3 ± 5.6 (33–62) years. Thirteen of them were diabetics (32.5%) and 27 (67.5%) were not diabetics.

There is a statistically significant reduction in hemoglobin levels at the first month after starting treatment ($p = 0.013$) and 9 months after the end of treatment ($p = 0.018$). Otherwise, the reduction at the other different treatment stages and follow-up is not significant.

As regards the platelet count, there is a statistically significant increase at the first month ($p = 0.003$) after onset of the treatment and 9 months after the end of the treatment ($p = 0.005$). There is a highly statistically significant increase in platelet count at 6 months after the end of treatment ($p < 0.001$); otherwise, the increase at the other different treatment stages is insignificant.

There is a statistically significant decrease in ALT levels at the first month after starting treatment ($p = 0.001$) than that before starting treatment and a statistically significant decrease after the end of treatment ($p - 0.004$); also, there is a highly statistically significant decrease in ALT at other different stages of treatment ($p < 00.1$), but there is no statistically significant change in AST levels at different stages of treatment or at follow-up. The same in AFP that shows no statistically significant change in its levels at different stages of treatment or after the end of treatment.

There is a highly statistically significant increase in serum albumin level after the end of the treatment ($p = 0.001$) and a statistically significant increase in serum albumin level at

3 months after the end of treatment (p = 0.019), at 6 months after the end of treatment (p = 0.04), and at 9 months after the end of treatment (0.004). As regards ALP, there is a statistically significant decrease in alkaline phosphatase level at 1 month after starting treatment (p = 0.002), after the end of treatment (p = 0.002), and 6 months after the end of treatment (p = 0.002) than that before starting treatment, while there is a highly statistically significant decrease in alkaline phosphatase levels at 3 months (p = 0.00) and at 9 months (p 0.00) after the end of the treatment.

There is a significant decrease in bilirubin levels at the end of treatment (p = 0.003), 6 months after treatment (p = 0.04), and 9 months after the end of treatment (p = 0.045), while there is no significant difference first month after starting treatment and 3 months after the end of treatment.

There is a highly statistically significant decrease in blood urea level at 3 months after the end of treatment (p = 0.001).

There is a statistically significant decrease in urea at the end of treatment (p = 0.005), 6 months after the end of treatment (p = 0.005), and 9 months after treatment (0.002), but there is no statistically significant difference in blood urea levels at 1 month after starting treatment; also, there is no statistically significant difference between serum creatinine levels at different stages of treatment and follow-up.

There is a highly statistically significant decrease in INR levels at the first month after starting treatment (p = 0.00). There is a significant decrease in INR levels at 3 months after the end of treatment (p = 0.002).

There is an insignificant decrease in INR levels after the end of treatment and 6 and 9 months after the end of treatment (Table 1).

All cases had negative PCR after the first month of treatment and continued till the end of follow-up (Table 2).

No ultrasonographic changes as regards hepatic focal lesion were detected during the course of treatment or after the course of treatment up to 9 months (Table 3).

Table 4 shows fibroscan results of the patients before treatment.

Discussion

This study included 40 patients who underwent living donor liver transplantation that started treatment at least 3 months following transplantation and no prior history of treatment of hepatitis C infection.

This study showed that 100% of patients achieved SVR after treatment of HCV with combined sofosbuvir and daclatasvir.

Poordad and his colleagues showed that 12 weeks of treatment with the pan-genotypic combination of daclatasvir with sofosbuvir and ribavirin achieved SVR12 rates of 83% and 94% in the advanced cirrhosis and post-transplantation cohorts, respectively [8].

Another study by Pellicelli and his colleagues evaluated the safety and efficacy of sofosbuvir and daclatasvir with or without RBV among 12 post-LT patients with severe recurrent HCV who were treated through an international compassionate use program. Three patients had fibrosing cholestatic HCV and 9 had cirrhosis. The mean MELD at baseline was 22 and the mean Child-

Table 1 Comparison between baseline and follow-up values of lab investigations of patients

	Baseline	During treatment				Follow-up					
		1 month	p value	EOT	p value	3 months	p value	6 months	p value	9 months	p value
Hemoglobin (g/dl)	11.5 ± 0.91	11.2 ± 0.77	0.013	11.4 ± 0.75	0.55	11.3 ± 0.69	0.45	11.3 ± 0.43	0.21	11.1 ± 0.58	0.018
Platelets	153.6 ± 39.4	184.1 ± 59.1	0.003	160.6 ± 36.2	0.43	157.3 ± 38.9	0.69	191.8 ± 36.2	< 0.001	179.7 ± 36.2	0.005
ALT (IU/l)	45.9 ± 15.2	35.8 ± 10.4	0.001	37.6 ± 7.9	0.004	34.3 ± 11.1	< 0.001	33.7 ± 12.4	< 0.001	32.6 ± 11.1	< 0.001
AST (IU/l)	36.8 ± 13.4	35.0 ± 7.1	0.35	33.7 ± 12.4	0.33	36.9 ± 8.6	0.98	38.5 ± 10.5	0.49	37.6 ± 7.9	0.64
AFP (ng/ml)	28.4 ± 17.05	28.9 ± 17.6	0.95	31.4 ± 18.9	0.54	35.3 ± 20.2	0.08	26.6 ± 14.8	0.64	22.6 ± 13.02	0.13
Albumin (g/dl)	3.23 ± 0.39	3.23 ± 0.35	0.49	3.6 ± 0.38	0.001	3.5 ± 0.42	0.019	3.4 ± 0.39	0.04	3.5 ± 0.45	0.004
ALP (IU/l)	132.8 ± 45.1	107.6 ± 11.5	0.002	103.5 ± 48.2	0.002	99.3 ± 14.9	< 0.001	107.6 ± 11.5	0.002	99.3 ± 14.9	< 0.001
Bilirubin (mg/dl)	1.07 ± 0.14	1.03 ± 0.15	0.28	0.99 ± 0.11	0.003	1.3 ± 1.7	0.08	0.99 ± 0.16	0.04	0.99 ± 0.20	0.045
Urea (mg/dl)	45.3 ± 16.9	40.0 ± 10.6	0.18	34.9 ± 10.7	0.005	34.3 ± 9.04	0.001	34.8 ± 7.7	0.005	34.6 ± 7.4	0.002
Creatinine (mg/dl)	0.91 ± 0.33	0.92 ± 0.25	0.99	0.93 ± 0.159	0.72	0.93 ± 0.16	0.52	0.96 ± 0.23	0.43	0.95 ± 0.24	0.65
INR	1.06 ± 0.13	0.92 ± 0.19	< 0.001	1.3 ± 1.6	0.63	0.93 ± 0.19	0.002	1.04 ± 0.14	0.36	1.03 ± 0.22	0.34

EOT end of treatment, *ALT* alanine aminotransferase, *AST* aspartate aminotransferase, *AFP* alpha fetoprotein, *ALP* alkaline phosphatase

Table 2 PCR changes during treatment

Item	Frequency	Percentage
PCR before		
Mean ± SD	366057.5 ± 376220.9	
Min–max	698–2000000	
PCR 1 month after starting treatment		
Positive	0	0
Negative	40	100
PCR after the end of treatment		
Positive	0	0
Negative	40	100
PCR 3 months after the end of treatment		
Positive	0	0
Negative	40	100
PCR 6 months after the end of treatment		
Positive	0	0
Negative	40	100
PCR 9 months after the end of treatment		
Positive	0	0
Negative	40	100

Pugh score was 10. During treatment, 3 deaths occurred: one due to rapidly progressive liver failure, one due to gastrointestinal bleeding, and one due to septic shock. Severe adverse events occurred among 4 of the remaining 9 patients and were attributed to the severity of the patients' underlying liver disease rather than directly to the antiviral treatment. The 9 patients who completed 24 weeks of treatment all had undetectable HCV RNA at the end of treatment. At the time the study was published, post-treatment virologic data was available for 5 patients, all of whom had achieved SVR (24). In this series as well as an additional case report describing the successful treatment of a patient with post-LT fibrosing cholestatic HCV with sofosbuvir and daclatasvir for 24 weeks, there were no apparent drug–drug interactions between DAA and tacrolimus [9].

Table 3 Ultrasonographic changes during the course of treatment

Item	Frequency	Percentage
US before treatment		
Splenomegaly	6	155
Normal	24	85
US 1 month after starting treatment		
HFL	0	0
No HFL	40	100
US after the end of treatment		
HFL	0	0
No HFL	40	100
US 3 months after the end of treatment		
HFL	0	0
No HFL	40	100
US 6 months after the end of treatment		
HFL	0	0
No HFL	40	100
US 9 months after the end of treatment		
HFL	0	0
No HFL	40	100

HFL hepatic focal lesion

Table 4 Fibroscan of the patients at baseline

Values	*N* (%)
F1	11 (27.5)
F2	29 (72.5)

F1 minimal fibrosis, *F2* fibrosis has occurred and spread inside the areas of the liver including blood vessels

High rates of virologic and clinical response were seen in 23 patients with post-LT fibrosing cholestatic HCV treated with sofosbuvir (n = 8) or sofosbuvir and daclatasvir (n = 15) based regimens [10].

An ongoing prospective multicenter study in France by Manns et al. evaluating the efficacy of sofosbuvir and daclatasvir with or without ribavirin has found high SVR rates in post-LT patients with aggressive recurrent HCV infection [11].

In a study by Suraweera and his colleagues, they reported data on 130 LT patients who underwent treatment for 12 or 24 weeks. The mean time period between LT and treatment was 74.2 (± 73.5) months. Eleven patients received sofosbuvir and daclatasvir without ribavirin for 12 weeks and had a response rate of 100% at the end of treatment as well as a SVR12 rate of 100%. Sixty-four patients underwent this same regimen for 24 weeks and had a response rate of 100% at the end of treatment and a SVR12 rate of 97%. Three patients received sofosbuvir and daclatasvir with ribavirin for 12 weeks; the end-of-treatment response rate was 67%, with a SVR12 rate of 67%. Fifty-two patients underwent the same regimen for 24 weeks and achieved an end-of-treatment response rate of 98% and a SVR12 rate of 96% [12].

The authors also concluded that ribavirin did not have a statistically significant influence on SVR and that further prognostic factors needed to be defined. Thirty patients were reported to have experienced severe side effects, with the most common being hematologic toxicity. Two patients died, 1 from diabetic coma and the other from HCV recurrence at 6 weeks post-treatment. Tacrolimus dosing was adjusted in 56% of patients, cyclosporine in 49% of patients, and everolimus in 38% of patients [12].

In the current study, the initial values of bilirubin, alkaline phosphatase, and liver enzymes were normal at baseline and improved during the treatment period and follow-up. No liver toxicity of the administered antivirals was observed. The values of albumin and platelets are significantly improved during treatment and follow-up.

Also, there were no changes in the ultrasonographic findings noted after starting treatment and there were no hepatic focal lesions detected during treatment or follow-up period.

The study regimen was compatible with multiple immunosuppressive regimens without dose adjustments, and there were no events of graft rejection.

In contrast, Price et al. found that regimens containing the NS3 protease inhibitors simeprevir or paritaprevir can have significant pharmacokinetic interactions with calcineurin inhibitors [13].

Adverse events during treatment were consistent with the underlying disease; no treatment-specific safety signals were apparent and no serious adverse events were detected due to treatment protocol.

According to data from eight studies being presented at *The International Liver Congress™ 2017* in Amsterdam, The Netherlands, there remains continued debate on whether patients are at risk of developing liver cancer after achieving sustained virological response (SVR) with a direct-acting antiviral (DAA) regimen for hepatitis C virus (HCV).

Despite Trépo and his colleagues found initially promising results, more than one study investigating genetic predisposition to liver cancer failed to identify any robust predictor of HCC development in HCV patients that can be used in clinical practice to optimize the management of patients with a liver cancer [14].

There was a decreased risk of HCC with antiviral treatment that was based on clinical trial data using INF-based regimens, but recently, results of studies linking the use of DAA therapy with an increased risk of HCC present an interesting dilemma for clinicians [15].

In the current study, no development of HCC was noted in the studied group.

Conclusion

In the current study, 40 patients were treated with combined sofosbuvir 400 mg and daclatasvir 60 mg for 24 weeks. All patients received treatment at least 3 months following transplantation. Forty patients (100%) have good response to treatment during treatment and during follow-up (SVR 12 was 100%). No abnormal side effects to treatment were detected; also, no drug–drug interactions were noted during treatment. No HCC was detected during treatment and follow-up.

Abbreviations

HCV: Hepatitis C virus; SVR: Sustained virological response; DAAs: Direct-acting antivirals; RBV: Ribavirin; ALT: Alanine aminotransferase; AST: Aspartate aminotransferase; AFP: Alpha fetoprotein; HCV PCR: Hepatitis C virus polymerase chain reaction; CBC: Complete blood count; INR: International normalized ratio; IQR: Interquartile range; ESLD: End-stage liver disease; LT: Liver transplantation; PEG-INF: Pegylated interferon; CNI: Calcineurin inhibitors; HCC: Hepatocellular carcinoma; SPSS: Statistical Package for Social Sciences; EOT: End of treatment

Acknowledgements

Not applicable

Authors' contributions

OAA selected the patients from Ain Shams University Specialized Hospital and El Maadi Military Hospital. WAY made the design for the study. AME and NMT contributed to the follow-up of the patients and analysis and interpretation of the data. EMS contributed to the data collection. All authors provided critical feedback and helped shape the research, analysis, and manuscript. All authors have read and approved the final manuscript.

Competing interests

The authors declare that they have no competing interests.

Author details

Division of Gastroenterology and Hepatology, Department of Internal Medicine, Faculty of Medicine, Ain Shams University, Cairo, Egypt. [2]Division of Nephrology, Department of Internal Medicine, Faculty of Medicine, Ain Shams University, Ramsis street 38, Abbasia, Cairo 11566, Egypt.

References

1. Jamieson N, McMaster P, O'Grady JG et al (2003) Evolution of liver transplantation in Europe: report of the European Liver Transplant Registry. Liver Transpl 9:1231–1243. https://doi.org/10.1016/j.lts.2003.09.018
2. Roche B, Samuel D (2007) Risk factors for hepatitis C recurrence after liver transplantation. J Viral Hepat 14(7):89–96. https://doi.org/10.1111/j.1365-2893.2007.00920.x
3. Berenguer M, Aguilera V, Prieto M (2008) Clinical benefits of antiviral therapy in patients with recurrent hepatitis C following liver transplantation. Am J Transplant 8(3):679–687. https://doi.org/10.1111/j.1600-6143.2007.02126.x
4. Coilly A, Roche B, Dumortier J et al (2014) Safety and efficacy of protease inhibitors to treat hepatitis C after liver transplantation: a multicenter experience. JHepatol 60:78–86
5. Lok AS (2013) HCV NS5A inhibitors in development. Clin Liver Dis 17(1):111–121. https://doi.org/10.1016/j.cld.2012.09.006
6. Fontana R, Hughes E, Bifano M (2013) Sofosbuvir and daclatasvir combination therapy in a liver transplant recipient with severe recurrent cholestatic hepatitis C. American Journal of Transplantation 13:1601–1605 https://doi.org/10.1111/ajt.12209
7. Mallet V, Gilgenkrantz H, Serpaggi J et al (2008) Brief communication: The relationship of regression of cirrhosis to outcome in chronic hepatitis C. Ann. Intern. Med. chapter 149:399–403. https://doi.org/10.7326/0003-4819-149-6-200809160-00006
8. Poordad F, Schiff E, Vierling J et al (2016) Daclatasvir with sofosbuvir and ribavirin for hepatitis C virus infection with advanced cirrhosis or post-liver transplantation recurrence. Hepatology 63(5):1493–1505 https://doi.org/10.1002/hep.28446
9. Pellicelli AM, Montalbano M, Lionetti R et al (2014) Sofosbuvir plus daclatasvir for post-transplant recurrent hepatitis C: potent antiviral activity but no clinical benefit if treatment is given late. Digestive and Liver Disease 46:923–927
10. Leroy V, Dumortier J, Coilly A et al (2015) Efficacy of sofosbuvir and daclatasvir in patients with fibrosing cholestatic hepatitis C after liver transplantation. Clin Gastroenterol Hepatol 13(11):1993–2001.e1-2. https://doi.org/10.1016/j.2015.05.030
11. Manns M, Reesink H, Berg T et al (2011) Rapid viral response of once-daily TMC435 plus pegylated interferon/ribavirin in hepatitis C genotype-1 patients: a randomized trial. AntiviralTherapy 16(7):1021–1033. https://doi.org/10.3851/IMP1894
12. Suraweera D, Sundaram V, Saab S (2016) Treatment of hepatitis C virus infection in liver transplant recipients. Gastroenterol. Hepatol 12(1):23–30
13. Price JC and Terrault NA (2015). Treatment of hepatitis C in liver transplant patients: interferon OUT, direct antiviral combos IN. Liver Transpl; (4)21:423-434. doi: https://doi.org/10.1002/lt.24080

14. Trépo E, Nahon P, Bontempi G et al (2014) Association between the PNPL A3 (rs738409 C>G) variant and hepatocellular carcinoma: evidence from a meta-analysis of individual participant data. Hepatology 59(6):2170–2177. https://doi.org/10.1002/hep.26767
15. Hirmatsu N, Oze T, Takehara T (2015) Suppression of hepatocellular carcinoma development in hepatitis C patients given interferon based antiviral therapy, Hepatol. Res 45(2):152–161. https://doi.org/10.1111/hepr.12393

19

A fish oil-rich diet leads to lower adiposity and serum triglycerides but increases liver lipid peroxidation in fructose-fed rats

Gabriel Perri Esteves[1*], Camila Sanches Manca[1], Hellen Paraguassú Veida-Silva[2], Paula Payão Ovidio[1], Héric Holland[1], Flávia Sayuri Matsuo[3], Mariana Kiomy Osako[3] and Alceu Afonso Jordao[1]

Abstract

Background: Consumption of refined carbohydrates has risen in recent years alongside chronic diseases such as type 2 diabetes mellitus, dyslipidemia, obesity, and non-alcoholic fatty liver disease (NAFLD). Fructose is a monosaccharide made widely available in industrialized products, capable of inducing excessive weight gain and liver steatosis in animal models, while omega-3 fatty acids, present in foods such as fatty fish and fish oil, have shown to inhibit genes related to lipogenesis and decrease cardiovascular risk. Therefore, our objective was to evaluate the impact of a high-fructose diet on weight gain, biochemical and oxidative stress parameters, and liver histology and investigate fish oil's potential protective role. Thirty male Wistar rats were divided into 3 groups: regular chow diet (CT), regular chow diet plus 20% fructose in drinking water (Fr), and a diet containing 10% fish oil plus 20% fructose in drinking water (FOFr). After 12 weeks, tissues of interest were collected for biochemical and histological analyses.

Results: Although fructose consumption did not lead to increased hepatic fat, it caused a significant increase in weight gain, white adipose tissue, and serum triglycerides in the Fr group, while fish oil promoted normalized serum triglycerides and even reduced adiposity in the FOFr group. Additionally, the inclusion of fish oil in the FOFr diet led to increased liver lipid peroxidation in the form of increased hepatic MDA.

Conclusions: It is concluded that fish oil can prevent important metabolic alterations caused by fructose consumption, but its dosage must be taken into account to prevent oxidative stress and potential liver damage.

Keywords: Oxidative stress, Lipid peroxidation, Omega-3 fatty acids, Fish oil, NAFLD, Fructose, Obesity

Background

The alarming increase in obesity prevalence around the world is a public health concern [1]. This pathological expansion of adipose tissue is accompanied by an inflammatory state and many comorbidities, such as type 2 diabetes (T2D), dyslipidemia, cardiovascular diseases (CVD), and non-alcoholic fatty liver disease (NAFLD) [2]. The latter is currently considered the most prevalent liver disease in the world, characterized by a higher than 5% fat deposition in the liver of individuals with no history of excessive alcohol intake. It is believed NAFLD progression occurs initially through increased lipid accumulation in the liver (the first "hit"), followed by oxidative stress and an increase in lipid peroxidation (the second "hit") [3] leading to its inflammatory form, non-alcoholic steatohepatitis (NASH), and possibly more serious liver diseases such as cirrhosis and hepatocellular carcinoma [4].

Oxidative stress is a condition in which unstable molecules known as reactive oxygen species (ROS) overwhelm antioxidant defenses, leading to potential damage of cellular constituents such as proteins, lipids, and DNA. ROS are

* Correspondence: gabipesteves3012@gmail.com
[1]Department of Health Sciences, Ribeirao Preto Medical School, University of Sao Paulo, São Paulo, Brazil

endogenously produced by the mitochondrial respiratory chain [5], as such, an increase in presence and oxidation of glucose and free fatty acids (FFA) can lead to increased generation of electron donors, resulting in ROS overproduction [6]. Furthermore, oxidative stress has been recognized as a contributor to the development of hypertension, inflammation, insulin resistance, and other chronic diseases [7].

A sedentary lifestyle and excessive energy intake, favored by the consumption of simple carbohydrates and energy-dense foods are major causes of obesity and NAFLD [8]. More specifically, fructose is a monosaccharide naturally present in fruits but made excessively available in industrialized products, and its role in the development of obesity and related comorbidities has been highly studied. After its intestinal absorption, fructose is rapidly transported into the liver via hepatic GLUT2 and is able to bypass important rate-limiting steps of glycolysis, therefore leading to an increase in triose phosphate intermediates at a faster rate than glucose, which can then be utilized in different pathways, including lipogenesis [9]. Additionally, fructose is able to interact with transcription factors such as SREBP1c and ChREBP, which are responsible for the expression of enzymes related to fatty acid synthesis and glycolysis [10, 11].

Fatty acids, another component of human diets, have been shown to interact with transcription factors and modulate lipogenesis [12]. Fish oil, a compost rich in marine omega-3 (n-3) polyunsaturated fatty acids (PUFAs), is known to have anti-inflammatory properties, as well as being able to reduce hepatic triglycerides (TG), fatty acid synthesis, and adipose cell size [3, 13]. On the other hand, excessive incorporation of n-3 fatty acids into cell membranes raises its peroxidizability index due to an increase in sites susceptible to lipid peroxidation, which can result in membrane glycolipid, phospholipid, and cholesterol peroxidation [14, 15].

Therefore, considering the important increase in the consumption of industrialized products and in the prevalence of obesity and its related comorbidities, the aim of this study was to evaluate the effects of a marine n-3 fatty acid-rich diet in fructose-fed rats in terms of liver, biochemical, and oxidative stress parameters.

Methods

Animals and diet

All procedures were approved by the Ribeirão Preto Medical School's Ethics Committee of Animal Experimentation (protocol number 185/2017). Thirty male Wistar rats were obtained from the Central Animal House of Ribeirão Preto Campus, University of São Paulo, Brazil, and kept in a 12-h light/12-h dark cycle, at an average temperature of 22 °C. Animals weighed an average of 200 g upon arrival and were randomly assigned to 3 groups (n = 10). The control group (CT) was fed a regular chow diet (Nuvilab Cr-1®, Nuvital Nutrientes S/A, Table 1) and tap water. The fructose (Fr) group was fed a regular chow diet and water containing 20% fructose. The fish oil-fructose group (FOFr) also received water containing 20% fructose but had its diet altered to contain 10% fish oil. Fish oil was acquired from Campestre Industry and Trade of Vegetable Oils (São Bernardo do Campo, Brazil).

Animals were weighed 3 times a week while also receiving fresh chow and water. Diet and water intake were also recorded every 2 days. After 12 weeks, animals were euthanized through decapitation following a 12-h fast. Blood was immediately collected and then centrifuged at 4 °C, and serum was stored at − 80 °C. Liver tissue was removed, weighed, and sampled for histological, oxidative stress, and total fat analyses and later stored at − 80 °C. Retroperitoneal and epididymal fat tissues were also collected and weighed.

Hepatic histology

For histological analysis, hepatic tissues were dissected, fixed in 10% neutral buffered formalin, and embedded in paraffin according to standard procedures. Tissue sections of 5 μm thickness were stained with hematoxylin and eosin (H&E). Histological images were captured using the Scanscope (Olympus BX61VS).

Biochemical analyses

Fish oil's fatty acids were determined using gas chromatography (Shimadzu, Europe, Duisburg, Germany), fitted with an SP2560 column (100 m, 0.25 mm, 0.20 μm). Helium was used as the carrier gas (1.6 ml/min flux), and a mix of methyl esters fatty acids were utilized as a standard (Supelco 37 Component FAME Mix).

Total fat was quantified through Bligh and Dyer's [16] method utilizing 500 mg samples of hepatic tissue. Lipid peroxidation was assessed through the quantification of serum and hepatic malondialdehyde (MDA) following Gérard-Monnier et al.'s proposed method [17]. Reduced glutathione (GSH) was determined though Sedlak and Lindsay's [18] method. Hepatic α-tocopherol concentration was measured according to the method proposed by

Table 1 Nutritional composition of used standard chow diet and modified fish oil diet

Nutritional composition (100 g)	Standard chow diet (CT)[1]	Modified fish oil diet (FOFr)
Energy content	336 Kcal	392.4 Kcal
Carbohydrates	53 g (63%)	47.7 g (49%)
Proteins	22 g (26%)	19.8 g (21%)
Lipids	4 g (11%)	13.6 g (30%)

[1]Nutritional information was obtained from Nuvilab Cr-1® (Nuvital Nutrientes S/A) product label

Arnaud et al. [19] utilizing a high-performance liquid chromatograph (Shimadzu Europe, Duisburg, Germany) equipped with a C-18 column (Shimpack CLC-ODS 4.6 × 25 cm) and a 4 mm × 1 cm precolumn. The mobile phase was made by acetonitrile/dichloromethane/methanol (70/20/10) solution. Transaminases alanine aminotransferase (ALT) and aspartate aminotransferase (AST), total serum cholesterol, and serum TG were determined through commercial kits (Labtest Diagnóstica S.A., Brazil). Free fatty acids (FFAs) were determined through a quantitative colorimetric assay (BioAssay Systems, Hayward, CA, USA).

Statistical analysis

Data was subjected to ANOVA variance analysis with Tukey's post hoc test (GraphPad Software, San Diego, CA, USA), with a significance level set at $p < 0.05$. Data is presented as means ± standard deviation.

Results

Table 2 shows the fatty acid composition of the fish oil utilized in the experiment, presenting a higher amount of n-3 fatty acids compared to n-6 fatty acids, and a significant amount of EPA and DHA, therefore demonstrating the FOFr diet indeed had an increased marine n-3 fatty acid content.

Table 2 Percentage of fatty acids in utilized fish oil

Structure	%
14:0	6.3
16:0	23.6
16:1	6.7
17:0	0.9
17:1	0.9
18:0	5.3
18:1n9c	12.1
18:2n6c	14.3
18:3n3	2.2
20:1n9	ND
20:2	0.6
20:3n6	0.2
21:0	0.2
20:3n3	0.1
20:4n6	1.4
20:5n3 (EPA)	9.6
22:1n9	0.3
24:0	1.2
22:6n3 (DHA)	12.6
Others	12.6
n-6	15.9
n-3	24.5

ND not detected, *n-6* polyunsaturated omega-6 fatty acids, *n-3* polyunsaturated omega-3 fatty acids

Table 3 shows consumption data regarding food, fluid (and therefore, fructose), and calorie intake. Food intake was similarly reduced in groups consuming fructose (Fr and FOFr). While fluid intake remained the same between CT and Fr, it was reduced in the FOFr group, leading to a subtle, albeit significant reduction in fructose intake compared to the Fr group. Curiously, total calorie intake was the same between experimental groups.

Figure 1 shows the initial and final body weight. Initially, body weight was the same between experimental groups. After 12 weeks, animals from the Fr showed significantly increased body weight, and FOFr had a similar weight to CT.

Figure 2 presents data regarding body composition. Retroperitoneal fat was significantly increased in the Fr group, and similar between CT and FOFr, while epididymal fat was reduced only in the FOFr group. When combined, total body fat was significantly lower in the FOFr group and higher in the Fr group. Additionally, liver weight corrected according to animal weight did not differ between animals.

As for biochemical parameters (Fig. 3), serum TG was found to be elevated in the Fr group and normalized in the FOFr group. Additionally, total serum cholesterol was lower in the group consuming fish oil. No significant differences were seen in total hepatic fat, free fatty acids, or in the hepatic enzymes AST and ALT.

Figure 4 shows data regarding oxidative stress parameters. While serum MDA and GSH were not significantly different between groups, there was an important increase in hepatic MDA in the FOFr group. Hepatic GSH was also found to be significantly increased, but only in the Fr group. Additionally, hepatic α-tocopherol was found to be significantly reduced in FOFr animals. Finally, Fig. 5 displays H&E staining of liver samples, showing no significant difference between groups.

Discussion

In the present study, fructose consumption in water led to lower diet intake, causing caloric intake to be very similar between experimental groups. Indeed, previous research has shown that animals are capable of altering

Table 3 Food, fluid, fructose, and calorie intake

Variables	CT	Fr	FOFr
Food intake (g/day)	35 ± 2.3	21 ± 2.3^{a}	19 ± 3.3^{a}
Fluid intake (ml/day)	67 ± 5.1	66 ± 8.1	54 ± 3.2^{ab}
Fructose intake (g/day)	-	13.1 ± 1.5	10.9 ± 0.53^{b}
Total calorie intake (kcal/day)	124 ± 8.1	124 ± 10.2	122 ± 8.5

Values are mean ± SD. Superscript letters are significantly different
[a]A significant difference when compared to the CT group
[b]A significant difference when compared to the Fr group

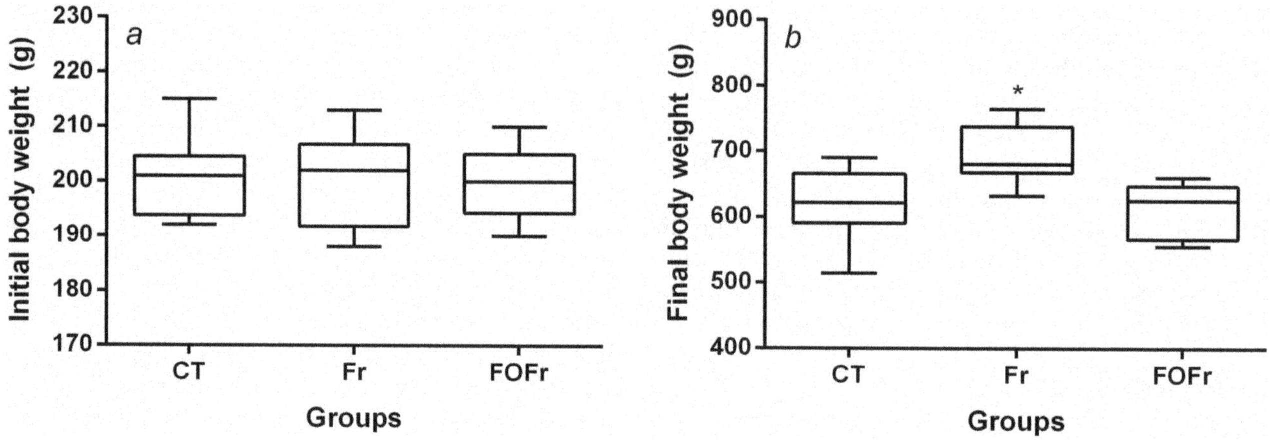

Fig. 1 Body weight. **a** Initial body weight and **b** final body weight. Values are mean ± SD. Asterisk indicates a significant difference between groups ($P < 0.05$)

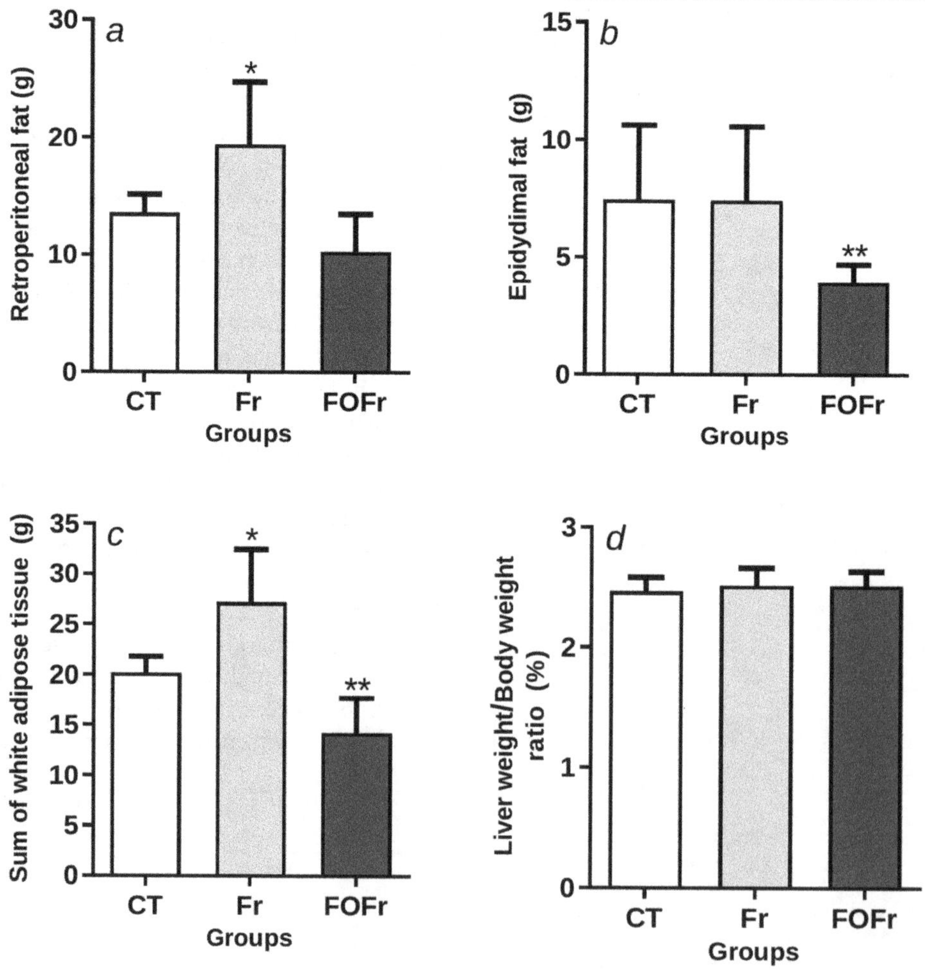

Fig. 2 Body composition. **a** Retroperitoneal fat, **b** epididymal fat, **c** sum of adipose tissues, and **d** liver weight corrected by animal weight. Values are mean ± SD. Asterisk indicates a significant difference when compared to CT and FOFr. Double asterisk indicates a significant difference when compared to CT and Fr ($P < 0.05$)

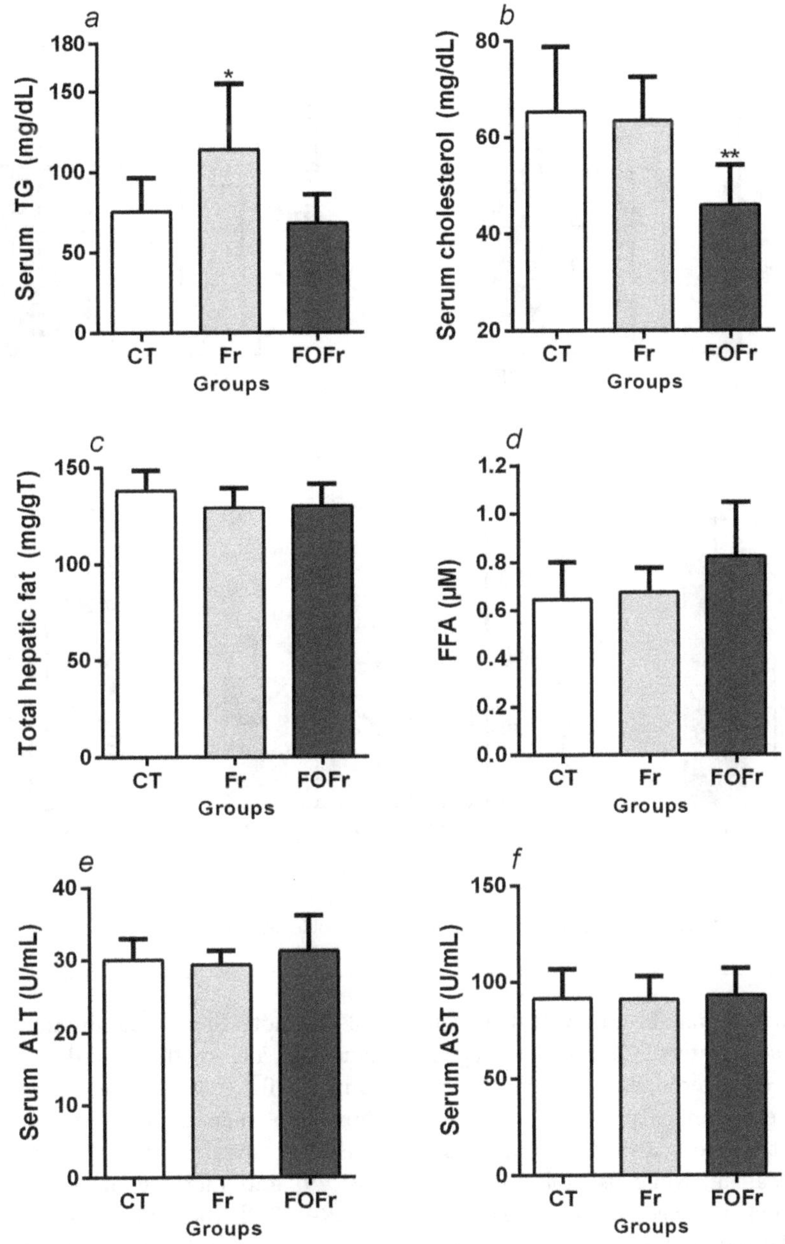

Fig. 3 Biochemical parameters. **a** Serum triglycerides, **b** serum total cholesterol, **c** total hepatic fat, **d** free fatty acids, and **e** serum ALT and **f** AST. Values are mean ± SD. Asterisk indicates a significant difference when compared to CT and FOFr. Double asterisk indicates a significant difference when compared to CT and Fr ($P < 0.05$)

their food intake to maintain similar energy intake when consuming fructose in water [20, 21], although not always being sufficient to compensate for the additional calories from fructose [22, 23]. Equal energy ingestion may suggest that differences in weight gain and biochemical parameters seen in this study were due to fructose and fish oil's significant effects on lipid metabolism and not due to a more energy-dense diet. Also, water intake remained the same between CT and Fr groups, and decreased slightly in the FOFr group, leading to marginally smaller fructose intake. In similar studies, animals receiving water in fructose tend to have increased water intake, which in turn leads to a higher daily fructose intake [20, 21]. It is unclear why water intake did not increase in our experiment; however, that may have protected animals from developing more serious metabolic complications, such as liver steatosis. Decreased fructose intake in the FOFr group presents a limitation of our study; however, since this decrease was subtle, fish oil can still be partially implicated in the positive changes seen in FOFr animals, such as normalized serum

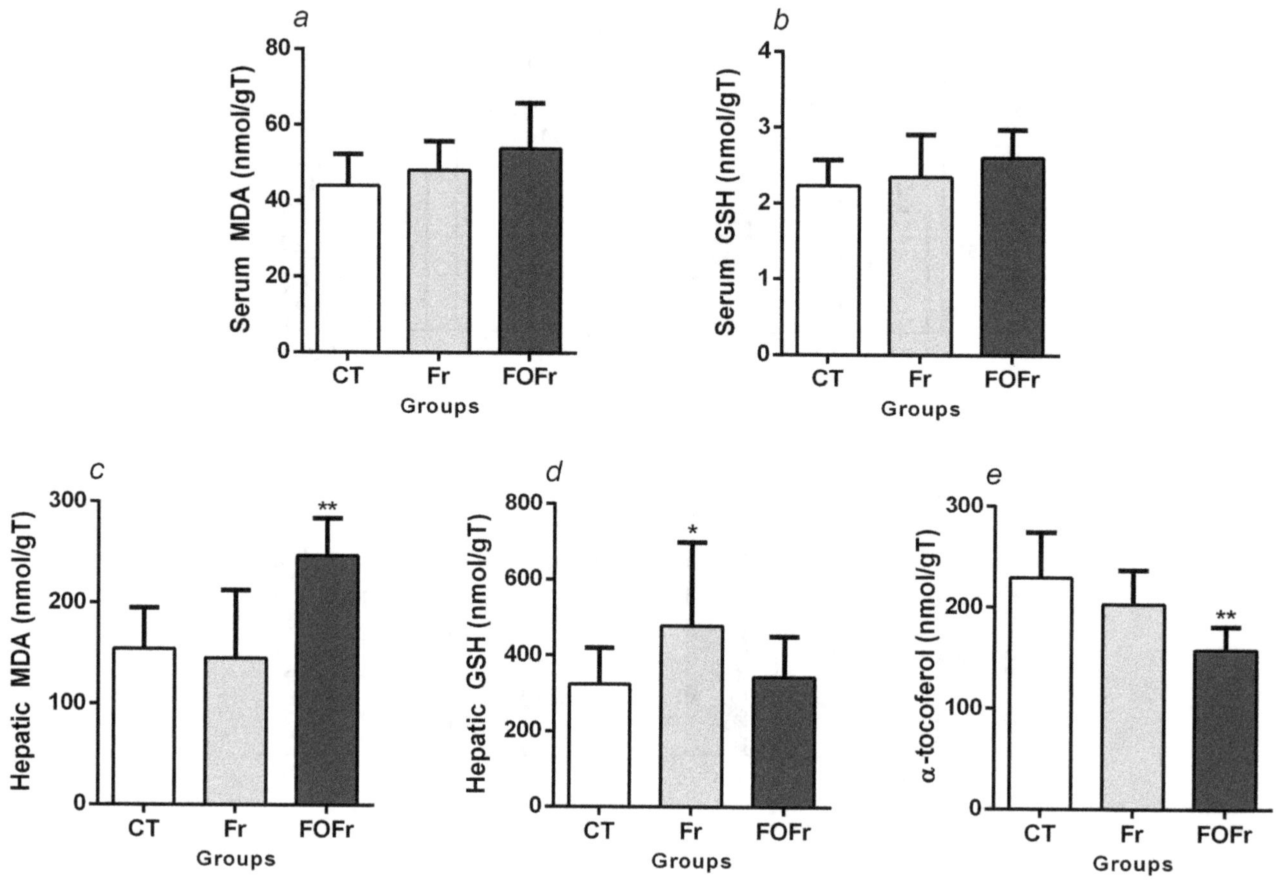

Fig. 4 Oxidative stress parameters. **a** Serum MDA, **b** serum GSH, **c** hepatic MDA, **d** hepatic GSH, and **e** hepatic α-tocopherol. Values are mean ± SD. Asterisk indicates a significant difference when compared to CT and FOFr. Double asterisk indicates a significant difference when compared to CT and Fr ($P < 0.05$)

TGs and reduced adiposity. It may be the case that diets that are rich in lipids, such as the FOFr, lead to higher satiety and therefore reduced water intake, as seen in experiments offering high-fat diets to animals [24].

Fructose ingestion led to increased weight gain, mainly in terms of retroperitoneal fat, while fish oil prevented these changes and further reduced serum cholesterol and epididymal fat. Although fat deposition stems mainly from positive energy balance, fructose is known to have an important impact on lipid synthesis. Since fructose bypasses rate-limiting steps of glycolysis, it is rapidly metabolized in the liver into substrates that can be used for acetyl-CoA production and eventually for lipogenesis. Fructose-derived substrates also activate ChREBP, which further increases metabolic pathways such as glycolysis and fructolysis. Additionally, by inducing hyperinsulinemia [25], fructose promotes SREBP1-c activation [26], leading to increased expression of lipogenic enzymes such as fatty acid synthase and acetyl-CoA carboxylase [27]. Since intrahepatic lipids increase when their production surpasses hepatic lipid output [9], perhaps fructose ingested by rats in our experiment did not promote lipid accumulation in the liver but led to increased TG synthesis and its storage in fat tissue. In contrast, fish oil and marine n-3 fatty acids have been shown to reduce fatty acid synthesis by suppressing SREBP-1c expression and preventing LXRα activation [28, 29] and increase lipolysis by upregulating hepatic PPAR-α [30], therefore hindering TG synthesis and fat storage. In a similar experiment, the addition of fish oil in the animal diet failed to attenuate an increase in serum TGs due to fructose consumption 30 days after fructose ingestion in water was initiated [21]. It would seem therefore that fish oil is more efficient at preventing the development of elevated serum TGs rather than treating it, since in the aforementioned experiment fish oil ingestion started alongside fructose addition in water.

Although fructose is implicated in hepatic lipogenesis, no liver alterations were seen in our experiment, such as liver steatosis, fibrosis, increased liver weight, or increased hepatic enzymes. Indeed, multiple protocols are employed to study NAFLD in the literature [31–35], differing in terms of fructose concentration, experiment length, and animal model, making the comparison between heterogeneous

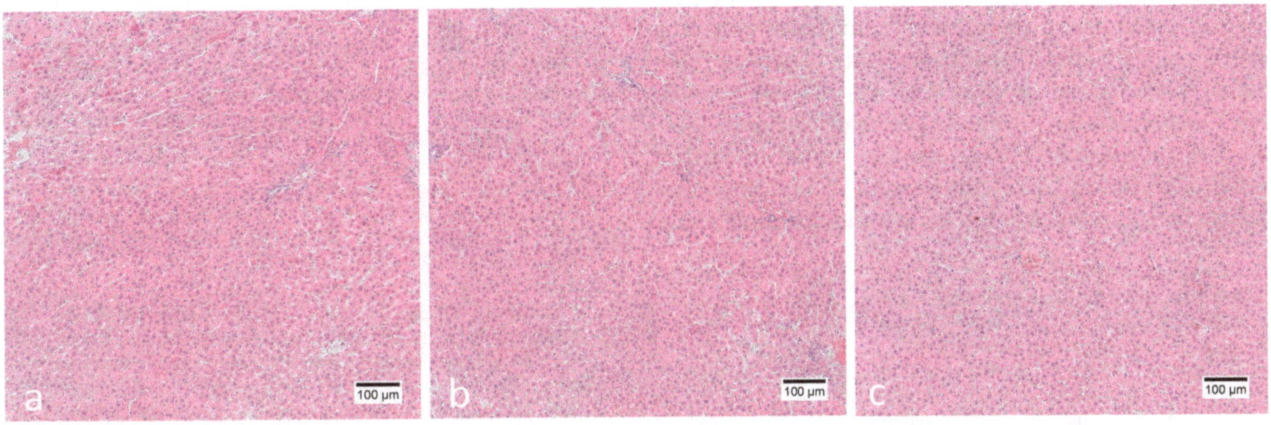

Fig. 5 Histological analysis from liver samples of rats consuming regular chow, fructose, or fructose and fish oil. **a** Liver histology of CT group. **b** Liver histology of Fr group. **c** Liver histology of FOFr group

data a difficult task. In similar experiments that utilized Wistar rats receiving fructose in drinking water, increased hepatic lipid accumulation was seen after 8 weeks of fructose consumption [35], and liver injury consisting of hepatocyte degeneration and hyperemia were seen after 24 weeks [34]. Even though water intake data was not available in these previous studies, it can be hypothesized that the extent to which fructose can lead to hepatic injury and lipid accumulation depends heavily on the experiment's duration and water intake, which directly impacts fructose intake. As discussed previously, since water intake was not increased in the Fr group, as opposed to what is seen in similar experiments [20, 21], fructose intake was limited. Other methods that circumvent this limitation can be used to induce NAFLD and obesity in animals, such as including fructose in the actual diet alongside saturated fat [36–38], leading to an increased fructose intake and a stronger stimulus to provoke metabolic alterations, given the effects of saturated fats on the onset of inflammation and weight gain in animal models [39, 40].

Fish oil also led to increased hepatic MDA and reduced hepatic α-tocopherol in the FOFr group, suggesting there was a significant increase in lipid peroxidation in the liver and that hepatic α-tocopherol, a fat-soluble antioxidant which acts as a hydrogen donor, was significantly depleted. It has been described that the susceptibility for free radical damage increases alongside the number of double bonds in fatty acids present in tissues [15]. As such, the incorporation of a significant amount of n-3 fatty acids such as EPA and DHA in the liver, which are available in fish oil and abundant in double bonds, can potentially lead to increased lipid peroxidation, and thus pose a threat to overall hepatic health. Oxidative stress is now recognized as a significant part in the development of many metabolic conditions such as chronic inflammation and hypertension [7], and in the liver, it is directly implicated in alcoholic hepatic diseases [41]. Therefore, these findings raise concerns regarding the safety of fish oil when ingested at such high dosages.

Experiments in which a fructose-rich diet containing 10% fish oil was given to rats also saw an increase in lipid peroxidation in the form of increased liver and serum TBARS, leading to significant DNA damage [42]. Later, the same group showed that a 5% dosage of fish oil could still ameliorate metabolic alterations of a fructose-enriched diet without increasing lipid peroxidation [43]. It would seem, therefore, that as the diet's fish oil content rises, so does hepatic lipid peroxidation, but at a given proportion, fish oil retains its therapeutic properties without favoring oxidative stress. Curiously, hepatic GSH was increased in the Fr group, a result that is not seen in other experiments [42, 43]. This change may have protected these animals from oxidative stress, given that MDA levels were normal in the Fr group. The ratio of reduced glutathione to oxidized glutathione (GSH/GSSG) is an effective method to assess the redox state of glutathione in tissues, which unfortunately was not present in our experiment. It would be important to utilize this analysis in future experiments, possibly shedding more light on this specific alteration found in animals consuming fructose.

Conclusions

Obesity and its comorbidities affect an ever-growing number of patients around the world. As such, it is fundamental to study its causes and different therapeutic options. In our experiment, we found that fructose ingestion through water led to increased weight gain and increased adiposity and serum triglycerides, without causing liver injury or steatosis. The inclusion of fish oil in the diet prevented such alterations and further decreased serum cholesterol and fat tissue. However, at such a dosage, it also led to increased hepatic lipid peroxidation. Considering fish oil is a widely available pharmaceutical agent, the present study raises concerns regarding its unadvised use by patients. Therefore, we propose that fish oil and its PUFAs may be suitable agents to prevent the metabolic effects of fructose ingestion, but an adequate dosage must be tested in further studies and clinical trials with the aim of avoiding deleterious changes while still retaining a therapeutic effect.

Abbreviations

NAFLD: Non-alcoholic fatty liver disease; MDA: Malondialdehyde; GSH: Reduced glutathione; ROS: Reactive oxygen species; FFA: Free fatty acids; SREBP1c: Sterol regulatory element-binding protein 1c; ChREBP: Carbohydrate-responsive element-binding protein; PUFA: Polyunsaturated fatty acid; ALT: Transaminases alanine aminotransferase; AST: Aspartate aminotransferase; LXRα: Liver X receptor alpha; PPAR-α: Peroxisome proliferator-activated receptor alpha; EPA: Eicosapentaenoic acid; DHA: Docosahexaenoic acid; TBARS: Thiobarbituric acid reactive substances

Acknowledgements

None.

Authors' contributions

GPE was responsible for manuscript elaboration and for conducting the project and worked on all of its stages. CSM and HPV-S assisted in animal handling and in discussions regarding the results. PPO and HH assisted in animal handling and biochemical assays. FSM and MKO assisted in histological procedures and result interpretation. AAJ is the main investigator responsible for the laboratory and supervised the project. All authors approved the final manuscript.

Competing interests

The authors declare that they have no competing interests.

Author details

[1]Department of Health Sciences, Ribeirao Preto Medical School, University of Sao Paulo, São Paulo, Brazil. [2]Department of Physiology, Ribeirao Preto Medical School, University of Sao Paulo, São Paulo, Brazil. [3]Department of Cell and Molecular Biology and Pathogenic Bioagents, Ribeirao Preto Medical School, University of Sao Paulo, São Paulo, Brazil.

References

1. Fruh SM (2017) Obesity: risk factors, complications, and strategies for sustainable long-term weight management. J Am Assoc Nurse Pract 29:S3–S14. https://doi.org/10.1002/2327-6924.12510
2. Cox AJ, West NP, Cripps AW (2015) Obesity, inflammation, and the gut microbiota. Lancet Diabetes Endocrinol 3:207–215. https://doi.org/10.1016/S2213-8587(14)70134-2
3. Castro GS, Calder PC (2018) Non-alcoholic fatty liver disease and its treatment with n-3 polyunsaturated fatty acids. Clin Nutr 37:37–55. https://doi.org/10.1016/j.clnu.2017.01.006
4. Milić S, Lulić D, Štimac D (2014) Non-alcoholic fatty liver disease and obesity: Biochemical, metabolic and clinical presentations. World J Gastroenterol 20:9330–9337. https://doi.org/10.3748/wjg.v20.i28.9330
5. Han D, Williams E, Cadenas E (2001) Mitochondrial respiratory chain-dependent generation of superoxide anion and its release into the intermembrane space. Biochem J 353:411. https://doi.org/10.1042/0264-6021:3530411
6. Brownlee M (2001) Banting Lecture 2004, the pathobiology of diabetic complications a unifying mechanism. Diabetes 51:7–18. https://doi.org/10.2337/diabetes.51.1.7
7. Matsuda M, Shimomura I (2013) Increased oxidative stress in obesity: implications for metabolic syndrome, diabetes, hypertension, dyslipidemia, atherosclerosis, and cancer. Obes Res Clin Pract 7:1–12. https://doi.org/10.1016/j.orcp.2013.05.004
8. Tappy L, Le KA (2010) Metabolic effects of fructose and the worldwide increase in obesity. Physiol Rev 90:23–46. https://doi.org/10.1152/physrev.00019.2009
9. Ter Horst KW, Serlie MJ (2017) Fructose consumption, lipogenesis, and non-alcoholic fatty liver disease. Nutrients 9:1–20. https://doi.org/10.3390/nu9090981
10. Iizuka K, Bruick RK, Liang G et al (2004) From the cover: deficiency of carbohydrate response element-binding protein (ChREBP) reduces lipogenesis as well as glycolysis. Proc Natl Acad Sci 101:7281–7286. https://doi.org/10.1073/pnas.0401516101
11. Aragno M, Tomasinelli CE, Vercellinatto I et al (2009) SREBP-1c in nonalcoholic fatty liver disease induced by Western-type high-fat diet plus fructose in rats. Free Radic Biol Med 47:1067–1074. https://doi.org/10.1016/j.freeradbiomed.2009.07.016
12. Jump DB, Botolin D, Wang Y et al (2006) Fatty acids and gene transcription. Scand J Food Nutr 50:5–12. https://doi.org/10.1080/17482970601069318
13. Lombardo YB, Chicco AG (2006) Effects of dietary polyunsaturated n-3 fatty acids on dyslipidemia and insulin resistance in rodents and humans. A review. J Nutr Biochem 17:1–13. https://doi.org/10.1016/j.jnutbio.2005.08.002
14. Ayala A, Muñoz MF, Argüelles S (2014) Lipid peroxidation: production, metabolism, and signaling mechanisms of malondialdehyde and 4-hydroxy-2-nonenal. Oxid Med Cell Longev 2014:1–31. https://doi.org/10.1155/2014/360438
15. Pamplona R, Portero-Otín M, Riba D et al (1998) Mitochondrial membrane peroxidizability index is inversely related to maximum life span in mammals. J Lipid Res 39:1989–1994
16. Bligh E, Dyer W (1959) A rapid method of total lipid extraction and purification. Can J Biochem Physiol 37:912–917
17. Gérard-Monnier D, Erdelmeier I, Régnard K et al (1998) Reactions of 1-methyl-2-phenylindole with malondialdehyde and 4-hydroxyalkenals. Analytical applications to a colorimetric assay of lipid peroxidation. Chem Res Toxicol 11:1176–1183. https://doi.org/10.1021/tx9701790
18. Sedlak J, Lindsay RH (1968) Estimation of total, protein-bound, and nonprotein sulfhydryl groups in tissue with Ellman's reagent. Anal Biochem 25:192–205. https://doi.org/10.1016/0003-2697(68)90092-4
19. Arnaud J, Fortis I, Blachier S, et al (1991) Simultaneous determination of retinol, α-tocopherol and β-carotene in serum by isocratic high-performance liquid chromatography. J Chromatogr B Biomed Sci Appl 572:103–116. https://doi.org/10.1016/0378-4347(91)80476-S
20. Mamikutty N, Thent ZC, Sapri SR et al (2014) The establishment of metabolic syndrome model by induction of fructose drinking water in male wistar rats. Biomed Res Int 2014:1–8. https://doi.org/10.1155/2014/263897
21. Sulis PM, Motta K, Barbosa AM et al (2017) Impact of fish oil supplementation and interruption of fructose ingestion on glucose and lipid homeostasis of rats drinking different concentrations of fructose. Biomed Res Int:2017. https://doi.org/10.1155/2017/4378328
22. Baena M, Sangüesa G, Hutter N et al (2014) Fructose supplementation impairs rat liver autophagy through mTORC activation without inducing endoplasmic reticulum stress. Biochim Biophys Acta - Mol Cell Biol Lipids 1851:107–116. https://doi.org/10.1016/j.bbalip.2014.11.003
23. Vilà L, Roglans N, Perna V et al (2011) Liver AMP/ATP ratio and fructokinase expression are related to gender differences in AMPK activity and glucose intolerance in rats ingesting liquid fructose. J Nutr Biochem 22:741–751. https://doi.org/10.1016/j.jnutbio.2010.06.005
24. Poudyal H, Campbell F, Brown L (2010) Olive leaf extract attenuates cardiac, hepatic, and metabolic changes in high carbohydrate–, high fat–fed rats. J Nutr 140:946–953. https://doi.org/10.3945/jn.109.117812
25. Iizuka K, Horikawa Y (2008) ChREBP: a glucose-activated transcription factor involved in the development of metabolic syndrome. Endocr J 55:617–624. https://doi.org/10.1507/endocrj.K07E-110
26. Miyazaki M, Dobrzyn A, Man WC et al (2004) Stearoyl-CoA desaturase 1 gene expression is necessary for fructose-mediated induction of lipogenic gene expression by sterol regulatory element-binding protein-1c-dependent and independent mechanisms. J Biol Chem 279:25164–25171. https://doi.org/10.1074/jbc.M402781200
27. Ferré P, Foufelle F (2007) SREBP-1c transcription factor and lipid homeostasis: Clinical perspective. Horm Res 68:72–82. https://doi.org/10.1159/000100426
28. Howell G, Deng X, Yellaturu C et al (2009) N-3 polyunsaturated fatty acids suppress insulin-induced SREBP-1c transcription via reduced trans-activating capacity of LXRα. Biochim Biophys Acta - Mol Cell Biol Lipids 1791:1190–1196. https://doi.org/10.1016/j.bbalip.2009.08.008
29. Sekiya M, Yahagi N, Matsuzaka T et al (2003) Polyunsaturated fatty acids ameliorate hepatic steatosis in obese mice by SREBP-1 suppression. Hepatology 38:1529–1539. https://doi.org/10.1016/j.hep.2003.09.028
30. Deckelbaum RJ, Worgall TS, Seo T (2006) N-3 fatty acids and gene expression. Am J Clin Nutr 83:1520–1525. https://doi.org/10.2307/3976938

31. Abd El-Haleim EA, Bahgat AK, Saleh S (2016) Resveratrol and fenofibrate ameliorate fructose-induced nonalcoholic steatohepatitis by modulation of genes expression. World J Gastroenterol 22:2931–2948. https://doi.org/10.3748/wjg.v22.i10.2931
32. Chaturvedi A, Ravishankar B, Rao N, Mudugaru R (2016) Evaluation of metabolic syndrome signs in two different animal models. Pharmacol Toxicol Biomed Reports 2:41–44. https://doi.org/10.5530/ptb.2016.2.5
33. Moura RF, Ribeiro C, de Oliveira JA et al (2008) Metabolic syndrome signs in Wistar rats submitted to different high-fructose ingestion protocols. Br J Nutr 101:1178–1184. https://doi.org/10.1017/S0007114508066774
34. Pektas MB, Yücel G, Koca HB et al (2017) Dietary fructose-induced hepatic injury in male and female rats: influence of resveratrol. Drug Res (Stuttg) 67: 103–110. https://doi.org/10.1055/s-0042-118386
35. Mamikutty N, Thent ZC (2015) Haji Suhaimi F (2015) Fructose-drinking water induced nonalcoholic fatty liver disease and ultrastructural alteration of hepatocyte mitochondria in Male wistar rat. Biomed Res Int. https://doi.org/10.1155/2015/895961
36. Lee JS, Jun DW, Kim EK et al (2015) Histologic and metabolic derangement in high-fat, high-fructose, and combination diet animal models. Sci World J 2015. https://doi.org/10.1155/2015/306326
37. Fakhoury-Sayegh N, Trak-Smayra V, Khazzaka A et al (2015) Characteristics of nonalcoholic fatty liver disease induced in wistar rats following four different diets. Nutr Res Pract 9:350–357. https://doi.org/10.4162/nrp.2015.9.4.350
38. Jegatheesan P, Beutheu S, Freese K et al (2016) Preventive effects of citrulline on Western diet-induced non-alcoholic fatty liver disease in rats. Br J Nutr 116:191–203. https://doi.org/10.1017/S0007114516001793
39. Maric T, Woodside B, Luheshi GN (2014) The effects of dietary saturated fat on basal hypothalamic neuroinflammation in rats. Brain Behav Immun 36: 35–45. https://doi.org/10.1016/j.bbi.2013.09.011
40. Rocha-Rodrigues S, Rodríguez A, Gonçalves IO et al (2017) Impact of physical exercise on visceral adipose tissue fatty acid profile and inflammation in response to a high-fat diet regimen. Int J Biochem Cell Biol 87:114–124. https://doi.org/10.1016/j.biocel.2017.04.008
41. Cichoz-Lach H, Michalak A (2014) Oxidative stress as a crucial factor in liver diseases. World J Gastroenterol 20:8082–8091. https://doi.org/10.3748/wjg.v20.i25.8082
42. Castro GS, Santos RA, Portari GV et al (2012) Omega-3 improves glucose tolerance but increases lipid peroxidation and DNA damage in hepatocytes of fructose-fed rats. Appl Physiol Nutr Metab 37:233–240. https://doi.org/10.1139/h11-154
43. Castro GS, Deminice R, Simões-Ambrosio LMC et al (2015) Dietary docosahexaenoic acid and eicosapentaenoic acid influence liver triacylglycerol and insulin resistance in rats fed a high-fructose diet. Mar Drugs 13:1864–1881. https://doi.org/10.3390/md13041864

20

High efficacy of low-dose albumin infusion in the prevention of paracentesis-induced circulatory dysfunction

Ayman Alsebaey*, Eman Rewisha and Imam Waked

Abstract

Background: Large-volume paracentesis (LVP) is a main pillar in treating patients with tense ascites. Without plasma expanders use, paracentesis-induced circulatory dysfunction (PICD) is a common complication with decreased survival. The aim was to compare low-dose albumin (2 g/L ascitic fluid removed n = 85) with standard-dose albumin (6 g/L ascitic fluid removed, n = 25) for prevention of PICD. Liver function tests, urea, creatinine, CBC, and abdominal ultrasonography were done. Plasma renin activity (PRA) was measured at baseline and on the 6th day post-LVP. The delta change (**Δ**) = day 6 variable minus baseline variable value. PICD was defined as increase in PRA of > 50% of the baseline value.

Results: Patients in low-dose albumin group were mainly Child B compared with Child C (85.9% vs. 52%; p = 0.001), underwent less paracentesis volume (9.78 ± 3.56 vs. 12.52 ± 3.6 L; p = 0.001), but had higher baseline PRA (859.62 ± 1151.34 vs. 165.93 ± 95.34 pg/mL; p = 0.001). In both groups, the PRA increased at day 6 compared with the baseline (1141.57 ± 1433.01 vs. 859.62 ± 1151.34 pg/mL; p = 0.01) and (192.21 ± 80.99 vs. 165.93 ± 95.34 pg/mL; p = 0.01) respectively. Both groups were comparable for **Δ** PRA (281.95 ± 851.4 vs. 26.28 ± 30.2 pg/mL; p = 0.102) and PRA percent increase (10.97 ± 30.77 vs. 12.57 ± 14.87; p = 0.844). They had comparable PICD incidence (24.7% vs. 12%; p = 0.27). Females were more liable for PICD occurrence than males (OR 2.91, 95% CI 1.125–7.547, p = 0.028) and so Child B patients than Child C (OR 8.4, 95% CI 1.072–65.767, p = 0.043).

Conclusion: Low-dose albumin infusion is comparable to the standard-dose albumin for the prevention of PICD.

Keywords: Large-volume paracentesis, Ascites, Albumin, Paracentesis-induced circulatory dysfunction, Plasma renin activity

Background

Liver cirrhosis is the final station of many liver diseases. Clinically, it may be compensated then after a variable period being decompensated. The development of ascites is the main sign of decompensation [1]. Actually, ascites develops in 50% of the patients within 10 years of liver cirrhosis diagnosis. Ascites is associated poor survival where 50% of the patients survive for 2–5 years [2].

Clinically, ascites is classified into 3 grades. The 1st and the 2nd one can be managed by salt restriction and diuretics, but the 3rd degree "tense" ascites is managed by large-volume paracentesis (LVP) followed by diuretics. About 20% of the patients who were diuretic responder will be diuretic resistant [3, 4].

Refractory ascites is a condition that is seen in 10% of patients with ascites. It is due to resistance to diuretics "diuretic-resistance ascites" or contraindication for diuretics "diuretic-intractable ascites". Until now, the main arms for the treatment of patients with tense or refractory ascites is LVP or transjugular intrahepatic portosystemic shunt (TIPS). Liver transplantation is the best solution. In fact, TIPS is associated with decreased demand for paracentesis, for nutritional improvement, and may be for survival benefit though it is associated with increased risk of encephalopathy. So, LVP is still the first option especially that TIPS is not widely available [4, 5].

Paracentesis-induced circulatory dysfunction (PICD) is a complication of LVP that is less seen if paracentesis is less

* Correspondence: aymanalsebaey@liver.menofia.edu.eg
Department of Hepatology and Gastroenterology, National Liver Institute, Menoufia University, Shebeen El-Koom 32511, Egypt

than 5 L. It is related to marked activation of the renin-angiotensin and sympathetic nervous systems over the levels before paracentesis. It is preventable by plasma expanders use especially human albumin (6–8 g/L ascitic fluid removed). PICD is associated with rapid re-accumulation of ascites, dilutional hyponatremia, hepatorenal syndrome, and decreased survival [6].

Albumin is not a simple plasma expander but has other advantages as detoxification of reactive oxygen and nitrogen species, endothelial stabilization and platelet anti-aggregation, and modulation of the immune and inflammatory responses [7]. The main drawback is that the drug is costly, so searching for alternatives is highly warranted [8].

This study aimed to compare low-dose albumin (2 g/L ascitic fluid removed) to standard-dose albumin (6 g/L ascitic fluid removed) for the prevention of PICD.

Methods

In our previous study [8], we compared terlipressin (3 mg IV), hydroxyethyl starch (HES 130/0.4; 8 g/L ascitic fluid removed), oral midodrine (5–10 mg daily), low-dose albumin (2 g/L ascitic fluid removed), and standard-dose albumin (6 g/L ascitic fluid removed) for PICD prevention. All groups were equal for PICD development. In this study, we could increase the number of patients in low-dose albumin group.

This study was conducted in National Liver Institute hospitals, hepatology, and gastroenterology department, Menoufia University. Prior institutional review board approval was acquired, and then an informed consent was obtained from all enrolled patients.

Patients who were requiring LVP for tense ascites (n = 110) were included in the study. Liver cirrhosis was diagnosed according to the clinical, laboratory, and abdominal ultrasonography findings [9].

Patients with the following criteria were included: tense ascites requiring LVP, age 18–70 years old, absence of cardiac disease, respiratory disease, hepatic encephalopathy, sepsis, spontaneous bacterial peritonitis, renal impairment (serum creatinine > 1.5 mg/dL), and gastrointestinal hemorrhage within 7 days before the study. All patients were on a low-sodium diet (34 mmol/day) for at least 7 days outpatient before inclusion in the study.

On day 0, a baseline workup, including body weight, mean arterial pressure (MAP), heart rate, electrocardiogram, liver tests (bilirubin, albumin, AST, ALT, alkaline phosphatase), and renal function tests (urea and creatinine), were conducted. Blood samples were collected after an overnight fast and bed rest for at least 30 min in the supine position for measuring PRA. Blood samples were put into chilled ethylenediaminetetraacetic acid tubes, centrifuged at 2500 rpm for 10 min at − 3 °C, and stored at − 20 °C. Total paracentesis was then done under local anesthesia and strict aseptic conditions.

Patients were categorized into 2 groups: low-dose albumin (2 g/L ascitic fluid removed; n = 85) and standard-dose albumin (6 g/L ascitic fluid removed; n = 25). Human albumin (20%; infusion solution; DRK-Blutspendedienst NSTOB 31830 Springe; each 1000 ml containing 200 g of human albumin) was used. Fifty percent of the dose was given within 2 h and the remainder 6 h after the procedure if more than 150 mL was infused to avoid pulmonary edema.

From day 1 to day 5, the patients were monitored daily for body weight, daily urine output volume, blood pressure, heart rate, and development of complications. On the day of hospital discharge (day 6), blood pressure, heart rate, and weight were recorded. Electrocardiogram, renal, and liver function tests were done, and blood was collected for PRA. Changes of the effective arterial blood volume were evaluated by measuring plasma rennin activity (PRA) on the day of paracentesis (day 0; baseline) and on the day of hospital discharge (day 6).

The primary end point was taken as development of PICD that was defined as an increase in PRA of > 50% of the baseline value [10]. PRA was laboratory measured in accord with Alsebaey et al [8].

Statistical analysis

Data was statistically analyzed using IBM® SPSS® Statistics® version 21 for Windows (IBM Corporation, Armonk, New York, USA). Data are expressed as mean ± standard deviation for parametric data, number with column percentage for nominal data, and the range for non-parametric data. All p values are two tailed, with values < 0.05 considered statistically significant. Comparisons between two groups were performed using the Student's t test for parametric data, and Mann-Whitney test for nonparametric data. Comparisons of the variables treatment induced change in the same group were performed using the paired t test for parametric data and Wilcoxon signed ranks test for nonparametric data. Chi-squared test (χ^2) and Fisher exact test for categorical data analysis. Univariate and multivariate binary logistic regression was done for detecting the predictors of PICD.

Results

Table 1 shows the baseline data in both groups. There was a statistically significant difference ($p < 0.05$) between both groups as regards the Child Pugh class, paracentesis volume, baseline serum albumin, and baseline PRA.

Patients who underwent low-dose albumin infusion post-paracentesis were mainly Child Pugh class B in contrast to patients in the other group (85.9% vs. 52%; p = 0.001), underwent less average paracentesis volume (9.78 ± 3.56 (7–25 L) vs. 12.52 ± 3.6 (6–20 L); p = 0.001), less baseline serum albumin (2.20 ± 0.36 vs. 2.55 ± 0.6 g/dL; p = 0.002), but higher baseline PRA (859.62 ± 1151.34 vs. 165.93 ± 95.34 pg/mL; p = 0.001).

Table 1 Comparison of the baseline parameters in both groups

		Low-dose albumin $N = 85$	Standard-dose albumin $N = 25$	p
Age (years)		53.19 ± 8.55	51.60 ± 6.84	0.397
Sex	Male	50 (58.8%)	9 (36%)	0.067
	Female	35 (41.2%)	16 (64%)	
Etiology	HCV	80 (93%)	22 (91.7%)	1
	Non-HCV	6 (7%)	2 (8.3%)	
Child Pugh class	Child B	73 (85.9%)	13 (52%)	0.001
	Child C	12 (14.1%)	12 (48%)	
PICD	None	64 (75.3%)	22 (88%)	0.27
	PICD	21 (24.7%)	3 (12%)	
Weight, kg		90.56 ± 11.26	87.08 ± 14.18	0.252
MAP, mmHg		78.98 ± 6.40	77.58 ± 5.81	0.358
Heart rate, beat/minute		83.70 ± 13.73	83.12 ± 5.24	0.84
Paracentesis, L		9.78 ± 3.56	12.52 ± 3.60	0.001
Total bilirubin, mg/dL		3.04 ± 2.65	2.78 ± 1.59	0.643
Total protein, g/dL		6.38 ± 0.93	6.33 ± 1.21	0.836
Albumin, g/dL		2.20 ± 0.36	2.55 ± 0.60	0.002#
AST, U/L		53.48 ± 26.78	72.32 ± 48.92	0.106#
ALT, U/L		35.48 ± 27.80	35.84 ± 24.11	0.954
ALP, U/L		104.21 ± 132.88	119.24 ± 103.15	0.604
GGT, U/L		47.66 ± 46.11	52.95 ± 68.15	0.66
Hemoglobin, g/dL		10.36 ± 1.32	10.12 ± 1.98	0.319#
WBCs, 10^9/L		6.90 ± 9.27	4.98 ± 2.55	0.309
Platelets, 10^9/L		82.14 ± 33.32	83.60 ± 38.47	0.853
INR		1.62 ± 0.51	1.55 ± 0.28	0.495
Urea, mg/dL		55.35 ± 30.48	38.16 ± 17.07	0.003#
Creatinine, mg/dL		0.95 ± 0.27	0.85 ± 0.36	0.103#
Sodium, mmol/L		123.25 ± 13.85	128.16 ± 6.03	0.088
Potassium, mmol/L		4.28 ± 0.69	4.20 ± 0.58	0.636
Child Pugh score		10.36 ± 1.26	9.88 ± 1.56	0.113
MELD		15.24 ± 4.41	15.28 ± 4.11	0.964
MELD Na		22.88 ± 4.12	21.88 ± 4.02	0.285
PRA, pg/mL		859.62 ± 1151.34	165.93 ± 95.34	0.001#

PICD paracentesis-induced circulatory dysfunction, *MAP* mean arterial pressure, *PRA* plasma renin activity, *HCV* hepatitis C virus, *MELD* model for end-stage liver disease
#Mann–Whitney *U* test

The other parameters did not show statistically significant difference ($p > 0.05$), namely age, sex, weight, MAP, heart rate, serum bilirubin, serum total protein, AST, ALT, ALP, GGT, hemoglobin, WBCs, platelets, INR, blood urea, serum creatinine, sodium, potassium, MELD, and MELD Na score.

The delta change (Δ) = day 6 variable value minus baseline variable value. Positive delta means higher day 6 value than baseline and vice versa. There was a statistically significant difference ($p < 0.05$) between both groups as regards the Δ weight and Δ blood urea (Table 2). Patients underwent low-dose albumin infusion post-paracentesis had less drop in the weight (− 4.35 ± 7.02 vs. − 10.64 ± 3.67 kg; $p = 0.001$) but higher blood urea increase (14.96 ± 23.84 vs. 3.72 ± 10.62 mg/dL; $p = 0.005$).

Delta MAP, heart rate, serum bilirubin, serum total protein, serum albumin, AST, ALT, ALP, GGT, hemoglobin, WBCs, platelets, INR, serum creatinine, sodium, potassium, model of end-stage liver disease (MELD), and MELD Na score did not show a statistically significant difference ($p > 0.05$) between both groups.

Table 2 Comparison of treatment induced changes in both groups

	Low-dose albumin N = 85	Standard-dose albumin N = 25	p
Δ Weight, kg	– 4.35 ± 7.02	– 10.64 ± 3.67	0.001#
Δ MAP, mmHg	– 1.59 ± 9.29	– 1.19 ± 6.09	0.699#
Δ Heart rate, beat/minute	2.07 ± 14.14	0.80 ± 3.18	0.523#
Δ Total bilirubin, mg/dL	0.15 ± 0.89	0.12 ± 0.59	0.756#
Δ Total protein, g/dL	– 0.12 ± 0.49	– 0.28 ± 0.85	0.249
Δ Albumin, g/dL	– 0.01 ± 0.19	2.35 ± 11.56	0.65#
Δ AST, U/L	– 0.95 ± 24.65	0.80 ± 25.02	0.756
Δ ALT, U/L	– 2.34 ± 24.98	2.44 ± 12.10	0.358
Δ ALP, U/L	– 12.06 ± 114.57	– 31.12 ± 106.93	0.46
Δ GGT, U/L	– 1.72 ± 20.57	– 7.86 ± 72.38	0.486
Δ Urea, mg/dL	14.96 ± 23.84	3.72 ± 10.62	0.005#
Δ Creatinine, mg/dL	0.14 ± 0.35	0.06 ± 0.29	0.348#
Δ Sodium, mmol/L	–1.84 ± 17.39	– 2.72 ± 1.43	0.8
Δ Potassium, mmol/L	0.07 ± 0.69	– 0.14 ± 0.64	0.166
Δ MELD	0.79 ± 3.46	0.12 ± 1.59	0.145#
Δ PRA, pg/mL	281.95 ± 851.4	26.28 ± 30.2	0.102#
PRA percent increase	10.97 ± 30.77	12.57 ± 14.87	0.844#

Δ indicates day 6 values to day 1 value
MAP mean arterial pressure, *PRA* plasma renin activity
#Mann–Whitney *U* test

Tables 1 and 2 and Figs. 1 and 2 showed the PICD studied parameters. Patients in the low-dose albumin group had higher baseline PRA (859.62 ± 1151.34 vs. 165.93 ± 95.34 pg/mL; p = 0.001) (Table 1). In both low-dose and standard-dose albumin groups, the PRA increased at day 6 compared with the baseline (1141.57 ± 1433.01 vs. 859.62 ± 1151.34 pg/mL; p = 0.01) and (192.21 ± 80.99 vs. 165.93 ± 95.34 pg/mL; p = 0.01) respectively (Fig. 1). Both the low-dose and standard-dose albumin groups were comparable for Δ PRA (281.95 ± 851.4 vs. 26.28 ± 30.2 pg/mL; p = 0.102) (Table 2, Fig. 1), and PRA percent increase (10.97 ± 30.77 vs. 12.57 ± 14.87; p = 0.844) respectively (Fig. 1). By application of the PICD definition [10], both low-dose and standard-dose albumin groups had comparable PICD incidence (24.7% vs. 12%; p = 0.27) (Fig. 2).

The univariate binary regression analysis (Table 3) showed that females were more liable for PICD occurrence than males (OR 2.91, 95% CI 1.125–7.547, p = 0.028) and so Child Pugh class B patients than class C (OR 8.4, 95% CI: 1.072–65.767, p = 0.043). The multivariate binary regression found also that females were more liable for PICD occurrence than males (OR 3.07, 95% CI: 1.155–8.162, p = 0.025) and so Child Pugh class B patients than class C (OR 8.92, 95% CI: 1.120–71.118, p = 0.039).

On comparison of the two current studies groups with previously published data [8] as shown in Table 4 and Fig. 3, all groups namely terlipressin, HES 130/0.4, midodrine, low-dose albumin, and standard-dose albumin were equal in the prevention of PICD (p > 0.05).

Discussion

The main concept of PICD pathogenesis is circulatory disturbance that develops after LVP if plasma expanders are not used. Immediately after LVP, there is decreased abdominal pressure, increased venous return, increased cardiac output, and suppression of the renin-angiotensin-sympathetic system. After 12 h, if no plasma expanders are used, the opposite occurs with marked activation of the renin-angiotensin-sympathetic system with reduced cardiac output. PICD may not be mere circulatory derangement [6]. In fact, Carl et al [11] in a small study (n = 10) hypothesized that LVP-induced hypotension increased bacterial translocation, innate immune activation that is responsible of vasodilation and subsequent PICD development.

PICD development is unrelated to the paracentesis flow rate [12]. Sersté et al [13] accused Beta blockers in the development of PICD in a small number study (n = 10). PICD can be prevented by either plasma expanders or finding other solutions to avoid or replace LVP which is the accused factor.

Regarding avoiding LVP, TIPS is a good solution since it modifies the pathogenesis of ascites and improves the quality of life and survival. Unfortunately, the increased

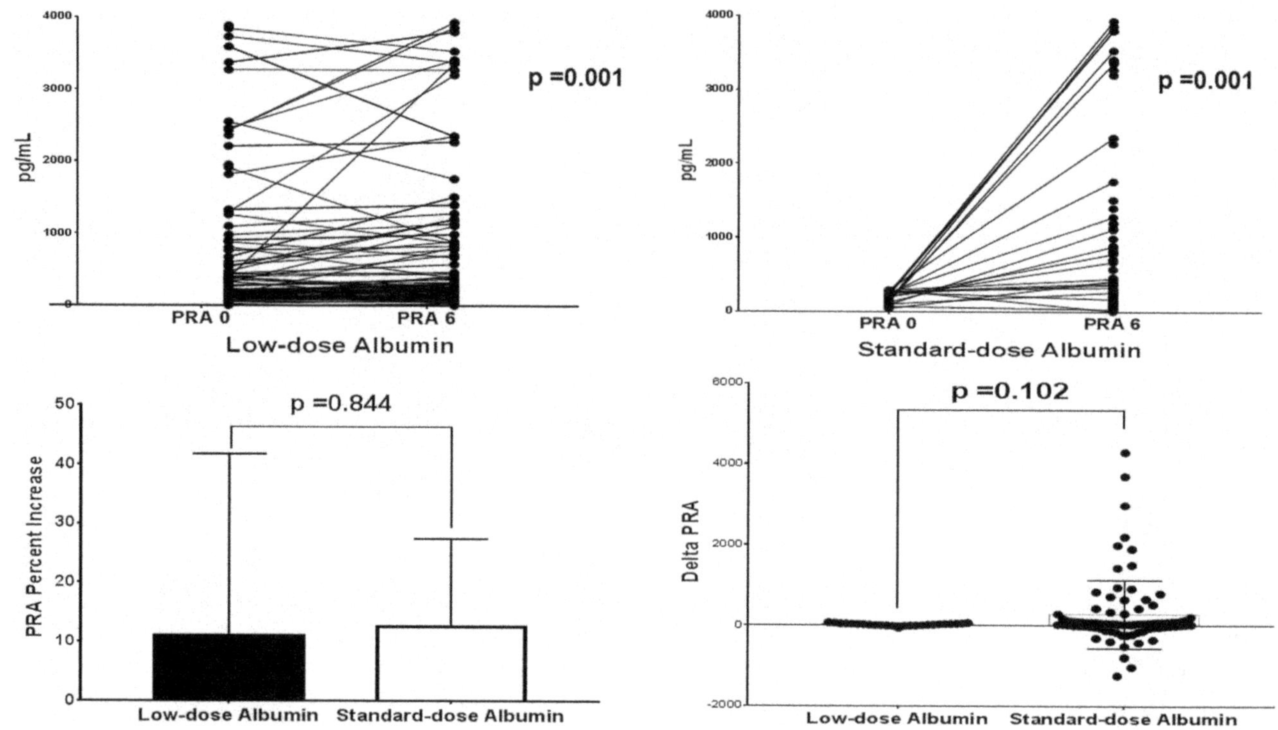

Fig. 1 Plasma renin activity (PRA) panel (days 0 and 6, delta change, percent increase) in low- and standard-dose albumin (Mann–Whitney *U* test and Wilcoxon signed ranks test)

incidence of hepatic encephalopathy is a drawback [4]. Permanent-tunneled peritoneal catheter is a new modality to avoid LVP [14]. It is not associated with renal impairment but further studies are needed. Alfa pump is another new modality "low flow pump system" for the treatment of refractory ascites [15–17]. It pumps the ascitic fluid through a valve to the urinary bladder and gets out by urination. It is considered continuous low-volume paracentesis. It decreased the ascites grade and the LVP times [15, 16]. Bureau et al [17] compared alfa pump to standard of care LVP with albumin replacement. Patients who underwent alfa pump had a marked decreased need for LVP, improved quality of life, and nutritional status but unfortunately increased the adverse effects especially early acute kidney injury. Both groups had the same survival. The enthusiasm for alfa pump will fades with the small number study (n = 10) by Solà et al [18]. They followed up the patients for 1 year with measure of the glomerular filtration rate by isotopes, blood pressure, and activity of vasoconstrictor

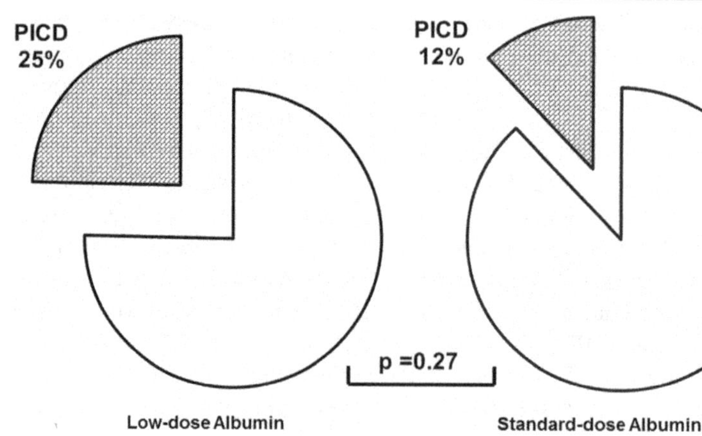

Fig. 2 Incidence of paracentesis circulatory dysfunction (PICD) in low- and standard-dose albumin

Table 3 Univariate and multivariate analysis of predictors of PICD occurrence

	Univariate				Multivariate			
	B	*p*	OR	95% CI	*B*	*p*	OR	95% CI
Age	− 0.01	0.737	0.99	0.937–1.047				
Females	1.07	0.028	2.91	1.125–7.547	1.12	0.025	3.07	1.155–8.162
Child Pugh B	2.13	0.043	8.40	1.072–65.767	2.19	0.039	8.92	1.120–71.118
MAP, mmHg	0.03	0.505	1.03	0.940–1.133				
Low-dose albumin	0.88	0.187	2.41	0.654–8.857				
Paracentesis liters	0.00	0.970	1.00	0.883–1.127				
Total bilirubin	− 0.06	0.545	0.94	0.768–1.149				
Albumin	0.41	0.408	1.51	0.567–4.038				
Urea	0.01	0.238	1.01	0.994–1.023				
Creatinine	0.28	0.725	1.32	0.281–6.216				
Sodium	− 0.03	0.183	0.97	0.937–1.012				
MELD	− 0.01	0.919	0.99	0.895–1.105				
MELD Na	0.00	0.942	1.00	0.899–1.122				

MAP mean arterial pressure, *OR* odds ratio, *CI* confidence interval, *MELD* model for end-stage liver disease, *Na* sodium

systems. The patients had significant decreased glomerular filtration rate at the 6th month and marked increase of PRA and norepinephrine concentration, with increased incidence of acute kidney injury. These features actually mimic PICD.

Tan et al [19] studied subtotal LVP not exceeding 8 L with using standard-dose albumin (6 g/L ascitic fluid removed; n = 57) as a method for PICD prevention. They used plasma active renin instead of PRA. PICD was detected in 40.3% of patients. The MAP decreased at day 6 compared with the baseline in patients with and without PICD. Though they had comparable baseline and day 6, creatinine with no renal impairment was noted. These patients were followed up 24 months. They had comparable serial creatinine values; same risk of hospitalization, spontaneous bacterial peritonitis, other infections, or gastrointestinal bleeding; and finally same survival.

IV albumin infusion (6–8 g/L ascitic fluid removed) is the standard of care plasma expander to prevent PICD. But it is associated with increased cost, so finding alternatives is warranted. Various drugs were studied like terlipressin [8, 20–23], noradrenaline [20, 24], midodrine [8, 25–27], synthetic colloids [8, 28–34], and saline [35, 36]. Our previous study [8] is the first study to our knowledge that did head-to-head drug comparison. All previous studies compared the used drug, e.g., terlipressin to the standard of care IV albumin. In our previous study, we compared terlipressin, midodrine, HES 130/0.4, and low-dose albumin (2 g/L ascitic fluid removed) to the standard-dose albumin (6 g/L ascitic fluid removed). The incidence of PICD was comparable in all groups, suggesting that albumin alternatives could be used.

Why returning back to albumin? The study of Carl et al [11] suggested that there are bacterial translocation and innate immune activation that play a role in PICD development. Since albumin has antioxidant, immunomodulatory effect in addition to increased oncotic pressure [37], it will be the preferred drug in such condition. To skip the high cost of albumin, using low doses may be of benefit.

Alessandria et al [38] was the first researcher who suggested the use of low-dose albumin. She compared low-dose albumin (4 g/L ascitic fluid removed; n = 35) with standard-dose albumin (8 g/L ascitic fluid removed; n = 35). Both groups were comparable for PICD development (14% vs 20%) respectively and 6-month survival or recurrence of ascites. The second study was conducted by Alsebaey et al [8]. One arm was low-dose albumin (2 g/L ascitic fluid removed; n = 25) which is the lowest tested dose compared with other studies [38, 39]. The

Table 4 Comparison of different treatment protocols for the PICD prevention

		Terlipressin	HES 130/0.4	Midodrine	Low-dose albumin	Standard-dose albumin	*p*
		N (%)	*N* (%)	*N* (%)	*N* (%)	*N* (%)	
PICD	None	23 (92%)	23 (92%)	20 (80%)	64 (75.3%)	22 (88%)	0.153
	PICD	2 (8%)	2 (8%)	5 (20%)	21 (24.7%)	3 (12%)	

PICD paracentesis-induced circulatory dysfunction

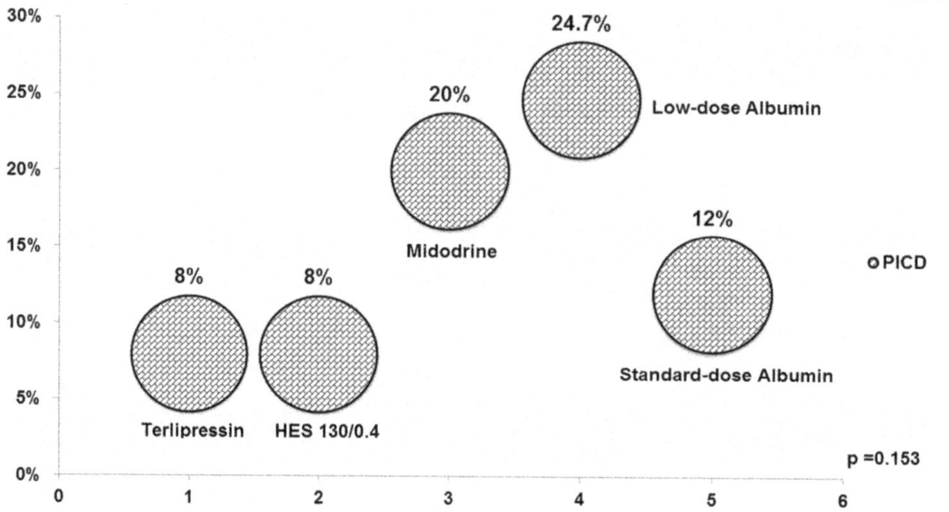

Fig. 3 Incidence of paracentesis circulatory dysfunction (PICD) in different groups, namely terlipressin, HES 130/0.4, midodrine, and low- and standard-dose albumin

PICD incidence in low-dose albumin was comparable to standard-dose albumin (6 g/L ascitic fluid removed; n = 35), HES 130/0.4, midodrine, and terlipressin. The third study was conducted by Hussain et al [39] on the utility of low-dose albumin (4 g/L ascitic fluid removed) on the prevention of paracentesis induced renal impairment. Actually, he did not measure PRA; he just followed up serum creatinine and sodium. Furthermore, he did not have arm of standard-dose albumin. He compared the utility of low-dose albumin in the prevention of renal impairment in patients who underwent low-volume paracentesis (6.2 ± 1 L) and large-volume paracentesis (10.4 ± 1.5 L). Few patients developed renal impairment (4.62% vs. 6.45%) respectively.

In the current study, only blood urea increased from baseline to the 6th day especially in the low-dose albumin compared with the standard-dose albumin in contrast to creatinine which was not affected. The PRA increased in both groups, but the delta change and the percent increase were comparable in both groups. In addition, the PICD development was comparable in both groups. Females and Child Pugh class B patients were more liable for PICD development. When we compared the current two arms with the old arms in our previous study [8], the incidence of PICD was comparable in the five groups, namely terlipressin, HES 130/0.4, low-dose albumin (2 g/L ascitic fluid removed), and the standard-dose albumin (6 g/L ascitic fluid removed).

The limitations of the current study are being single center experience, have relative small number of patients, and have absence of longitudinal follow-up to calculate the incidence of renal impairment, infections, bleeding, and importantly the survival.

Conclusion

Low-dose albumin infusion is comparable to the standard-dose albumin for the prevention of PICD. Furthermore, it is equivalent to terlipressin, midodrine, and HES 130/0.4 for PICD prevention.

Abbreviations

LVP: Large-volume paracentesis; MAP: Mean arterial pressure; MELD: Model of end stage liver disease; PICD: Paracentesis-induced circulatory dysfunction; PRA: Plasma renin activity; TIPS: Transjugular intrahepatic portosystemic shunt

Acknowledgements

None

Authors' contributions

Data collection was contributed by AA, HMA, and MAE. Study design was done by AA, HMA, and MAE. Manuscript writing and final revision was performed by AA. All authors have read and approved the final manuscript.

Competing interests

Imam Waked is an investigator and/or speaker for Abbvie, Gilead Sciences, Janssen, Marcyrl, Onxio, and Pharco. The rest of the authors declare that they have no competing interests.

References

1. D'Amico G, Garcia-Tsao G, Pagliaro L (2006) Natural history and prognostic indicators of survival in cirrhosis: a systematic review of 118 studies. J Hepatol 44:217–231
2. Kawaratani H, Fukui H, Yoshiji H (2017) Treatment for cirrhotic ascites. Hepatol Res 47:166–177
3. Solà E, Solé C, Ginès P (2016) Management of uninfected and infected ascites in cirrhosis. Liver Int 36:109–115
4. Annamalai A, Wisdom L, Herada M, Nourredin M, Ayoub W, Sundaram V et al (2016) Management of refractory ascites in cirrhosis: are we out of date? World J Hepatol 8:1182–1193
5. Salerno F, Guevara M, Bernardi M, Moreau R, Wong F, Angeli P et al (2010) Refractory ascites: pathogenesis, definition and therapy of a severe complication in patients with cirrhosis. Liver Int 30:937–947
6. Sola-Vera J, Such J (2004) Understanding the mechanisms of paracentesis-induced crculatory dysfunction. Eur J Gastroenterol Hepatol 16:295–298

7. Caraceni P, Angeli P, Prati D, Bernardi M, Alessandria C, Riggio O et al (2016) AISF-SIMTI position paper: the appropriate use of albumin in patients with liver cirrhosis. Dig Liver Dis 48:4–15
8. Alsebaey A, Abdel-Razek W, Bassuni A, Rewisha E, Khalil M, Waked I (2013) Prevention of paracentesis-induced circulatory dysfunction: could we use other albumin alternatives? Egyptian Liver Journal 3:118–125
9. Schuppan D, Afdhal NH (2008) Liver cirrhosis. Lancet 371:838–851
10. Ruiz-del-Arbol L, Monescillo A, Jimenez W, Garcia-Plaza A, Arroyo V, Rodes J (1997) Paracentesis-induced circulatory dysfunction: mechanism and effect on hepatic hemodynamics in cirrhosis. Gastroenterology 113:579–586
11. Carl DE, Ghosh S, Cheng J, Gehr TWB, Stravitz RT, Sanyal A (2014) Post-paracentesis circulatory derangements are related to monocyte activation. Liver Int 34:1001–1007
12. Elsabaawy MM, Abdelhamid SR, Alsebaey A, Abdelsamee E, Obada MA, Salman TA et al (2015) The impact of paracentesis flow rate in patients with liver cirrhosis on the development of paracentesis induced circulatory dysfunction. Clin Mol Hepatol 21:365–371
13. Sersté T, Francoz C, Durand F, Rautou P-E, Melot C, Valla D et al (2011) Beta-blockers cause paracentesis-induced circulatory dysfunction in patients with cirrhosis and refractory ascites: a cross-over study. J Hepatol 55:794–799
14. Solbach P, Höner zu Siederdissen C, Taubert R, Ziegert S, Port K, Schneider A et al (2017) Home-based drainage of refractory ascites by a permanent-tunneled peritoneal catheter can safely replace large-volume paracentesis. Eur J Gastroenterol Hepatol 29:539–546
15. Bellot P, Welker M-W, Soriano G, von Schaewen M, Appenrodt B, Wiest R et al (2013) Automated low flow pump system for the treatment of refractory ascites: a multi-center safety and efficacy study. J Hepatol 58:922–927
16. Thomas MN, Sauter GH, Gerbes AL, Stangl M, Schiergens TS, Angele M et al (2015) Automated low flow pump system for the treatment of refractory ascites: a single-center experience. Langenbeck's Arch Surg 400:979–983
17. Bureau C, Adebayo D, de Rieu MC, Elkrief L, Valla D, Peck-Radosavljevic M et al Alfapump system vs. large volume paracentesis for refractory ascites: a multicenter randomized controlled study. J Hepatol
18. Solà E, Sanchez-Cabús S, Rodriguez E, Elia C, Cela R, Moreira R et al (2017) Effects of alfapump™ system on kidney and circulatory function in patients with cirrhosis and refractory ascites. Liver Transpl 23:583–593
19. Tan HK, James PD, Wong F (2016) Albumin may prevent the morbidity of paracentesis-induced circulatory dysfunction in cirrhosis and refractory ascites: a pilot study. Dig Dis Sci 61:3084–3092
20. Abdullah MH, Saleh SM, Morad WS Terlipressin versus norepinephrine to counteract intraoperative paracentesis induced refractory hypotension in cirrhotic patients. Egyptian Journal of Anaesthesia
21. Singh V, Kumar R, Nain CK, Singh B, Sharma AK (2006) Terlipressin versus albumin in paracentesis-induced circulatory dysfunction in cirrhosis: a randomized study. J Gastroenterol Hepatol 21:303–307
22. Moreau R, Asselah T, Condat B, de Kerguenec C, Pessione F, Bernard B et al (2002) Comparison of the effect of terlipressin and albumin on arterial blood volume in patients with cirrhosis and tense ascites treated by paracentesis: a randomised pilot study. Gut 50:90–94
23. Lata J, Marecek Z, Fejfar T, Zdenek P, Bruha R, Safka V et al (2007) The efficacy of terlipressin in comparison with albumin in the prevention of circulatory changes after the paracentesis of tense ascites--a randomized multicentric study. Hepato-gastroenterology 54:1930–1933
24. Singh V, Kumar B, Nain CK, Singh B, Sharma N, Bhalla A et al (2006) Noradrenaline and albumin in paracentesis-induced circulatory dysfunction in cirrhosis: a randomized pilot study. J Intern Med 260:62–68
25. Singh V, Dheerendra PC, Singh B, Nain CK, Chawla D, Sharma N et al (2008) Midodrine versus albumin in the prevention of paracentesis-induced circulatory dysfunction in cirrhotics: a randomized pilot study. Am J Gastroenterol 103:1399–1405
26. Appenrodt B, Wolf A, Grunhage F, Trebicka J, Schepke M, Rabe C et al (2008) Prevention of paracentesis-induced circulatory dysfunction: midodrine vs albumin. A randomized pilot study. Liver Int 28:1019–1025
27. Hamdy H, ElBaz AA, Hassan A, Hassanin O (2014) Comparison of midodrine and albumin in the prevention of paracentesis-induced circulatory dysfunction in cirrhotic patients: a randomized pilot study. J Clin Gastroenterol 48:184–188
28. Planas R, Gines P, Arroyo V, Llach J, Panes J, Vargas V et al (1990) Dextran-70 versus albumin as plasma expanders in cirrhotic patients with tense ascites treated with total paracentesis. Results of a randomized study. Gastroenterology 99:1736 1744
29. Gines A, Fernandez-Esparrach G, Monescillo A, Vila C, Domenech E, Abecasis R et al (1996) Randomized trial comparing albumin, dextran 70, and polygeline in cirrhotic patients with ascites treated by paracentesis. Gastroenterology 111:1002–1010
30. Garcia-Compean D, Blanc P, Larrey D, Daures JP, Hirtz J, Mendoza E et al (2002) Treatment of cirrhotic tense ascites with Dextran-40 versus albumin associated with large volume paracentesis: a randomized controlled trial. Ann Hepatol 1:29–35
31. Moreau R, Valla DC, Durand-Zaleski I, Bronowicki JP, Durand F, Chaput JC et al (2006) Comparison of outcome in patients with cirrhosis and ascites following treatment with albumin or a synthetic colloid: a randomised controlled pilot trail. Liver Int 26:46–54
32. El-Ashry N, El-Damarawy M, Salem M, Mogawer S (2007) Large volume abdominal paracentesis effect on some humoral factors and cardiac performance in patients with liver cirrhosis and tense ascities. J Egypt Soc Parasitol 37:571–584
33. Abdel-Khalek EE, Arif SE (2010) Randomized trial comparing human albumin and hydroxyethyl starch 6% as plasma expanders for treatment of patients with liver cirrhosis and tense ascites following large volume paracentesis. Arab Journal of Gastroenterology 11:24–29
34. Nasr G, Hassan A, Ahmed S, Serwah A (2010) Predictors of large volume paracantesis induced circulatory dysfunction in patients with massive hepatic ascites. J Cardiovasc Dis Res 1:136–144
35. Cabrera J, Inglada L, Quintero E, Jimenez W, Losada A, Mayor J et al (1991) Large-volume paracentesis and intravenous saline: effects on the renin-angiotensin system. Hepatology 14:1025–1028
36. Sola-Vera J, Minana J, Ricart E, Planella M, Gonzalez B, Torras X et al (2003) Randomized trial comparing albumin and saline in the prevention of paracentesis-induced circulatory dysfunction in cirrhotic patients with ascites. Hepatology 37:1147–1153
37. Spinella R, Sawhney R, Jalan R (2016) Albumin in chronic liver disease: structure, functions and therapeutic implications. Hepatol Int 10:124–132
38. Alessandria C, Elia C, Mezzabotta L, Risso A, Andrealli A, Spandre M et al (2011) Prevention of paracentesis-induced circulatory dysfunction in cirrhosis: standard vs half albumin doses. A prospective, randomized, unblinded pilot study. Dig Liver Dis 43:881–886
39. Hussain W, Khalid AB, Usmani T, Ghufran A, Shah H (2015) Low dose albumin for the prevention of renal impairment following large volume paracentesis in cirrhosis. Pakistan Journal of Medical Sciences 31:592–596

21

The diagnostic value of diffusion-weighted imaging in differentiating benign from malignant hepatic lesions

Reza Javadrashid[1], Abolhassan Shakeri Bavil Olyaei[1], Mohammad Kazem Tarzamni[1], Roghayeh Razzaghi[1], Javad Jalili[1], Shahryar Hashemzadeh[2], Mohammad Mirza-Aghazadeh-Attari[3], Ali Kiani Nazarlou[4] and Armin Zarrintan[4*]

Abstract

Background: Diffusion-weighted imaging (DWI) is a novel imaging technique with growing application in onco-imaging. This modality evaluates the diffusion of water molecules in various tissues, which is restricted in hyper cellular regions such as malignant tissue. Apparent diffusion co-efficient (ADC) is a method which can quantify the degree of restriction in tissues and can have diagnostic roles in characterization of hepatic lesions. In this study, 93 patients with proven hepatic lesions were included. These patients had undergone initial evaluation via ultrasonography and dynamic CT scan, and had a definite diagnosis confirmed by biopsy. These patients underwent DW imaging and ADC values of their lesions were calculated. Patients were divided into two groups, benign and malignant groups, based on their biopsy results; and ADC values of hepatic lesions were compared in the two groups.

Results: The two groups were gender matched. There was a significant difference in the age distribution between the two groups. Mean ADC values for benign and malignant hepatic lesions were 1.58 ± 0.35 (10^{-3} mm^2/s) and 0.87 ± 0.16 (10^{-3} mm^2/s), respectively. There was a statistically significant differences between benign and malignant hepatic lesions (p value $< 10^{-3}$). DW imaging had a sensitivity of 97.6% and specificity of 98.7% in detecting malignant hepatic lesions from benign ones ($p = 0.0001$, AUC = 0.99).

Conclusion: DW MRI imaging can differentiate malignant and benign liver lesions with high sensitivity and specificity using ADC values generated; furthermore, each subgroup of hepatic lesions could be determined based on ADC values.

Keywords: (DWI) Diffusion weighted, Hepatic mass, MRI

Background

Diffusion-weighted (DW) magnetic resonance imaging (MRI) was initially introduced in the middle of the 1990s and has since gained clinical significance in human pathologies. This imaging technique relies on variances in diffusion of water molecules in intracellular and intercellular spaces [1]. Initial efforts were made to utilize DW-MRI in stroke patients, as DW-MRI was theoretically able to diagnose stroke in seconds [2]. Success in these initiatives led researchers to focus on other applications of DW MRI in imaging, including onco-imaging [3]. Studies have shown that malignant tissue differs significantly from normal tissue in cellular architecture, cellular density, and extracellular matrix composition [4]. This causes the water molecules to have an altered diffusion pattern compared to normal tissue, which can be detected by DW-MRI. More so, different cancers arising from different tissues and cancers varying in stage also have different cellular structure, making them distinguishable in DW imaging [5]. Many studies have indeed shown this in cancers of the breast, brain, head and neck, colon, and the hepatobiliary system [6].

* Correspondence: zarrintanarmin@gmail.com
[4]Department of Radiology, Imam Reza Hospital, Tabriz University of Medical Sciences, Tabriz, Iran

Many malignant and benign lesions comprising of cystic lesions, solid primary tumors, metastasis, patches of fibrosis, vascular lesions, and infectious lesions can be found in the liver and distinguishing them may be a diagnostic challenge [7, 8]. DW-MRI has shown beneficence in distinguishing the aforementioned lesions, but question remains regarding the sensitivity and specificity of this modality in diagnosing malignant lesions [9] and if DW MRI is able to distinguish between benign lesions of the liver and normal tissue. Previous studies have aimed to examine the efficacy of DW MRI in diagnosing liver masses, but no consensus exists regarding the routine use of DWI in detecting neoplastic lesions, as no definite cut-off point is set for values generated by DWI imaging, such as apparent diffusion coefficient (ADC) which is used for quantitative analysis of hepatic lesion [10]. Also, there are ambiguities regarding the optimal technical specifications for hepatic lesions, as different studies have reported DW images with varying *b* values [11]. This study aims to study the sensitivity and specificity of DW imaging in diagnosing benign and malignant hepatic lesions and to examine whether an ADC value could be determined as a cutoff value to diagnose benign lesions from malignant ones.

Methods

Patients

In this prospective study, which was conducted between June 2016 and April 2019, in a tertiary referral center, a total of 93 patients with 118 liver masses were included. All patients had gone under initial evaluation by ultrasonography or dynamic CT scan of the liver. Then DWI MRI was performed for all patients. Inclusion criteria consisted of being above 18 years, having at least one lesion in the liver, having a definite pathologic diagnosis of the lesion (either by biopsy or fulfilling radiologic criteria), and being followed up for at least 6 months. Exclusion criteria consisted of patients who underwent chemotherapy before MRI imaging, inability of the patient to withstand the conditions necessary for performing an MRI, and lack of will to participate in the study.

In considering the results of ultrasonography, liver dynamic CT scan and biopsies, patients were categorized to five groups including liver hemangioma, liver focal nodular hyperplasia (FNH), liver metastasis, cholangiocarcinoma, and hepatocellular carcinoma (HCC). Patients were also divided into two main groups of those with benign hepatic lesions (including liver hemangioma and FNH) and patients with malignant hepatic lesion (including liver metastasis, cholangiocarcinoma, and HCC). Other liver lesions were not included, such as hepatic fibrosis and infectious cysts or secondary hemorrhages in primary lesions, as our goal was to study the role of DW imaging in differentiating mass-like lesions which are not suitably diagnosed using ultrasonography and CT scan.

Imaging technique

MR imaging was performed utilizing 1.5-T MR systems (Siemens Medical Solutions, Erlangen, Germany) at the MRI ward of our medical educational center. Single-shot spin-echo (SE) echo-planar technique combined with fat suppression was performed according to these technical specifications: matrix 128 × 128, field of view 36cm × 36cm, section thickness 8 mm, and gap 2 mm and scan time 3–4 min. The *b* values of 0 and 1000 s/mm^{-2} were applied in three orthogonal directions and combined to provide isotropic images. The ADC of the region of interest was calculated using workstation.

Ethical considerations

All patients being included in this study had signed written informed consent forms. This article was approved in the local ethics committee of the tertiary medical center in which it was performed. This study was performed according to the Helsinki declaration. Personal information, including imaging findings were not disclosed to any third party.

Statistical analysis

Statistical analysis was performed using Statistical Package for the Social Sciences (SPSS Version 19, Chicago, USA). Chi-square test was used to compare ADC values of malignant and benign lesions, while Student *T* test was used to compare quantitative data. Power of the study was set at 80% and a *p* value less than 0.05 was considered significant.

Results

Ninety three patients were included in this study. These patients had 118 distinct liver masses. The follow-up of the patients showed that 42 masses were malignant, while 76 where benign. Of all the patients, 73 had only a single lesion in their liver, of which 42 were malignant and 31 were benign, 15 and 5 patients had two and three lesions in their livers, respectively, which were all benign. Demographics of the patients and types of lesions are summarized in Table 1.

The highest ADC value was recorded for a hemangioma (2.86 × 10^{-3} mm^2/s), while the lowest value recorded was for a metastasis (0.49 × 10^{-3} mm^2/s). ADC values for five categories of hepatic lesions are summarized in Table 2. The mean ADC value of all lesions combined was 1.3364 × 10^{-3} mm^2/s.

Table 1 Demographic information of patients being included in the study

Tumor type	Number of lesions	Male	Female	Age
Malignant lesion	42	30	12	57.34 ± 15.69
Benign lesion	31	18	33	46.14 ± 34/21

Table 2 Apparent diffusion coefficient values for detected lesions

	Number of lesions	Mean ADC value*	Standard deviation	Standard error	Confidence interval (95%)		Minimum ADC value *	Maximum ADC value *
Hemangioma	72	1.6134	0.34188	0.04029	1.5331	1.6938	0.85	2.86
FNH	4	1.1738	0.15593	0.07796	0.9256	1.4219	0.96	1.29
Metastasis	31	0.8451	0.16475	0.02959	0.7847	0.9056	0.49	1.31
Cholangiocarcinoma	7	0.9809	0.10885	0.04114	0.8802	1.0815	0.78	1.11
HCC	4	0.9435	0.07911	0.03955	0.8176	1.0694	0.86	1.04
Total	118	1.3364	0.45189	0.04160	1.2541	1.4188	0.49	2.86

**ADC* apparent diffusion coefficient (10^{-3} mm^2/s)

The mean ADC values for benign and malignant lesions was 1.58 ± 0.35 (10^{-3} mm^2/s) and 0.87 ± 0.16 (10^{-3} mm^2/s), respectively. The mean ADC value was significantly higher in benign lesions ($p = 0.001$). ADC measurement had a sensitivity of 97.6% and specificity of 98.7% in differentiating malignant lesions from benign ones. Positive predictive value was 97.61% and negative predictive value was 98.68 %. Positive likelihood ratio was 75.07, and negative likelihood ratio was 0.02.

The cutoff value in differentiating benign and malignant lesions was 1.1×10^{-3}. Figure 1 shows the ROC curve for ADC values. Figure 2 shows mean ADC values for each of the five types of liver masses studied. Figure 3 shows the differences between the mean ADC values between the benign and malignant groups. Figures 4, 5, and 6 demonstrate examples of imaging findings.

Discussion

In the present study, the application of DW-MRI in differentiating malignant masses of the liver was examined. We found that DW-MRI was indeed a suitable method to distinguish malignant lesions and that ADC values

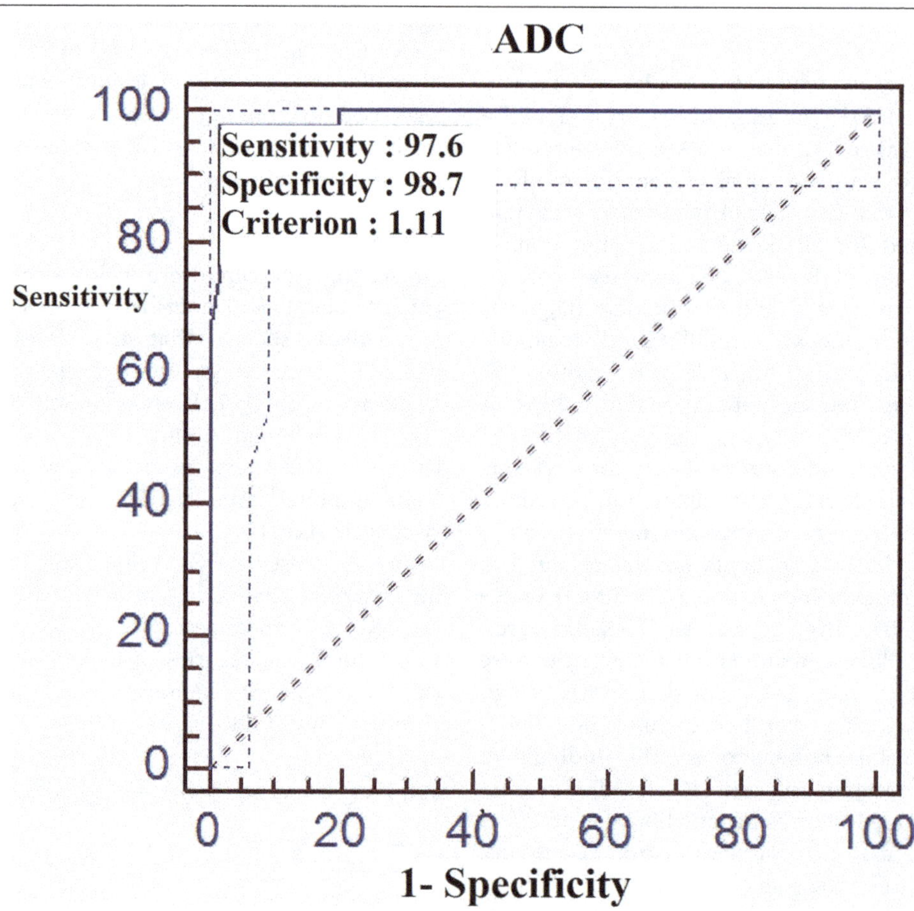

Fig. 1 ROC curve of ADC values for diagnosing malignant lesion

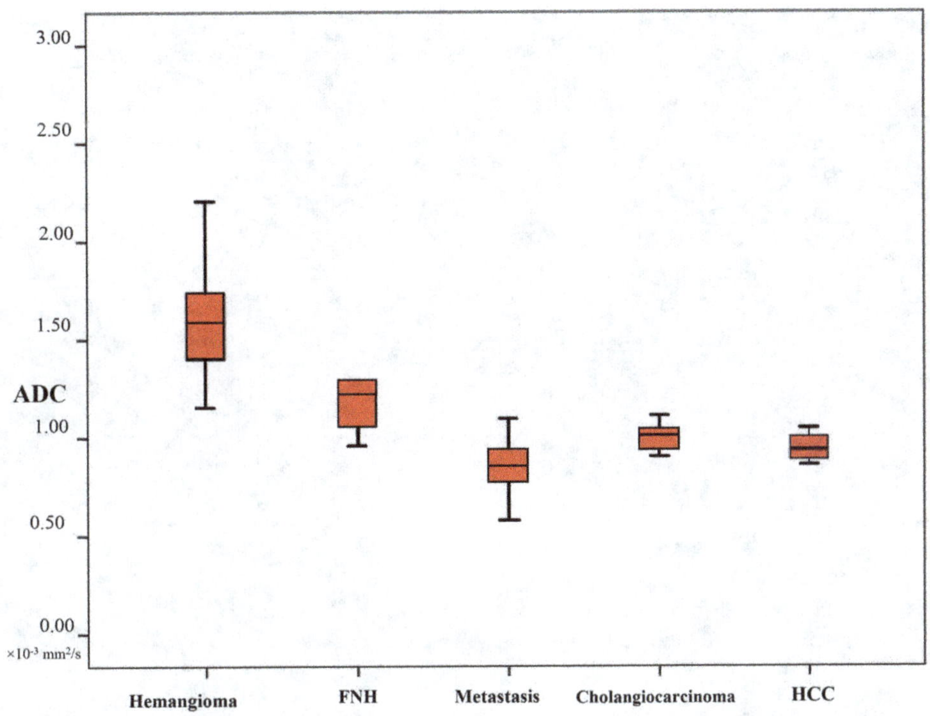

Fig. 2 Box and whisker plots of ADC values for different groups of liver masses

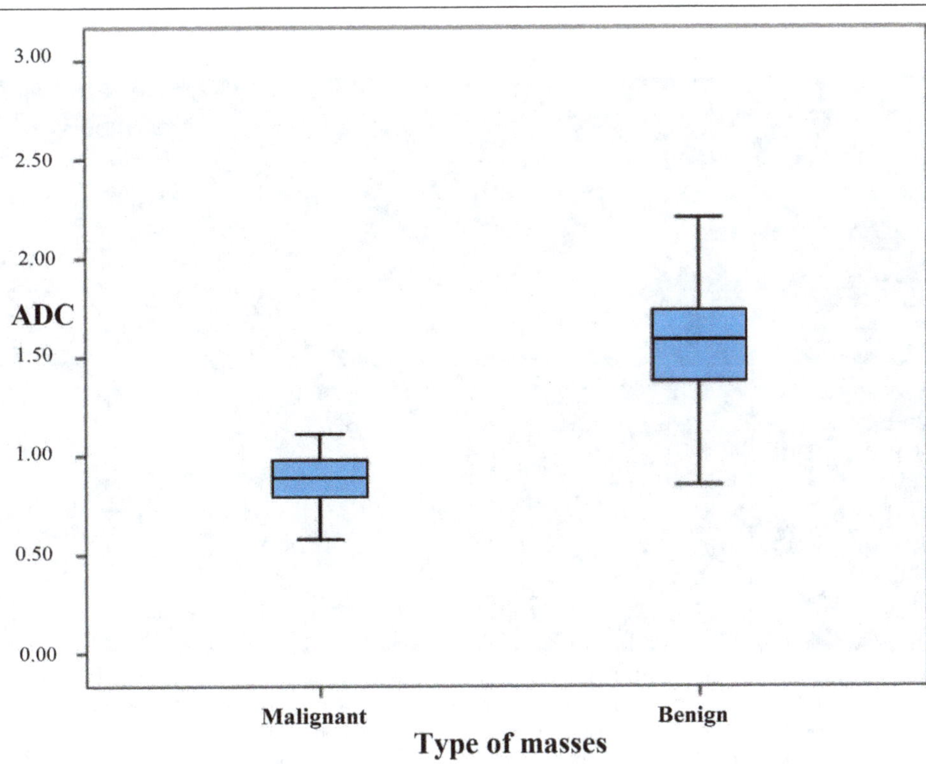

Fig. 3 Box and whisker plots of ADC values for malignant and benign lesions

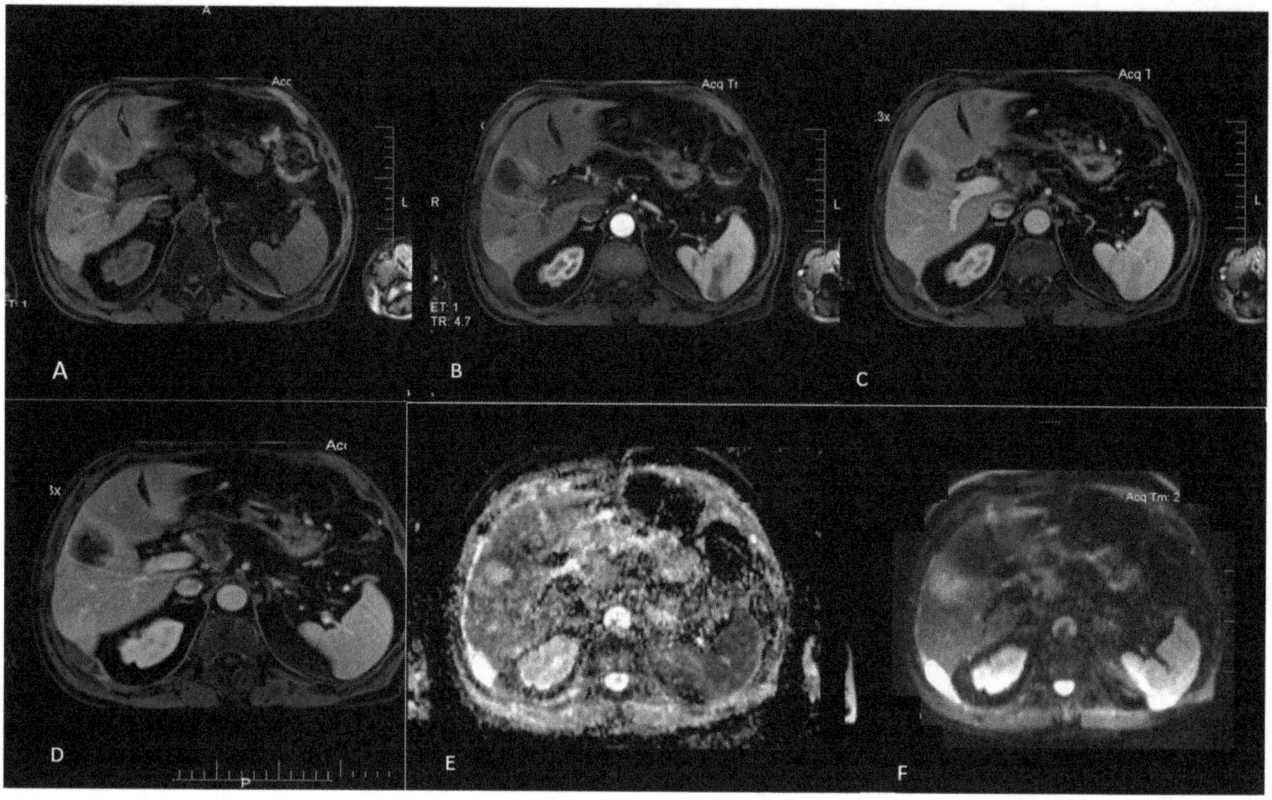

Fig. 4 Tri-phasic MRI of a patient with pancreatic cancer, presenting with liver metastasis. **a** pre-contrast T1 sequence. **b** Arterial phase T1 sequence. **c** venous phase T1 sequence. **d** Interstitial phase T1 sequence. As it can be seen, the lesion is hypo-intense in T1 sequences with evident ring enhancement. **e** ADC map showing restricted diffusion (ADC value:0.8 × 10^{-3} mm^2/s). **f** DWI imaging of the liver in *b* value of 800 s/mm^2

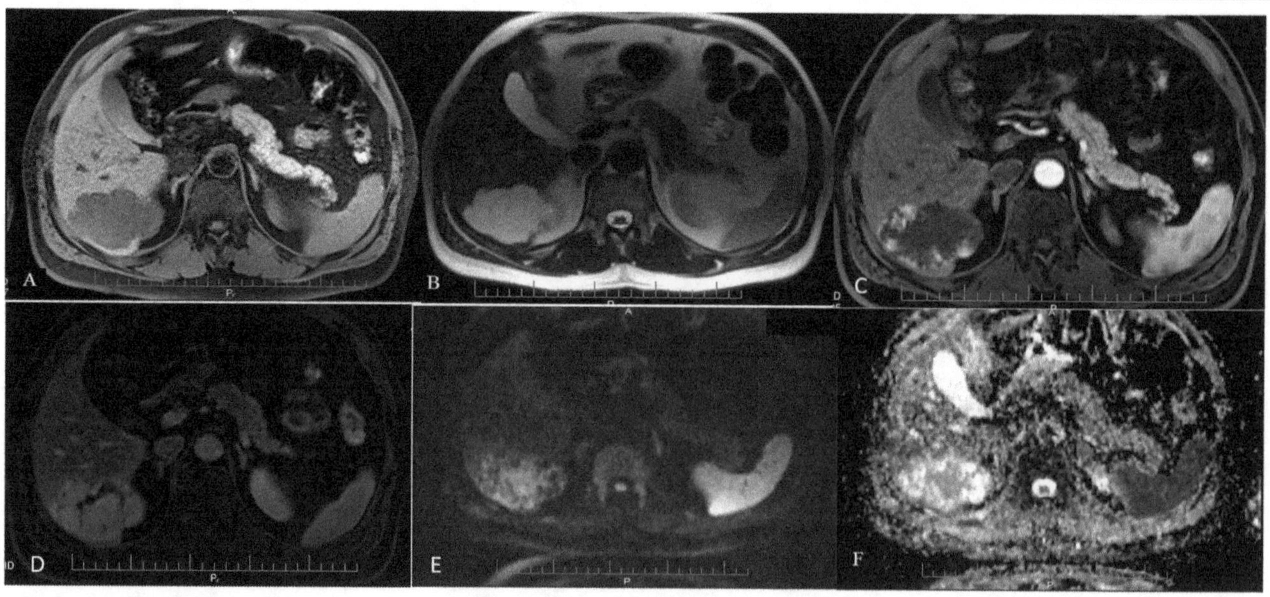

Fig. 5 a T1 sequence showing a hypo-intense lesion. **b** T2 HASTE sequence: There is a large oval mass at the right lobe of the liver, which is hyper intense compared to liver parenchyma. **c** Post gadolinium T1-weighted sequences at arterial phase. The image shows that the mass has nodular peripheral enhancement. **d** Post gadolinium T1-weighted sequences at delayed phase: The mass shows more peripheral centripetal enhancement compared to arterial phase. **e** DWI in *b* value of 800 s/mm^2. The ADC value of the lesion was 1.53 × 10^{-3} mm^2/s. **f** ADC map of the liver. The aforementioned findings are suggestive of hemangioma

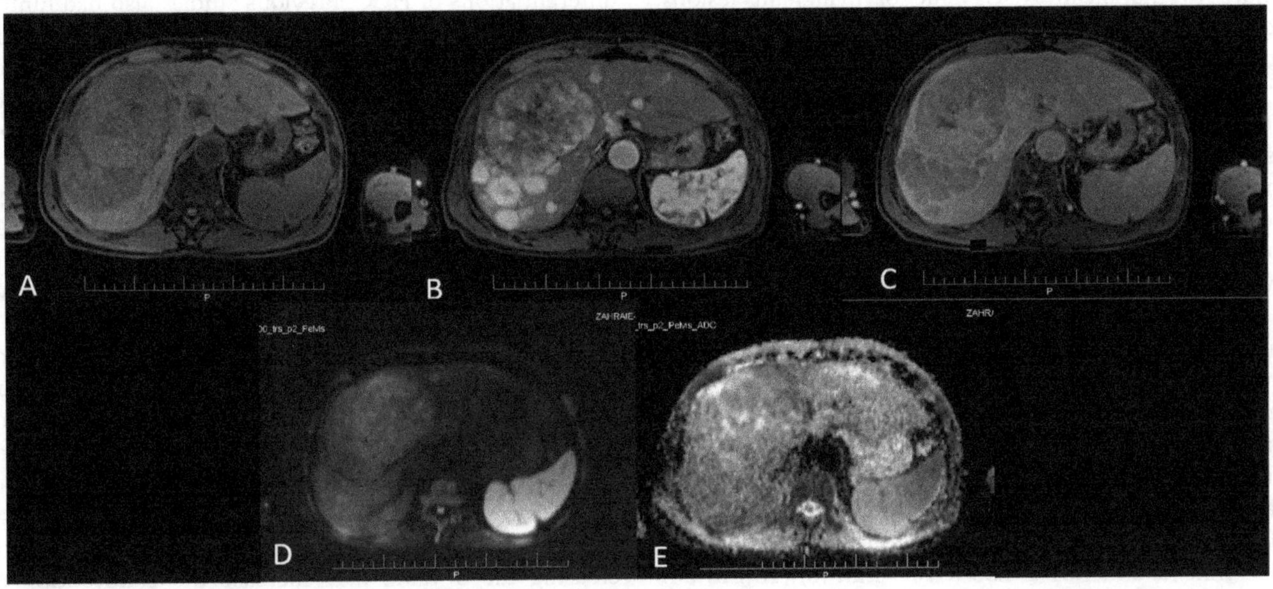

Fig. 6 An HCC in a 67-year-old patient with long standing cirrhosis. **a** The lesion in T1 with no contrast, shows a hypo intense mass. **b** Arterial phase, shows rapid hyper-enhancement. **c** Delayed phase, showing rapid washout. **d** DWI in *b* value of 800 s/mm^2. The ADC value of the lesion equaled to 0.93 × 10^{-3} mm^2/s. **e** ADC map of the liver

could even be used to distinguish specific lesions. Our results revealed that the ADC value is significantly higher in benign hepatic lesion compared to malignant ones. In this study, the cutoff point of 1.1 × 10^{-3} was determined to differentiate between benign and malignant hepatic lesions.

Histopathologic studies have shown that various liver lesions have characteristic findings in pathological examination and unique cellular architecture. Malignant lesions such as hepatocellular carcinoma and metastasis are composed of a dense formation of cells tightly packed within an absent or minimal stroma, while focal nodular hyperplasia is composed of normal-looking hepatocytes imbedded in a rich fibrous mesh with considerably more extracellular space, and hemangiomas are composed of vascular spaces with an abundant stroma. These histopathologic variances could hypothetically be witnessed in DW MRI, as water molecules could move freely in less dense cellular structures such as those of benign lesions, resulting in increased values of ADC, which could be useful in differentiating between them and malignant lesions. This hypothesis could also be true for differentiating various malignant lesions from each other. This is shown best by grading of astrocytoma using ADC values [12].

Application of DW MRI in hepatic lesion detection is also possible. Initial results have been contradictory, and no definite suggestions have been made, but primary results have shown that low *b* values could be beneficial in lesion detection, while increasing the *b* value could assist in lesion classification.

Experimental evidence in this regard is given by Testa et al., where DW MRI was used to classify 188 masses in 67 adults. Of all the lesions, 105 were metastatic lesions, 37 were hemangiomas, 42 were cysts, 2 were adenomas, and 2 were nodular hyperplasia. This study showed that the average ADC for metastasis was 1.0 × 10^{-3} mm^2/s (CI 0.8–1.3), 1.4 × 10^{-3} mm^2/s (CI 1.1–1.7) for solid benign lesions and 2.4 × 10^{-3} mm^2/s (CI 2.1–2.6) for cystic lesions. The cutoff value for distinguishing metastatic lesions from benign solid lesions was reported to be 1.2 × 10^{-3} mm^2/s, and 1.5 × 10^{-3} mm^2/s for all benign lesions, including cysts. The accuracy of DW MRI in detecting malignant lesions from non-malignant solid lesions was 71%, and 78% if cysts were included. A study performed by Kilickesmez et al. also studied the efficacy of DW MRI in diagnosing malignant lesions from benign lesions. They included benign entities such as simple liver cysts, hydatid cysts, and hemangiomas. Most of the lesions included were of the aforementioned, while a smaller number of malignant lesions were also included. The authors suggested that there was a significant difference between the ADC values of hepatic lesions and normal liver parenchyma, and also between hemangiomas and HCCs or metastasis [13]. This study provides practical evidence regarding the use of DW in liver masses, but the low number of malignant lesions, and high number of normal liver tissue limits its generalizability (65 normal liver specimens were included compared to 13 metastases and 13 HCCs). This study does not include FNHs and cholangiocarcinomas, entities which theoretically would have closer ADC values to the mean ADC value of malignant lesions, compared to the ADC value of cystic lesions (which is considerably higher).

In regard to previous studies, it is noteworthy to mention that diagnosing cystic lesions is not of a challenge as those of diagnosing solid benign and malignant masses, and not including cysts could reveal the true efficacy of DW imaging in detecting liver lesions. The same could also be said regarding fibrotic lesions of the liver, which have distinct radiological appearances [14].

A large number of malignant hepatic lesions are metastasis from distant sites and differentiating between these lesions and non-malignant hepatic lesions is of great importance, especially in patients effected by a primary tumor in another organ. Parikh et al. found that there was no significant difference between the ADC values of benign hepatic lesions, metastatic lesions, and HCC (ADC = $1.49 \pm 0.49 \times 10^{-3}$ mm^2/s, $1.50 \pm 0.42 \times 10^{-3}$ mm^2/s, and $1.31 \pm 0.33 \times 10^{-3}$ mm^2/s) [15]. In our study, there was a significant difference between the ADC values of non-malignant lesions and metastasis. This could be because of utilizing *b* values up to 1000, compared to Parikh et al. where only *b* values of 0, 100, and 500 were used. Also, use of non-DWI MRI imaging could be beneficial in increasing the sensitivity of MRI in detecting malignant metastatic lesions.

A meta-analysis by Xia et al. published in 2010 focused on the efficacy of DW MRI in diagnosing hepatic lesions, and reported that indeed DW MRI would be of beneficence, but the exact sensitivity and specificity would vary greatly based on the diagnostic implication, as differentiating between normal hepatic masses and metastasis would be easier than differentiating focal nodular hyperplasia from low-grade hepatocellular carcinoma. The authors suggested that more studies would be needed to determine exact imaging protocols incorporating DW MRI, and that more studies were needed to determine the efficacy in differentiating various malignant lesions from each other [16]. In our study, metastasis, HCC, and cholangiocarcinoma had almost identical ADC values, which was in concordance to other similar studies [17].

Ogihara et al. [18] utilized DW MRI to grade HCCs and examined which variables could be used to differentiate between high-grade and low-grade HCCs. They studied 83 patients with 100 histologically diagnosed HCCs. They used DW MRI with a *b* value of 1000 and retrospectively matched radiologic findings with histopathologic findings. They found that in *b* values of 800 and 1000, ADC was not significantly different between well and poorly differentiated HCCs and it could only be used in differentiating well differentiated HCCs from moderately and poorly differentiated HCCs, while relative contrast ratio (RCR) and contrast-to-noise ratio (CNR) could be used to differentiate between all three differentiations of HCC. Previous studies also had hinted that non-ADC values could be utilized in determining the differentiation of tumors, but no consensus exists regarding the best strategy to determine the grading of malignant tumors based on ADC or any other parameters [19, 20].

As mentioned, the growing role of DWI MRI has been encountered with challenges, including technical difficulties and limitations. T2 shine effect is defined as the hyper intensity of tissue with normal diffusion in DW imaging which is caused by long T2 decay time. T2 shine effect depends on the intrinsic characteristics of the lesions being imaged, and can depend on cellular structure, lesion size, and even anatomical location of the lesion [21]. This effect is especially important in lesions such as hemangiomas, where DW imaging may mislead towards hyper-cellular lesions, including malignant lesions. Experimental studies have shown that increasing the *b* value may increase the contribution of cellularity of the lesion to signal intensity, while decreasing that of T2 shine effect [22].

More challenges may also arise in utilizing DW imaging alongside previously established imaging guidelines, such as Liver Imaging Reporting and Data System (LI-RADS) [23]. This imaging guideline is effectively introduced in order to enable radiologists to distinguish HCC from non-malignant lesions in patients with chronic conditions such as cirrhosis which are regarded as risk factors for HCC, and no further interpretation is suggested for distinguishing other malignant lesions (excluding lesions such as confluent hepatic fibrosis which may be classified as possibly malignant lesions) [24]. In contrast, DW is used to distinguish all sorts of malignant lesions from benign ones, and as mentioned, no consensus exists regarding its role in the diagnosis of HCC alone, as a clinical entity. In this study, we not only included patients with established risk factors for HCC, but also included those with otherwise no clinically proven risk factor, who had a liver mass with an unknown diagnosis. Serious questions remain regarding the efficient use of DW alongside these guidelines (cost efficacy, specificity of combined diagnostic plans and availability issues), but evidence suggests that DW could be used as a supplementary diagnostic technique in LR3-5 lesions, and can also increase the sensitivity of the LI-RADS in detecting HCC lesions [25, 26].

The present study was conducted in a single tertiary center, which limits the extent to which the results could be generalized. In this study, we concluded only five subgroups of hepatic lesions, which had similar appearances in CT scan and sonographic imaging, so our results do not indicate the beneficence of DW imaging in diagnosing other sorts of liver pathologies, including cysts and fibrotic lesions. If these lesions were included, a dramatic change may have occurred in mean ADC values of benign lesions, and the analysis may have yielded a different result. More so, some lesions with borderline ADC values such as secondary hemorrhages in adenomas and high-density cysts were not included, which may further limit generalizability.

Conclusion

DW MRI can differentiate benign and malignant hepatic lesions based on ADC values calculated in various b values, especially high b values. More so, different hepatic lesions have a distinct mean ADC profile which can be used to further differentiate subgroups of benign and malignant lesions. Importantly, non-ADC parameters of DW imaging could also be used in this regard, although our study does not focus on this topic. More studies performed on hepatic lesions could better determine the mean ADC values for various lesions, and future meta-analysis of these studies could determine clear, evidence-based cutoffs for differentiating various lesions.

Abbreviations

ADC: Apparent diffusion coefficient; DWI: diffusion-weighted imaging; FNH: Focal nodular hyperplasia; HCC: Hepatocellular carcinoma; MRI: Magnetic resonance imaging

Acknowledgements

We would like to thank the radiology staff of the medical educational center in which the case underwent diagnostic imaging. This study was done as a thesis for receiving a specialty degree in radiology, done by Dr. Roghayeh Razzaghi. This study was in part supported by Tabriz University of Medical Sciences.

Authors' contributions

RJ, ASB, and MKT did the data collection, manuscript preparation, approval of the final version, interpretation of imaging findings and study conception. RR and JJ did the data collection, obtaining the informed consent, study conception, and approval of the final version of the study. SH did the data collection, patient selection, and approval of the final version of the study. MMAA did the study conception, manuscript preparation, systemic search of the literature, statistical analysis, and approval of the final version of the study. AKN did the data collection, manuscript preparation, statistical analysis, and approval of the final version of the study. AZ did the data collection, manuscript preparation, study conception, and approval of the final version of the manuscript.

Competing interests

The authors declare that they have no competing interests.

Author details

[1]Radiology Department, Medical Radiation Sciences Research Group, Imam Reza Hospital, Tabriz University of Medical Sciences, Tabriz, Iran. [2]General and Vascular Surgery Department, Imam Reza Hospital, Tabriz University of Medical Sciences, Tabriz, Iran. [3]Aging Research Institute, Tabriz University of Medical Sciences, Tabriz, Iran. [4]Department of Radiology, Imam Reza Hospital, Tabriz University of Medical Sciences, Tabriz, Iran.

References

1. Song KD, Kim SH, Lim HK, Jung S-H, Sohn I, Kim HS (2015) Subcentimeter hypervascular nodule with typical imaging findings of hepatocellular carcinoma in patients with history of hepatocellular carcinoma: natural course on serial gadoxetic acid-enhanced MRI and diffusion-weighted imaging. Eur Radiol 25(9):2789–2796
2. Okorie CK, Ogbole GI, Owolabi MO, Ogun O, Adeyinka A, Ogunniyi A (2015) Role of diffusion-weighted imaging in acute stroke management using low-field magnetic resonance imaging in resource-limited settings. West Afr J Radiol. 22(2):61–66
3. Padhani AR, Koh D-M, Collins DJ (2011) Whole-body diffusion-weighted MR imaging in cancer: current status and research directions. Radiology. 261(3):700–718
4. He L, Long LR, Antani S, Thoma GR (2012) Histology image analysis for carcinoma detection and grading. Comp Methods Programs Biomed. 107(3):538–556
5. Chilla GS, Tan CH, Xu C, Poh CL (2015) Diffusion weighted magnetic resonance imaging and its recent trend—a survey. Quantitative imaging in medicine and surgery. 5(3):407
6. Malayeri AA, El Khouli RH, Zaheer A, Jacobs MA, Corona-Villalobos CP, Kamel IR et al (2011) Principles and applications of diffusion-weighted imaging in cancer detection, staging, and treatment follow-up. Radiographics. 31(6):1773–1791
7. Robinson P (2002) Indeterminate liver lesions in cancer. Cancer Imaging. 2(2):130
8. Mergo PJ, Ros PR (1998) Benign lesions of the liver. Radiologic Clinics of North America. 36(2):319–331
9. Saito K, Tajima Y, Harada TL (2016) Diffusion-weighted imaging of the liver: current applications. World journal of radiology. 8(11):857
10. Hasan NMA, Zaki KF, Alam-Eldeen MH, Hamedi HR (2016) Benign versus malignant focal liver lesions: diagnostic value of qualitative and quantitative diffusion weighted MR imaging. Egypt J Radiol Nucl Med. 47(4):1211–1220
11. Yang D-w, Wang K-y, Yao X, Ye H-Y, Jiang T, Liu Y et al (2016) Diffusion-weighted imaging with two different b-values in detection of solid focal liver lesions. BioMed Res Int 2016:8128207
12. Darbar A, Waqas M, Enam SF, Mahmood SD (2018) Use of preoperative apparent diffusion coefficients to predict brain tumor grade. Cureus 10(3):e2284-e
13. Kilickesmez O, Bayramoglu S, Inci E, Cimilli T (2009) Value of apparent diffusion coefficient measurement for discrimination of focal benign and malignant hepatic masses. Journal of medical imaging and radiation oncology. 53(1):50–55
14. Obmann VC, Mertineit N, Berzigotti A, Marx C, Ebner L, Kreis R et al (2018) CT predicts liver fibrosis: prospective evaluation of morphology- and attenuation-based quantitative scores in routine portal venous abdominal scans. PloS one. 13(7):e0199611
15. Parikh T, Drew SJ, Lee VS, Wong S, Hecht EM, Babb JS et al (2008) Focal liver lesion detection and characterization with diffusion-weighted MR imaging: comparison with standard breath-hold T2-weighted imaging. Radiology. 246(3):812–822
16. Xia D, Jing J, Shen H, Wu J (2010) Value of diffusion-weighted magnetic resonance images for discrimination of focal benign and malignant hepatic lesions: a meta-analysis. J Magn Resonan Imaging. 32(1):130–137
17. Ergelen R, Sahin C, Bal H, Tuney D (2016) Diffusion-weighted MRI: in differential diagnosis of liver masses
18. Ogihara Y, Kitazume Y, Iwasa Y, Taura S, Himeno Y, Kimura T et al (2018) Prediction of histological grade of hepatocellular carcinoma using quantitative diffusion-weighted MRI: a retrospective multivendor study. The British journal of radiology. 91(1084):20170728
19. Nakanishi M, Chuma M, Hige S, Omatsu T, Yokoo H, Nakanishi K et al (2012) Relationship between diffusion-weighted magnetic resonance imaging and histological tumor grading of hepatocellular carcinoma. Annals of surgical oncology. 19(4):1302–1309
20. Le Moigne F, Boussel L, Haquin A, Bancel B, Ducerf C, Berthezene Y et al (2014) Grading of small hepatocellular carcinomas (≤ 2 cm): correlation between histology, T2 and diffusion-weighted imaging. Br J Radiol. 87(1041):20130763
21. Duran R, Ronot M, Kerbaol A, Van Beers B, Vilgrain V (2014) Hepatic hemangiomas: factors associated with T2 shine-through effect on diffusion-weighted MR sequences. Eur J Radiol 83(3):468–478
22. Inan N, Kilinc F, Sarisoy T, Gumustas S, Akansel G, Demirci A (2010) Diffusion weighted MR imaging in the differential diagnosis of haemangiomas and metastases of the liver. Radiol Oncol. 44(1):24–29
23. Chernyak V, Fowler KJ, Kamaya A, Kielar AZ, Elsayes KM, Bashir MR et al (2018) Liver Imaging Reporting and Data System (LI-RADS) version 2018: imaging of hepatocellular carcinoma in at-risk patients. Radiology. 289(3):816–830

24. Faria SC, Ganesan K, Mwangi I, Shiehmorteza M, Viamonte B, Mazhar S et al (2009) MR imaging of liver fibrosis: current state of the art. Radiographics. 29(6):1615–1635
25. Patella F, Pesapane F, Fumarola EM, Emili I, Spairani R, Angileri SA et al (2018) CT-MRI LI-RADS v2017: a comprehensive guide for beginners. J Clin Transl Hepatol 6(2):222
26. Basha MAA, Refaat R, Mohammad FF, Khamis ME, El-Maghraby AM, El Sammak AA et al (2019) The utility of diffusion-weighted imaging in improving the sensitivity of LI-RADS classification of small hepatic observations suspected of malignancy. Abdom Radiol 44(5):1773–1784

Renal resistive index in non-alcoholic fatty liver disease as an indicator of early renal affection

Hossam El-Din A. Mahmoud[1], Wael A. Yousry[1], Shereen A. Saleh[1*], Mohamed El Badry[2], Ahmed Hussein[3], Mostafa Hassan Ali[4] and Hazem M. El-Hariri[5]

Abstract

Background: Nonalcoholic fatty liver disease (NAFLD) is a possible risk factor for chronic kidney disease (CKD). Renal resistive index (RRI) which is a ratio of peak systolic and end diastolic velocity can test arterial stiffness and endothelial renal dysfunction. The aim of the work is to detect the relation between NAFLD and RRI as an indicator of early renal affection and its relation to the disease severity. This study included 150 subjects divided into 3 groups: patients with NASH, simple steatosis, and control group (50 patients each). All patients were subjected to full history taking, clinical examination, laboratory investigations, abdominal ultrasound examination, and RRI measurement.

Results: 6.0% of NASH patients had significant fibrosis by NAFLD fibrosis score. RRI was significantly higher in NASH patients with fibrosis (mean = 0.74) than NASH patients without fibrosis (mean = 0.65) and patients with simple steatosis (mean = 0.63). It was the lowest in normal controls (mean = 0.61). There were significant correlations between RRI and age, BMI, serum lipids, liver enzymes, and NAFLD fibrosis score. Multiple linear regression analysis found that age and serum cholesterol were significant independent factors of increased RRI ($p < 0.0001$). RRI showed low diagnostic performance in differentiation between NASH and simple steatosis using ROC curve.

Conclusion: RRI was significantly higher in NASH patients with and without hepatic fibrosis. RRI correlates significantly with NAFLD fibrosis score. RRI can be used as an indicator of early renal affection in patients with NAFLD.

Keywords: NAFLD, NASH, RRI, CKD

Background

Non-alcoholic fatty liver (NAFLD) is a fatty infiltration of the liver (steatosis) diagnosed by imaging or histology with or without inflammation or fibrosis in the absence of other causes of hepatic fatty infiltration. NAFLD is subcategorized to simple hepatic steatosis and nonalcoholic steatohepatitis (NASH). Regarding simple hepatic steatosis, there is no evidence of inflammation, but in NASH, there is inflammation of the liver [1].

NAFLD is a worldwide health problem with prevalence of 6 to 35% [2]. Regarding sex distribution of NAFLD, studies are very different, and some studies suggest that it is more prevalent in males [3], while others suggest that it is more prevalent in females [4].

NAFLD patients (mainly NASH patients) often have at least one component of the metabolic syndrome (MS) [5]. Meanwhile, the MS is an important risk factor for cardiovascular disease (CVD) besides being common in NAFLD patients. There are recent data that support that NAFLD independently may contribute to increased risk of CVD [6].

On the other hand, chronic kidney disease (CKD) is an important health problem [7]. Nowadays, we know that cardiovascular diseases (CVD) are the main cause of morbidity and mortality in patients with CKD [8].

* Correspondence: shereen_saleh2014@hotmail.com
[1]Internal Medicine Department, Gastroenterology and Hepatology Unit, Faculty of Medicine, Ain Shams University, Abbassia, Cairo 11341, Egypt

Recently, NAFLD was considered as a probable risk factor for CKD development and progression [9].

CKD and NAFLD have convergent pathophysiological mechanisms and cardiometabolic risk factors. CKD and NAFLD pathogenesis may be due to insulin resistance (IR), rennin-angiotensin system (RAS) activation, oxidative stress, and inappropriate secretion of cytokines by the inflamed and steatotic liver. The expected link between the kidney and liver is seen in patients with liver cell failure (LCF) as hepatorenal syndrome [10]. Targher et al. performed two cross-sectional studies which declared that CKD prevalence is higher in NAFLD patients than in others without steatosis [11, 12].

Renal resistive index (RRI) is a semi-quantitative index obtained by Doppler evaluation of renal vascular bed. RRI = [(peak systolic velocity - end diastolic velocity) ÷ peak systolic velocity]. The value of RRI is in the range of 0.47–0.70, and it usually shows a difference between the two kidneys of less than 5–8% [13].

RRI role has been extensively investigated among various kidney diseases as an early test of arterial stiffness and endothelial dysfunction which may lead to severe end-organ disease, due to its known correlations with histological parameters, as tubulointerstitial lesions and glomerulosclerosis [14, 15].

The present study aimed to detect the relation between non-alcoholic fatty liver disease and renal resistive index as an indicator of early renal affection, with correlation between it and the disease severity.

Methods

This prospective observational case control study was conducted on 150 individuals. The enrolled individuals were divided into 3 groups. Group 1 included 50 patients with NASH with or without fibrosis, group 2 included 50 patients with simple steatosis, and group 3 included another 50 normal healthy individuals as controls.

All patients and controls (age > 18 years) were collected from the outpatient clinic of the Internal Medicine Department, Ain Shams University Hospitals, Cairo, Egypt, during the period from January 2016 to May 2016.

Detailed medical history taking and thorough physical examination were done to all participants and controls. They were subjected to laboratory workup, in the form of liver function tests including aspartate aminotransferase (AST), alanine aminotransferase (ALT), total and direct bilirubin (T. and D. Bil.), serum albumin, total proteins (total prot.), gamma glutamyl transferase (GGT), and alkaline phosphatase (ALP); viral markers including hepatitis B surface antigen (HBsAg) and hepatitis C antibodies (HCV Ab); lipid profile including total cholesterol, triglycerides (TG), low-density lipoproteins (LDL), and high-density lipoproteins (HDL); renal function tests including serum creatinine (SCr), blood urea nitrogen (BUN), serum sodium (Na), potassium (K), estimated glomerular filtration rate (eGFR), and complete urine analysis; and fasting blood glucose (FBG).

Radiological assessment, by a single professional radiologist, using an abdominal U/S was done for all patients and controls included in the study after fasting for 8 h. They were examined using ultrasound (U/S) equipment with color Doppler capability and 2.8–5 MHz convex linear transducer (LOGIQ P6, G E Medical Systems, USA) for the evaluation of liver size, capsular contour (smooth, coarse, lobulated), and parenchymal echogenicity. The kidney size, cortical thickness (not less than 10 mm), cortico-medullary differentiation, and echogenicity were assessed. The U/S equipment automatically calculated the RRI. Intra-renal resistance was recorded at interlobar arteries in three different regions of both kidney (superior, middle, and inferior zones), and the mean value was calculated. Then, a mean RRI was calculated derived from 6 measurements for each patient.

RRI formula: RRI = (peak systolic velocity - end diastolic velocity)/peak systolic velocity [16].

The sonographic picture of increased liver echogenicity together with normal or elevated liver enzymes was used for differentiation between simple steatosis and NASH, while the assessment of the presence of fibrosis in NAFLD non-invasively was done by calculating the NAFLD fibrosis score [17]. This score required the following data: age, body mass index (BMI), AST, ALT, albumin, platelet count, and fasting blood sugar.

NAFLD fibrosis score formula

$-1.675 + 0.037 \times \text{age (years)} + 0.094 \times \text{BMI (kg/m}^2) + 1.13 \times \text{IFG/diabetes (yes} = 1, \text{ no} = 0) + 0.99 \times \text{AST/ALT ratio} - 0.013 \times \text{platelet } (\times 10^9) - 0.66 \times \text{albumin (g/dL)}$.

The results were interpreted as follows:

- < -1.455: predictor of absence of significant fibrosis (F0-F2 fibrosis)
- ≥ -1.455 to ≤ 0.675: indeterminate score
- > 0.675: predictor of presence of significant fibrosis (F3-F4 fibrosis)

Patients with any structural or functional renal disease such as renal artery stenosis or acute or chronic renal diseases, patients receiving any nephrotoxic drugs, patients with diabetes mellitus or hypertension, and patients with any other liver diseases rather than NAFLD were excluded from the study. Controls were collected from those with irrelevant medical history, normal physical examination and body mass index, normal liver echogenicity, contour and size, normal liver and kidney function tests, and normal eGFR and urine analysis.

The study was performed according to the ethical guidelines of the 1975 Declaration of Helsinki. A written informed consent was obtained from all enrolled participants before enrolment to the study. This study was approved by the ethical committee of Faculty of Medicine, Ain Shams University.

Statistical methods

The collected data were coded, tabulated, and statistically analyzed using IBM SPSS statistics (Statistical Package for Social Sciences) software version 22.0, IBM Corp., Chicago, USA, 2013. Descriptive statistics were done using minimum and maximum of the range as well as mean ± SD (standard deviation) for quantitative normally distributed data, while it was done for qualitative data as number and percentage. Inferential analyses were done for quantitative variables using ANOVA test with post hoc Tukey test for more than two independent groups with normally distributed data. For qualitative data, inferential analyses for independent variables were done using chi square test for differences between proportions with post hoc Bonferroni test. Pearson correlation was used for numerical normally distributed data. ROC curve was used to evaluate the performance of different tests to differentiate between certain groups. Linear regression model was used to find out the independent factors affecting certain conditions. The level of significance was taken at P value < 0.05.

Results

Twenty-one, 24, and 26% of groups 1, 2, and 3 were males. The mean age of patients of groups 1, 2, and 3 was 51 ± 8.7, 49.1 ± 9.8, and 50.1 ± 10.5 years, respectively. BMI was significantly lower in the control group with no significant difference between NASH and simple steatosis groups (Table 1).

FBG and lipid profile were significantly higher, while HDL was significantly lower among the NASH group. Liver enzymes were significantly higher in NASH group with no significant difference between control and simple steatosis groups. Serum albumin was significantly higher in the control group with no significant difference between NASH and simple steatosis groups. Creatinine and BUN were within the normal ranges in all groups but showed significantly higher levels among NASH, followed by simple steatosis then the controls. eGFR was significantly highest in the control group with no significant difference between NASH and simple steatosis groups. RRI was significantly higher among NASH patients in comparison with the other two groups (Table 1).

NAFLD fibrosis score was significantly higher among NASH patients, followed by simple steatosis and lowest among controls. Higher number and percentage of patients with liver fibrosis were found in NASH patients (Table 2, Fig. 1).

There were significant positive correlations between RRI on one side and age and BMI on the other side. Also, there were significant positive correlations between RRI and cholesterol, triglycerides, ALT, AST, ALP, GGT, and liver fibrosis score. There was significant negative correlation between RRI and HDL. There was significant positive correlation between RRI and serum creatinine, and a significant negative correlation between RRI and eGFR. There was non-significant correlation between RRI and BUN, serum Na, and K (Table 3).

Age and cholesterol were found to be significant factors that increase RRI by logistic regression analysis (Table 4). RRI had significant low diagnostic performance in differentiation between NASH patients with or without fibrosis from patients with simple steatosis (Table 5, Fig. 2).

RRI was higher in NASH patients with fibrosis (mean = 0.74) than NASH patients without fibrosis (mean = 0.65) and patients with simple steatosis (mean = 0.63). It was the lowest in normal controls (mean = 0.61).

Discussion

The aim of this study was to find the relation between non-alcoholic fatty liver disease and renal resistive index as an indicator of an early renal affection with correlation between it and the disease severity determined by NAFLD fibrosis score.

In this study, there was no significant difference between the studied groups regarding demographic characteristics. These findings are consistent with Corey et al. who stated that there were no differences in mean age in NAFLD patients and others [18]. Higher body mass index was found in patients with NASH and simple steatosis in the current study. Fierbinteanu-Braticevici et al. stated that simple steatosis and NASH are associated with high BMI. They also found an association between old age and NASH [19]. On the other hand, Nugent and Younossi stated that NAFLD and NASH may be present in lean subjects having normal BMI and they may be absent in subjects having a high BMI [20].

Fasting blood glucose (FBG) was significantly higher in NASH group than simple steatosis and control groups in the current study. These results are consistent with Jimba et al. who found that NAFLD had a significant positive association with increasing FBG in non-diabetic individuals [21].

Total cholesterol, LDL, and TG were significantly higher, while HDL was significantly lower among NASH group than simple steatosis and control groups. These results are consistent with Puri et al., Miura and Ohnish, and Mahaling et al. who stated that, in NAFLD, serum total cholesterol, TG, and

Table 1 Comparison between the three groups regarding the studied variables using ANOVA test

Variables			Group 1 (*N* = 50)	Group 2 (*N* = 50)	Group 3 (*N* = 50)	*P*
BMI (kg/m^2)		Mean ± SD	29.3 ± 2.5	29.1 ± 1.6	22.0 ± 1.5	< 0.001*
		Range	24.0–34.3	25.5–34.5	18.2–24.5	
		HG	a	a	b	
FBG (mg/dL)		Mean ± SD	88.8 ± 5.6	84.4 ± 6.7	77.3 ± 5.9	< 0.001*
		HG	a	b	c	
Lipid profile	Cholesterol (mg/dL)	Mean ± SD	251.8 ± 38.1	224.8 ± 26.2	157.1 ± 27.1	< 0.001*
		HG	a	b	c	
	TG (mg/dL)	Mean ± SD	225.2 ± 59.2	198.8 ± 36.5	117.2 ± 17.5	< 0.001*
		HG	a	b	c	
	LDL (mg/dL)	Mean ± SD	194.8 ± 22.7	182.2 ± 16.3	106.2 ± 25.6	< 0.001*
		HG	a	a	b	
	HDL (mg/dL)	Mean ± SD	37.4 ± 4.1	41.1 ± 5.2	49.8 ± 10.8	< 0.001*
		HG	a	b	c	
	ALT (IU/L)	Mean ± SD	78.81 ± 17.8	25.7 ± 7.9	24.0 ± 7.2	< 0.001*
		HG	a	b	b	
	AST (IU/L)	Mean ± SD	69.4 ± 16.7	23.8 ± 6.9	23.4 ± 6.9	< 0.001*
		HG	a	b	b	
	ALP (IU/L)	Mean ± SD	128.1 ± 31.6	71.9 ± 23.7	61.9 ± 14.7	< 0.001*
		HG	a	b	b	
	GGT (IU/L)	Mean ± SD	75.1 ± 18.3	34.1 ± 8.1	31.8 ± 9.6	< 0.001*
		HG	a	b	b	
	D. Bil. (mg/dL)	Mean ± SD	0.60 ± 0.13	0.60 ± 0.12	0.62 ± 0.12	0.559
	T. Bil. (mg/dL)	Mean ± SD	0.16 ± 0.05	0.15 ± 0.05	0.15 ± 0.05	0.730
	Albumin (gm/dL)	Mean ± SD	4.04 ± 0.20	4.11 ± 0.21	4.22 ± 0.28	< 0.001*
		HG	a	a	b	
	Tot. Proteins (gm/dL)	Mean ± SD	7.29 ± 0.32	7.32 ± 0.34	7.36 ± 0.34	0.630
	Creatinine (mg/dL)	Mean ± SD	0.87 ± 0.11	0.73 ± 0.14	0.66 ± 0.13	< 0.001*
		HG	a	b	c	
	BUN (gm/dL)	Mean ± SD	14.9 ± 2.3	13.2 ± 2.9	11.5 ± 2.8	< 0.001*
		HG	a	b	c	
	eGFR (mL/min)	Mean ± SD	117.5 ± 5.1	118.8 ± 5.0	122.0 ± 5.3	< 0.001*
		HG	a	a	b	
	Na (mmol/L)	Mean ± SD	140.3 ± 2.3	140.2 ± 1.9	139.7 ± 1.8	0.294
	K (mmol/L)	Mean ± SD	4.13 ± 0.28	4.17 ± 0.31	4.07 ± 0.20	0.200
RRI	RRI	Mean ± SD	0.66 ± 0.04	0.63 ± 0.04	0.61 ± 0.04	< 0.001*
		Range	0.65–0.67	0.62–0.64	0.60–0.62	
		95% CI	0.65–0.67	0.62–0.64	0.60–0.62	
		HG	a	b	c	

CI confidence interval, *HG* homogenous groups (have the same letter by post hoc test). *Significant

LDL cholesterol show a stepwise increase from simple steatosis to NASH, while HDL cholesterol was lower in NASH patients followed by simple steatosis patients and highest in normal [22–24].

No significant difference was found between the studied groups regarding Na and K in the present study. Sun et al. and Tabbaa et al. stated that low serum potassium levels were associated with disease severity in NAFLD patients [25, 26].

ALT, AST, ALP, and GGT were significantly higher in NASH group with no significant difference between control and simple steatosis groups in the current study.

Table 2 NAFLD fibrosis score among the studied groups

Variables		Group 1 (*N* = 50)	Group 2 (*N* = 50)	Group 3 (*N* = 50)	*P*
Score	Mean ± SD	− 1.31 ± 0.95	− 2.15 ± 0.78	− 3.30 ± 0.74	^< 0.001*
	Range	− 3.50–0.68	− 4.00 to − 0.44	− 5.00 to − 1.8	
	HG	a	b	c	
Grade (*n*, %)	No fibrosis	31 (62.0%)	43 (86.0%)	50 (100.0%)	# 0.014*
	Intermediate score	16 (32.0%)	7 (14.0%)	0 (0.0%)	
	Fibrosis	3 (6.0%)	0 (0.0%)	0 (0.0%)	
	HG	a	b	c	

^ANOVA, #chi square test, *Significant

Frantzides et al. and Puri et al. stated that the values of AST and ALT were higher in NASH patients followed by simple steatosis patients and were the lowest in normal controls [22, 27]. Puri et al. stated that mean ALP was higher in NASH patients followed by NAFLD patients and was the lowest in normal controls [22]. Fierbinteanu–Braticevici et al. and Shen et al. found that GGT was high in NAFLD patients and increased with the severity of liver affection [20, 28].

In the present study, no significant difference was found between the study and control groups regarding serum bilirubin and total protein. Kwak et al., Hjelkrem et al., chang et al., and Tian et al. stated that serum bilirubin levels were inversely associated with NAFLD prevalence [29–32]. On the other hand, Puri et al. stated that total bilirubin was higher in NAFLD patients and increasing with the severity of liver affection [22].

Liver fibrosis score was significantly higher among NASH group. In NASH group, 62.0% of patients had no significant fibrosis, 32.0% of patients had indeterminate scores, and 6.0% of patients had significant fibrosis. In simple steatosis group, 86.0% of patients had no significant fibrosis, and 14.0% of patients had indeterminate scores. All the included subjects in the control group had no fibrosis. In agreement with the current study, Williams et al. stated that 7% of NAFLD patients who underwent liver biopsy had significant fibrosis [3]. Also, Wong et al. stated that the prevalence of significant fibrosis in NAFLD patients was 4% and unlikely to exceed 10% [33].

RRI was significantly higher in the NASH group than those with simple steatosis who were higher than the control group. In NASH patients, RRI was higher among those with hepatic fibrosis (mean = 0.74) than in those without fibrosis (mean = 0.65). Catalano et al. stated that they did not find a significant difference in RRI between NAFLD patients and normal controls. Also, they did not find a significant difference between NAFLD patients with normal levels of liver enzymes and those with high levels of liver enzymes [34].

In the current study, there were significant positive correlations between RRI and age, BMI, cholesterol, triglycerides, ALT, AST, ALP, GGT, and liver fibrosis. On the other hand, there was significant negative correlation between RRI and HDL. Using multiple linear regression analysis, age and cholesterol were found to be significant

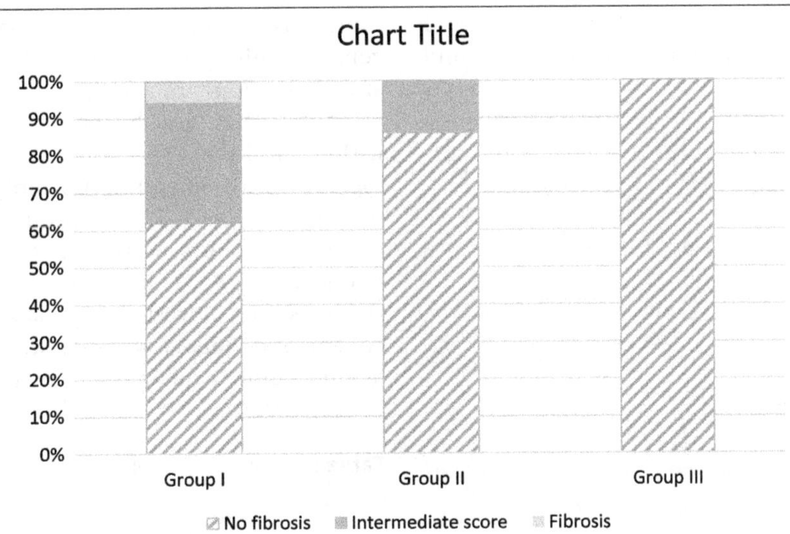

Fig. 1 Liver fibrosis among the studied groups

Table 3 Correlation between RRI and demographic and laboratory variables among the studied groups using Pearson correlation

Variables		Group 1 (*N* = 50)		Group 2 (*N* = 50)		Group 3 (*N* = 50)	
		r	*p*	*r*	*p*	*r*	*p*
Demographic	Age	0.634	< 0.001*	0.466	< 0.001*	0.644	< 0.001*
	BMI	0.826	< 0.001*	0.408	< 0.003*	0.648	< 0.001*
	FBG	0.102	0.480	0.109	0.449	0.040	0.784
Lipid profile	Cholesterol	0.405	0.004	0.344	0.014	0.513	< 0.001*
	TG	0.424	0.002*	0.303	0.047*	0.624	< 0.001*
	LDL	0.204	0.155	0.227	0.102	0.373	0.108
	HDL	− 0.443	< 0.001*	− 0.615	< 0.001*	− 0.314	0.026
Liver profile	ALT	0 12.428	0.002	0.449	< 0.001*	0.373	0.008
	AST	0.458	< 0.001*	0.376	0.007*	0.316	0.025*
	ALP	0.373	< 0.001*	0.338	0.016*	0.495	< 0.001*
	GGT	0.307	0.030*	0.416	0.003*	0.269	0.049*
	T. Bil	0.051	0.723	0.031	0.833	− 0.055	0.706
	D. Bil	− 0.004	0.978	0.031	0.830	− 0.063	0.665
	Albumin	− 0.584	< 0.001*	−0.467	< 0.001*	− 0.407	0.046
	Total protein	− 0.485	< 0.001*	−0.555	< 0.001*	− 0.415	0.019
Kidney functions	Creatinine	0.480	< 0.001*	0.356	0.011*	0.301	0.034*
	eGFR	− 0.593	< 0.001*	−0.512	< 0.001*	− 0.495	< 0.001*
Liver fibrosis	Score	0.851	< 0.001*	0.851	< 0.001*	0.532	< 0.001*

*Significant

independent factors of higher RRI. RRI showed low diagnostic performance in differentiation between patients with NASH and liver fibrosis and those with simple steatosis. Ponte et al. stated that higher BMI and age were associated with higher RRI values. Also, they stated that age is one of the significant determinants of the RRI in the general population, but they highlighted a nonlinear association between age and RRI [35].

The expanded and inflamed visceral adipose tissue mass is a source of multiple factors that are potentially involved in the process of atherogenesis and the development of insulin resistance, NAFLD, and possibly the cardiac and renal affection. These factors include free fatty acids (FFA), hormones, and proinflammatory adipocytokines [36]. Hepatic steatosis leads to subacute intrahepatic inflammation through activation of nuclear factor-κB pathways that exacerbate insulin resistance both locally in the liver and systematically [37]. NAFLD is associated with increased levels of circulating proinflammatory markers such as C reactive protein, interleukin (IL) 6, tumor necrosis factor (TNF)-α, and other hepatic acute-phase proteins, procoagulant factors as fibrinogen, plasminogen activator inhibitor-1, factor VIII, and adhesion molecules like vascular adhesion protein-1 that are likely to have been synthesized within the liver, especially in the presence of NASH, together with impaired fibrinolysis (e.g., high levels of PAI-1) [38]. These proinflammatory and procoagulant factors were found to be highest in patients with NASH, intermediate in those with simple steatosis, and lowest in age, sex, and weight-matched control individuals without steatosis [39]. These risk factors could explain the cardiac and renal affection in NAFLD.

Table 4 Linear logistic models for factors affecting RRI among the studied groups

Variables	B	SE	*p*	95% CI	R^2
Group 1					
Age	0.0042	0.0004	*< 0.001**	0.0033–0.0051	0.998
Cholesterol	0.0006	0.0001	*< 0.001**	0.0004–0.0008	
Group 2					
Age	0.0027	0.0007	*< 0.001**	0.0013–0.0040	0.995
Cholesterol	0.0007	0.0002	*0.004**	0.0002–0.0012	
Group 3					
Age	0.0024	0.0005	*< 0.001**	0.0014–0.0034	0.997
Cholesterol	0.0008	0.0002	*< 0.001**	0.0004–0.0011	

β regression coefficient, *SE* standard error, *CI* confidence interval, R^2 coefficient of determination, *significant

Table 5 Diagnostic performance of RRI in prediction of NASH

Groups	AUC	SE	*p*	95% CI
Group 1 from 2	0.692	0.054	*< 0.001**	0.586–0.798

AUC area under curve, *SE* standard error, *CI* confidence interval, *significant

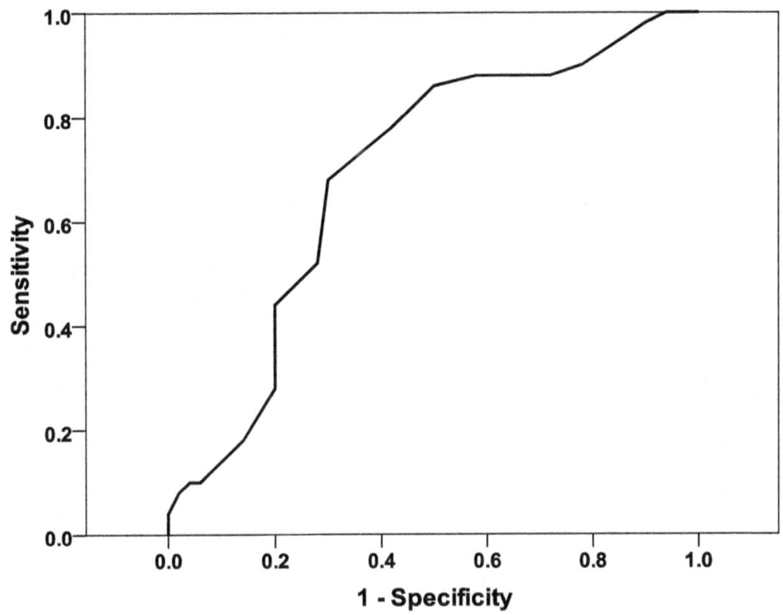

Fig. 2 ROC curve for RRI in differentiation between NASH patients and simple steatosis

Conclusion

NAFLD is associated with higher blood sugar, hazardous serum lipids, and liver enzymes. RRI was significantly higher in NASH patients with and without hepatic fibrosis. RRI correlated significantly with NAFLD fibrosis score, liver enzymes, and serum lipids.

Abbreviations

ALP: Alkaline phosphatase; ALT: Alanine aminotransferase; AST: Aspartate aminotransferase; CKD: Chronic kidney disease; CVD: Cardiovascular disease; D. Bil.: Direct bilirubin; FBG: Fasting blood glucose; GGT: Gamma glutamyl transferase; HBsAg: Hepatitis B surface antigen; HCV Ab: Hepatitis C antibodies; HDL: High-density lipoproteins; IFG: Impaired fasting glucose; IR: Insulin resistance; LCF: Liver cell failure; LDL: Low-density lipoproteins; MS: Metabolic syndrome; NAFLD: Nonalcoholic fatty liver disease; NASH: Nonalcoholic steatohepatitis; RAS: Rennin-angiotensin system; RRI: Renal resistive index; SD: Standard deviation; SPSS: Statistical Package for Social Sciences; T.Bil.: Total bilirubin; TG: Triglycerides

Acknowledgements

Not applicable.

Authors' contributions

Dr. 'HM' and Dr. 'WY' contributed in the revision of the work and in the acceptance of the final form of the manuscript. Dr. 'SS' contributed in conception and the design of the work, writing of the manuscript, and revision of the work. Dr. 'MEB' contributed in writing of the manuscript and revision of the work. Dr. 'AH' contributed in the conception and the design of the work together with performing the clinical part and revising the manuscript. Dr. 'MS' and 'HM' contributed in collection of the data and in performing the statistical part of the work. All authors have read and approved the manuscript.

Competing interests

None of the authors have any conflicts of interests or financial disclosures related to this work.

Author details

[1]Internal Medicine Department, Gastroenterology and Hepatology Unit, Faculty of Medicine, Ain Shams University, Abbassia, Cairo 11341, Egypt. [2]Tropical Medicine and Gastroenterology Department, Faculty of Medicine, Aswan University, Aswan, Egypt. [3]Diagnostic and Interventional Radiology Department, Faculty of Medicine, Ain Shams University, Cairo, Egypt. [4]Internal Medicine Department, Nephrology Unit, Ahmed Maher Hospital, Ministry of Health, Cairo, Egypt. [5]Department of Community medicine, National Research Centre, Dokki, Egypt.

References

1. Caldwell SH, Crespo DM (2004) The spectrum expanded: cryptogenic cirrhosis and the natural history of non-alcoholic fatty liver disease. J Hepatol 40:578–584
2. Lazo M, Hernaez R, Eberhardt MS, Bonekamp S, Kamel I, Guallar E, Koteish A, Brancati FL, Clark JM (2013) Prevalence of nonalcoholic fatty liver disease in the United States: the third national health and nutrition examination survey, 1988–1994. Am J Epidemiol 178:38–45
3. Williams CD, Stengel J, Asike MI, Torres DM, Shaw J, Contreras M, Landt CL, Harrison SA (2011) Prevalence of nonalcoholic fatty liver disease and nonalcoholic steatohepatitis among a largely middle-aged population utilizing ultrasound and liver biopsy: a prospective study. Gastroenterol 140: 124–131
4. Matteoni CA, Younossi ZM, Gramlich T, Boparai N, Liu YC, McCullough (1999) Nonalcoholic fatty liver disease: a spectrum of clinical and pathological severity. Gastroenterology 116:1413–1419
5. Rinella ME (2015) Nonalcoholic fatty liver disease: a systematic review. JAMA 313:2263–2273
6. Stepanova M, Younossi ZM (2016) Independent association between nonalcoholic fatty liver disease and cardiovascular disease in the US population. Clin Gastroenterol Hepatol 10:646–650
7. Locatelli F, Pozzoni P, Tentori F, Del Vecchio L (2003) Epidemiology of cardiovascular risk in patients with chronic kidney disease. Nephrol Dial Transplant 18:vii2–vii9
8. Hamad A, Khalil A, Connolly V, Ahmed MH (2012) Relationship between non-alcoholic fatty liver disease and kidney function: a communication between two organs that needs further exploration. Arab J Gastroenterol 13:161–165
9. Dowman JK, Tomlinson JW, Newsome PN (2011) Systematic review: the diagnosis and staging of non-alcoholic fatty liver disease and non-alcoholic steatohepatitis. Aliment Pharmacol Ther 33:525 540

10. Joachim IH, Sharma K (2010) Mechanisms linking obesity, chronic kidney disease, and fatty liver disease: the roles of fetuin-A, adiponectin, and AMPK. J Am Soc Nephrol 21:406–412
11. Targher G, Bertolini L, Chonchol M, Rodella S, Zoppini G, Lippi G, Zenari L, Bonora E (2010) Non-alcoholic fatty liver disease is independently associated with an increased prevalence of chronic kidney disease and retinopathy in type 1 diabetic patients. Diabetologia 53:1341–1348
12. Mikolasevic I, Racki S, Bubic I, Jelic I, Stimac D, Orlic L (2013) Chronic kidney disease and nonalcoholic fatty liver disease proven by transient elastography. Kidney Blood Press Res 37:305–310
13. Tublin ME, Bude RO, Platt JF (2003) The resistive index in renal Doppler sonography: where do we stand. Am J Roentgenol 180:885–892
14. Lerolle N, Guerot E, Faisy C, Bornstain C, Diehl JL, Fagon JY (2006) Renal failure in septic shock: predictive value of Doppler based renal arterial resistive index. Intensive Care Med 32:1553–1559
15. Spatola L, Andrulli S (2016) Doppler ultrasound in kidney diseases: a key parameter in clinical long-term follow-up. J Ultrasound 19:243–250
16. Bruno RM, Daghini E, Landini L, Versari D, Salvati A, Santini E, Di Paco I, Magagna A, Taddei S, Ghiadoni L, Solini A (2011) Dynamic evaluation of renal resistive index in normoalbuminuric patients with newly diagnosed hypertension or type 2 diabetes. Diabetologia 54:2430–2439
17. Angulo P, Hui JM, Marchesini G, Bugianesi E, George J, Farrell GC, Enders F, Saksena S, Burt AD, Bida JP, Lindor K, Sanderson SO, Lenzi M, Adams LA, Kench J, Therneau TM, Day CP (2007) The NAFLD fibrosis score: a noninvasive system that identifies liver fibrosis in patients with NAFLD. Hepatology 45:846–854
18. Corey KE, Misdraji J, Gelrud L, Zheng H, Chung RT, Krauss RM (2014) Nonalcoholic steatohepatitis is associated with an atherogenic lipoprotein subfraction profile. Lipids Health Dis 13:100
19. Fierbinteanu-Braticevici C, Baicus C, Tribus L, Papacocea R (2011) Predictive factors for nonalcoholic steatohepatitis (NASH) in patients with nonalcoholic fatty liver disease (NAFLD). J Gastrointestin Liver Dis 20:153–159
20. Nugent C, Younossi ZM (2007) Evaluation and management of obesity-related nonalcoholic fatty liver disease. Nat Clin Pract Gastroenterol Hepatol 4:432–441
21. Jimba S, Nakagami T, Takahashi M, Wakamatsu T, Hirota Y, Iwamoto Y, Wasada T (2005) Prevalence of non-alcoholic fatty liver disease and its association with impaired glucose metabolism in Japanese adults. Diabet Med 22:1141–1145
22. Puri P, Wiest MM, Cheung O, Mirshahi F, Sargeant C, Min HK, Contos MJ, Sterling RK, Fuchs M, Zhou H, Watkins SM, Sanyal AJ (2009) The plasma lipidomic signature of nonalcoholic steatohepatitis. Hepatology 50:1827–1838
23. Miura K, Ohnishi H (2012) Nonalcoholic fatty liver disease: from lipid profile to treatment. Clin J Gastroenterol 5:313–321
24. Mahaling DU, Basavaraj MM, Bika AJ (2013) Comparison of lipid profile in different grades of non-alcoholic fatty liver disease diagnosed on ultrasound. Asian Pac J Trop Biomed 3:907–912
25. Sun K, Lu J, Jiang Y, Xu M, Xu Y, Zhang J et al (2014) Low serum potassium level is associated with nonalcoholic fatty liver disease and its related metabolic disorders. Clin Endocrinol 80:348–355
26. Tabbaa A, Shaker M, Lopez R, Hoshemand K, Nobili V, Alkhouri N (2015) Low serum potassium levels associated with disease severity in children with nonalcoholic fatty liver disease. Pediatr Gastroenterol Hepatol Nutr 18: 168–174
27. Frantzides CT, Carlson MA, Moore RE, Zografakis JG, Madan AK, Puumala S, Keshavarzian A (2004) Effect of body mass index on nonalcoholic fatty liver disease in patients undergoing minimally invasive bariatric surgery. J Gastrointest Surg 8:849–855
28. Shen Z, Munker S, Luo F, Ma H, Yu C, Li Y (2015) Effect of non-alcoholic fatty liver disease on estimated glomerular filtration rate could be dependent on age. PLoS One 10:e0130614
29. Kwak MS, Kim D, Chung GE, Kang SJ, Park MJ, Kim YJ, Yoon JH, Lee HS (2012) Serum bilirubin levels are inversely associated with nonalcoholic fatty liver disease. Clin Mol Hepatol 18:383–390
30. Hjelkrem M, Morales A, Williams CD, Harrison SA (2012) Unconjugated hyperbilirubinemia is inversely associated with non-alcoholic steatohepatitis (NASH). Aliment Pharmacol Ther 35:1416–1423
31. Chang Y, Ryu S, Zhang Y, Son HJ, Kim JY, Cho J, Guallar E (2012) A cohort study of serum bilirubin levels and incident non-alcoholic fatty liver disease in middle aged Korean workers. PLoS One 7:e37241
32. Tian J, Zhong R, Liu C, Tang Y, Gong J, Chang J et al (2016) Association between bilirubin and risk of non-alcoholic fatty liver disease based on a prospective cohort study. Sci Rep 6:31006
33. Wong VW, Wong GL, Yip GW, Lo AO, Limquiaco J, Chu WC (2011) Coronary artery disease and cardiovascular outcomes in patients with non-alcoholic fatty liver disease. Gut 60:1721–1727
34. Catalano D, Trovato GM, Martines GF, Pirri C, Trovato FM (2011) Renal function and severity of bright liver. Relationship with insulin resistance, intrarenal resistive index, and glomerular filtration rate. Hepatol Int 5:822–829
35. Ponte B, Pruijm M, Ackermann D, Vuistiner P, Eisenberger U, Guessous I, Rousson V, Mohaupt MG, Alwan H, Ehret G, Pechere-Bertschi A, Paccaud F, Staessen JA, Vogt B, Burnier M, Martin PY, Bochud M (2014) Reference values and factors associated with renal resistive index in a family-based population study novelty and significance. Hypertension 63:136–142
36. Badman MK, Flier JS (2007) The adipocyte as an active participant in energy balance and metabolism. Gastroenterology 132:2103–2115
37. Yki-Jarvinen H (2010) Liver fat in the pathogenesis of insulin resistance and type 2 diabetes. Dig Dis 28:203–209
38. Adams LA, Anstee QM, Tilg H, Targher G (2017) Non-alcoholic fatty liver disease and its relationship with cardiovascular disease and other extrahepatic diseases. Gut 66(6):1138–1153
39. Northup PG, Argo CK, Shah N, Caldwell SH (2012) Hypercoagulation and thrombophilia in nonalcoholic fatty liver disease: mechanisms, human evidence, therapeutic implications, and preventive implications. Semin Liver Dis 32:39–48

23

Tacrolimus-induced posterior reversible encephalopathy syndrome presenting as left upper limb monoplegia, convulsions and sudden blindness

Mohamad-Sherif Mogawer[1], Mostafa EL-Shazly[2], Ayman Salah[2], Amany Abdel-Maqsod[1], Omar Abdelaziz[3], Ahmed Abdel-Ghani[1], Mahmoud Essam[4] and Abeer Awad Abdellatif[1*]

Abstract

Background: To report a case of sudden onset left upper limb monoplegia, convulsions, and bilateral blindness in a patient receiving tacrolimus for immunosuppression following living donor liver transplantation (LDLT) consistent with posterior reversible encephalopathy syndrome (PRES).

Case presentation: We report a case of a 64-year-old male patient on tacrolimus treatment following LDLT. On day 11, during his post-operative routine follow-up. The patient developed sudden onset of left upper limb monoplegia associated with attacks of convulsions and sudden bilateral blindness. MRI revealed multiple, bilateral cortical, and subcortical areas of high T2 and FLAIR signal intensity that did not show restricted diffusion. Findings were suggestive of posterior reversible encephalopathy syndrome (PRES). After the cessation of tacrolimus, vision was completely regained and all other neurologic symptoms were resolved, and follow-up MRI was normal. This case represents an uncommon presentation of tacrolimus toxicity.

Conclusion: Tacrolimus toxicity may present with PRES. Neurological deficits may be fully reversible with discontinuation of the drug; therefore, the early recognition and prompt management of this condition are of utmost importance.

Keywords: Tacrolimus, Left upper limb monoplegia, Convulsions, Sudden blindness, MRI brain, Posterior reversible encephalitis syndrome

Background

Nowadays, the liver transplantation is considered the standard therapy for acute and chronic liver failure. Survival rates have improved significantly in the last 25 years, achieving rates of 96% and 71% at 1 and 10 years after transplantation respectively [1]. This great success is mostly attributable to several advances one of which is the introduction of immunosuppressive agents like tacrolimus (FK506) [2].

It is important to recognize tacrolimus as a source of potential neurological and systemic toxicity and to promptly notify the patient and the transplant team. Tacrolimus toxicity has been described as optic neuropathy [3], as well as cortical blindness associated with bilateral occipital white matter lesions [4]. Tacrolimus has also been shown to cause biopsy proven demyelination [5]; named posterior reversible encephalopathy syndrome (PRES) [6], which is diagnosed by characteristic clinical findings which include headache, changes in mental state, and focal neurological deficits after exclusion of

* Correspondence: beero4a@yahoo.com
[1]Internal medicine department, Hepatogastroenterology and liver transplantation unit, Kasr Al-Ainy Hospital, faculty of medicine, Cairo University, Cairo University, Cairo, Egypt

other possible causes. There are also characteristic MRI and CT white matter lesions, but these are not always present as CT finding.

The aim of this case presentation is to raise the awareness of rare tacrolimus-induced side effects such as sudden bilateral blindness and serious neurological symptoms consistent with PRES.

Case presentation

A 64-year-old male underwent living donor liver transplantation for recurrent hepatocellular carcinoma (HCC) within the Milan criteria. He was not known to have a history of diabetes or hypertension. His donor was related (his sister), 40 years old, no past medical history, BMI = 27, liver biopsy showed 10–12% steatosis; graft to recipient weight ratio (GRWR) was 0.8%. PET scan was normal 1 month before transplantation.

On day 11, following liver transplantation and during regular daily assessment, painless left upper limb weakness (grade 0) was observed. Shortly after, an attack of status epilepticus started and followed by loss of consciousness (GCS less than 8). The patient was readmitted to ICU, sedated, and needed mechanical ventilated for 3 days due to his current conscious level and the state of status epilepticus. Convulsions were controlled with anticonvulsant treatment and a continuous infusion of midazolam; after that, the patient progressively regained normal conscious level and was weaned from the mechanical ventilation. Following regaining consciousness, the patient developed bilateral blindness. The neurological assessment revealed bilateral complete loss of vision with left upper limb monoplegia, other neurological examination was normal. Ophthalmologic examination revealed bilateral complete loss of vision up to no light perception. Pupils were non-reactive and pinpoint. Eye movements, intraocular tensions, fundus examination, and anterior slit-lamp examination were normal.

The patient's initial blood work-up included a complete blood count, chemistry panel including electrolytes, creatinine, liver function tests, and thyroid function tests and were all within normal ranges.

His medication included tacrolimus 2 mg twice a day since day 1 of transplantation. Tacrolimus blood level was 8.12 ng/ml (target therapeutic level in blood is 10–15 ng/mL) [7].

CT brain with contrast was normal. Magnetic resonance imaging (MRI) demonstrated bilateral, multifocal, cortical and subcortical areas of bright T2 and FLAIR signal intensity in the occipital and fronto-parietal regions. They show no diffusion restriction on DWI and ADC map. Those changes were consistent with atypical radiological features of posterior reversible encephalopathy syndrome (PRES) (Fig. 1). Also, atypical MRI findings that may be found with PRES could include diffusion restriction on DWI, post-gadolinium contrast enhancement on T1W images, and hemorrhage [8].

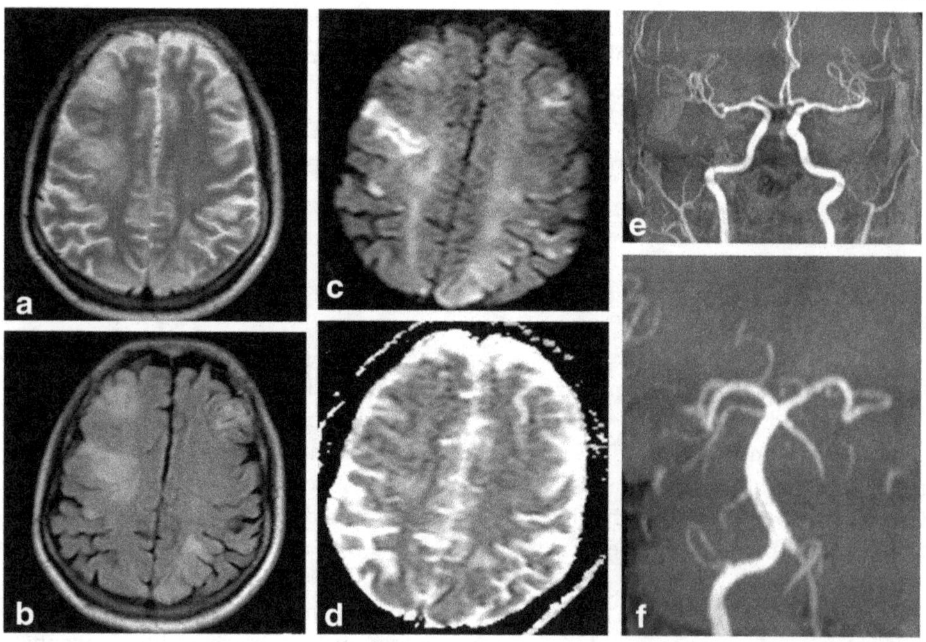

Fig. 1 MRI and MRA of the brain. **a**, **b** Axial T2 and FLAIR WIs demonstrate bilateral, cerebral, multifocal cortical, and subcortical areas of high signal intensity. **c**, **d** Axial diffusion WIs and ADC map at the same level showing no evidence of restricted diffusion. **e**, **f** MRA images showing normal appearance of the anterior and posterior circulation major vessels

He was not hypertensive and his workup excluded any infectious or metabolic causes.

Tacrolimus toxicity was considered the most probable suggested cause and accordingly was discontinued. Immunosuppressive regiment of was changed into mycophenolic acid 1000 mg three times a day and prednisone 40 mg daily. All manifestations including weakness and loss of vision progressively improved with complete normalization in a couple of weeks.

The patient had not had any further deterioration of his vision, attacks of convulsions, or weakness. His follow-up MRI 2 weeks later was completely normal.

Discussion

Posterior reversible encephalopathy syndrome (PRES) or reversible posterior leukoencephalopathy syndrome is a syndrome of clinical findings with characteristic neuroradiographic findings that was first described by Hinchey et al. [9]. It is a clinico-radiological syndrome that may present with one or a combination of headache, nausea, altered mental status, blurred vision, vision loss, and seizures. These symptoms were found in combination with neuroradiographic findings of edema of the posterior cerebral white matter. Although the exact pathophysiological mechanism is still unclear, numerous etiologies have been reported and include use of immunosuppressant medications, hypertensive encephalopathy, and eclampsia [8]; that is supposed to cause disruption in the BBB results in picture similar to that of vasogenic edema vs. cytotoxic edema [10].

Currently, there are no set diagnostic criteria for making the diagnosis of PRES; however, characteristic imaging findings in the setting of the above clinical presentations are consistent with the diagnosis. While changes may be present on CT, MRI is considered the best imaging modality to capture characteristic findings [11].

Our patient developed sudden onset of left upper limb weakness, convulsions, and blindness up to no light perception (symptoms consistent with PRES) while on oral tacrolimus therapy which promptly responded to discontinuation of accused medication. Although the patient did not have risk factors for optic neuropathy, the bilateral nature and concurrent PRES symptoms which resolved with the cessation of tacrolimus are consistent with tacrolimus-induced toxicity.

This can be explained by toxic effects of immunosuppressant medications on cells that may damage the endothelium of vessels and thus causing leakage of fluid into the brain parenchyma [12].

Tacrolimus is known to cause optic neuropathy and many mechanisms have been proposed including direct neurotoxic effect causing axonal swelling or a vascular mechanism [13].

It is important also to highlight that the tacrolimus toxicity can occur even within its therapeutic level [14] as occurred in our patient.

We find this association particularly important in an era of increased transplantation and immunosuppression use. Clinicians, including ophthalmologists, and neurologist should be aware of this association.

Herein, we portrayed a case of tacrolimus-induced side effect presenting with feature consistent of PRES.

Conclusion

It is important to raise the awareness of the possibility of tacrolimus-induced PRES as rare side effect following liver transplantation even within its therapeutic level. PRES generally has a good prognosis, prompt recognition, and management are important in preventing significant disease morbidity and mortality.

Abbreviations

LDLT: Living donor liver transplantation; PRES: Posterior reversible encephalopathy syndrome; HCC: Hepatocellular carcinoma; GRWR: Graft to recipient weight ratio

Acknowledgements

We would like to acknowledge our great Kasr Al Ainy Hospital, and its workers, nurses, and staff members, for all the support and help in this study and throughout our careers.

Authors' contributions

MS analyzed and interpreted the patient data regarding the liver disease and the transplant from the surgical point of view. MS and AS analyzed and interpreted the patient data regarding the liver disease and the transplant from the surgical point of view. AA participated in revising the manuscript and general supervision of the research group. OA analyzed and interpreted the patient data regarding the radiological data. AG participated in writing the manuscript and general supervision of the research group. ME collected the data. AAA was a major contributor in writing the manuscript. All authors read and approved the final manuscript.

Competing interests

The authors declare no potential competing interests.

Author details

[1]Internal medicine department, Hepatogastroenterology and liver transplantation unit, Kasr Al-Ainy Hospital, faculty of medicine, Cairo University, Cairo University, Cairo, Egypt. [2]General surgery department and liver transplantation unit, Kasr Al-Ainy Hospital, faculty of medicine, Cairo University, Cairo, Egypt., Cairo University, Cairo, Egypt. [3]Diagnostic and intervention Radiology department, Kasr Al-Ainy Hospital, Faculty of Medicine, Cairo University, Egypt., Cairo university, Cairo, Egypt. [4]Tropical Medicine Department, and liver transplantation unit, Kasr Al-Ainy Hospital, Faculty of Medicine, Cairo University, Cairo, Egypt.

References

1. Adam R, Karam V, Delvart V, O'Grady J, Mirza D, Klempnauer J et al (2012) Evolution of indications and results of liver transplantation in Europe. A report from the European Liver Transplant Registry (ELTR). J Hepatol 57:675–688
2. Dutkowski P, De Rougemont O, Mullhaupt B, Clavien PA (2010) Current and future trends in liver transplantation in Europe. Gastroenterology 138:802–809 e1–e4

3. Brazis PW, Spivey JR, Bolling JP, Steers JL (2000) A case of bilateral optic neuropathy in a patient on tacrolimus (FK506) therapy after liver transplantation. Am J Ophthalmol. 129(4):536–538
4. Kommana S (2019) S, Bains U, Fasula V, Henderer J: A Case of Tacrolimus-Induced Posterior Reversible Encephalopathy Syndrome Initially Presenting as a Bilateral Optic Neuropathy. Case Rep Ophthalmol 10:140–144. https://doi.org/10.1159/000496916
5. Venneti S, Moss HE, Levin MH, Vagefi MR, Brozena SC, Pruitt AA et al (2011) Asymmetric bilateral demyelinating optic neuropathy from tacrolimus toxicity. J Neurol Sci. 301(1-2):112–115
6. Wong R, Beguelin GZ, de Lima M, Giralt SA, Hosing C, Ippoliti C et al (2003) Tacrolimus-associated posterior reversible encephalopathy syndrome after allogeneic haematopoietic stem cell transplantation. Br J Haematol. 122(1): 128–134
7. Jia JJ, Lin BY, He JJ et al (2014) "Minimizing tacrolimus" strategy and long-term survival after liver transplantation. World J Gastroenterol. 20(32):11363–11369. https://doi.org/10.3748/wjg.v20.i32.11363
8. Bartynski WS (2008) Posterior reversible encephalopathy syndrome, part 1: Fundemental imaging and clinical features. AJNR Am J Neuroradiol. 29(6): 1036–1042
9. Hinchey J, Chaves C, Appignani B et al (1996) A reversible posterior leukoencephalopathy syndrome. N Engl J Med. 334:494–500
10. Anderson RC, Patel V, Sheikh-Bahaei N et al (2020) Posterior Reversible Encephalopathy Syndrome (PRES): Pathophysiology and Neuro-Imaging. Front Neurol 11:463. Published 2020 Jun 16. https://doi.org/10.3389/fneur.2020.00463
11. Schwartz RB, Jones KM, Kalina P et al (1992) Hypertensive encephalopathy: findings on CT, MR imaging, and SPECT imaging in 14 cases. AJR Am J Roentgenol. 159:379–383
12. Ito Y, Arahata Y, Goto Y et al (1998) Cisplatin neurotoxicity presenting as reversible posterior leukoencephalopathy syndrome. AJNR Am J Neuroradiol. 19:415–417
13. Helwig U, Müller M, Hedderich J, Schreiber S (2012) Corticosteroids and immunosuppressive therapy influence the result of QuantiFERON TB Gold testing in inflammatory bowel disease patients. J Crohn's Colitis. 6(4):419–424
14. Sikma MA, van Maarseveen EM, van de Graaf EA, Kirkels JH, Verhaar MC, Donker DW, Kesecioglu J, Meulenbelt J (2015) Pharmacokinetics and Toxicity of Tacrolimus Early After Heart and Lung Transplantation. Am J Transplant. 15(9):2301–2313. https://doi.org/10.1111/ajt.13309 Epub 2015 Jun 4. PMID: 26053114

Role of circulating miRNA-17-3P as a potential diagnostic biomarker for sporadic colon cancer in Egyptian cohort

Mohamed Ahmed Abdel Aziz[1*], Ezzat Ali Ahmed[1], Amany Ahmed Elbanna[1], Reham Abdel Halim[2], Khloud Salahuddin Afifi[1] and Hanan Hosny Nouh[1]

Abstract

Background: Cancer colon is one of the leading causes of death and MiRNAs are incorporated in biological pathways that affect tumorigenesis as proved by multiple studies. The present study aimed to investigate whether miR-17-3p is elevated in the plasma free samples of colon cancer patients in correlation with other tumor markers (CEA, CA19.9).

Results: MiRNA 17-3P plasma free sample levels were significantly elevated in the plasma free samples of colon cancer patients compared with healthy controls ($P < 0.001$); on the other hand, serum levels of CA19.9 were significantly higher in colon cancer patients compared to healthy controls while serum levels of CEA were found to be of no statistical significance.

Conclusion: The detection miRNA-17-3p may be considered of clinical value for the detection of colon cancer; also, CA19.9 detection was found to significantly increase the sensitivity and specificity of a colon cancer diagnosis.

Keywords: miR-17-3p, Carcinoembryonic antigen, CA19.9, Colon cancer, Diagnostic biomarker

Background

All over the world, colon cancer is estimated to be the 2nd most common type of cancer in females (614,000 cases representing ~ 9.2% of all cancers) and the 3rd most common type in males (746,000 cases representing ~ 10.0% of the total). Early detection of patients with cancer has a favorable outcome with treatment, with the 5-year survival rates exceeding 70%. For several decades, colonoscopy has been used as the first choice for screening of early-stage colon cancer; but because of its invasive character, patients show low compliance in the clinical setting. Thus, cost-effective and non-invasive biomarkers with high sensitivity and specificity are essentially required to help early detection of colon cancer [1].

* Correspondence: m.aziz.git@gmail.com
[1]Department of Internal Medicine, Faculty of Medicine, Alexandria University, Alexandria, Egypt

Recently detected microRNAs (miRNAs) are endogenous, small, non-coding evolutionarily conserved RNA (~ 22–25 nucleotide length), also referred as micro-coordinators of gene expression that have been revealed to be an efficient method to study the biology of various diseases and to be used as a novel diagnostic and prognostic biomarkers with a great level of specificity and sensitivity. Additionally, miRNAs are characterized by a high degree of stability so they could be isolated from body fluids and tissues and can be measured easily [2].

MiRNAs are incorporated in various biological pathways that may affect tumorigenesis and progression and also may function as oncogenes or tumor suppressors, based on the downstream effects produced by the affected miRNA. Although the miRNA function is not completely understood yet, they have been accompanied by various important molecular pathways that have been related to carcinogenesis and tumor progression as proved by multiple experimental models and clinical studies that were carried out on different types of cancer, including colon cancer [2].

MiRNAs have been assumed to be a potential reliable biomarker for screening of cancer because they are highly stable and can be measured easily using the common laboratory methods. In 2015, Kara et al. [3] conducted a study aiming to evaluate the expression profile of some cancer-related genes and their regulatory miRNA molecules. In this study, they used a high-throughput real-time PCR method on 54 colon cancer patients and normal colon tissue samples of 42 healthy controls. Their results revealed that a wide range of miRNA types, including miRNA-17-3p were significantly deregulated in colon cancer. They strongly concluded the possible involvement of novel cancer-related genes and their regulatory miRNAs in colon cancer physiopathology along with the probability of using this miRNA as a biomarker for early detection of colon cancer.

A lot of studies have thrown the light on the role of various biomarkers in the progression and diagnosis of colon cancer. These markers include CEA and CA19.9. Recently, the gene encoding CEA has been categorized as a member of the immunoglobulin supergene family that includes gene encoding for adhesion molecules as intercellular adhesion molecule 1(ICAM-1), major histocompatibility (MHC) antigen, and lymphocyte function-associated antigen [4].

The application of CEA as a marker for the diagnosing of colon cancer is limited because it is neither sensitive nor specific, mainly at the onset of the disease. At a cutoff of 2.5 μg/L, the range of sensitivity is about 30–80% according to the stage of the disease. But, as concluded by Fletcher, in symptomatic patients, the sensitivity of CEA is more elevated than asymptomatic subjects as the symptomatic group usually has more advanced disease [5].

CA19-9 is a Sialylated Lewis antigen of the MUC1 protein [6]. The American Society of Oncology does not encourage the use of CA19-9 because it is less sensitive in asymptomatic, non-advanced cases of colon cancer giving false negative results. Also, it is present in non-cancer cases (false positive) [7].

CA19-9 is less specific in colon cancer as it may be found in various types of tumors such as pancreatic, gastric cancers and hepatocellular carcinoma, as well as in benign cases such as bile duct diseases as obstruction of the bile duct. Besides, subjects who do not have the Lewis antigen "(a blood type antigen on RBCs) who represent approximately 10% of the Caucasian population," do not express CA19-9, even if they have large tumors. This is due to a deficiency of a fucosyl transferase enzyme which is required for the production of CA19-9 and the Lewis antigen [7]. Both CEA and CA19-9 biomarkers are considered of prognostic value better than a diagnostic tool.

The present study aimed to investigate whether miR-17-3p is elevated in the blood of colon cancer patients with different stages and assess their role as a novel biomarker for this type of cancer, and if there is any role of this biomarker in staging in correlation with other well-known tumor markers (CEA, CA19.9).

Methods

Patients

Peripheral blood samples were obtained from 50 newly diagnosed colon cancer Egyptian patients who were attending the outpatient clinics at the Alexandria Main University Hospital, Gastroenterology unit (Alexandria, Egypt) between 2016 and 2018. An additional 25 peripheral blood samples were obtained from age- and sex-matched healthy volunteers as control group patients were classified based on TNM and pathological staging system into two groups (group A: 25 patients with stage II/III and group B: 25 patients with stage VI), and patients did not receive any line of treatment before sample withdrawing.

Sample collection

Peripheral blood samples were collected into plain vacuum tubes. Immediately after collection of the samples, a 2-step centrifugation protocol was performed at room temperature (1800 g for 10 min, then 3000 g for 10 min) to get platelet-poor, cell-free plasma. Aliquots were frozen in – 80 °C till further processing, and miR-16 was used as the endogenous control.

Relative quantification of microRNA- 17-3-p expression

Total RNA including miRNA was purified from the cell-free plasma samples and was done using the miRNeasy extraction kit (Qiagen, Germany).QIAzol. Single-stranded cDNA was produced from purified samples of RNA using the TaqMan® MicroRNA RT Kit with miRNA primers specific for miRNA-17-3-p (ID 000392) and miR-16(ID 000391) (Applied Biosystems, USA) according to the manufacturer's protocol. Real-time PCR (260) for relative quantifications of miRNA 17-3P was performed on the Stratagene mx3005p qPCR system. PCR reaction mix was prepared as summarized in Table 1.

Table 1 qPCR reaction mix

PCR reaction mix components	Volume (μL)/ 20-μL Reaction	Final concentration
TaqMan universal master mix II, with no UNG, 2×	10.0	1×
TaqMan MicroRNA Assay (20×)	1.0	1×
cDNA/DNA template + RNase free water	9.0	1 to 100 ng
Total volume	20.0	–

Data analysis

The cycle threshold (Ct) values were assessed using the SDS 2.0.1 software (Applied biosystems). The average expression levels of miR-17-3p were normalized via miR-16 (Applied biosystems) as a reference gene, and subsequently, the $2^{-\Delta\Delta CT}$ method was applied.

Serum CEA determination

CEA was assayed using an immune radiometric assay (ADVIA Centaur XP (Siemens Diagnostics, Tarrytown, NY, USA), and the threshold for a positive result was 10 ng/ml. The assay was performed based on the manufacturer's instructions.

Serum CA19.9 determination

CA19.9 was assayed with an immunoradiometric assay (ADVIA Centaur XP (Siemens Diagnostics, Tarrytown, NY, USA)), and the threshold for a positive result was 37 ng/ml. The assay was carried out based on the manufacturer's instructions

Statistical analysis of the data

Data were fed to the computer and analyzed using the IBM SPSS software package version 20.0. (Armonk, NY: IBM Corp). Qualitative data were described using the number and percentage. Quantitative data were described using range (minimum and maximum), mean, standard deviation (SD), and median. The significance of the obtained results was judged at the 5% level.

Results

Table 2 shows the comparison between patients and controls as regards demographic data. There were no differences between patients and controls regarding gender distribution, as both had 56% females and 44% males. The mean age was 50.18 ± 13.24 for the patient's group; however; it was 48.24 ± 15.06 for the control group. There were no significant statistical differences between patients and controls as regards gender or age distribution.

Table 2 Baseline characteristics of the study population

	Patients (***n*** = 50)		Control (***n*** = 25)		Test of sig.	*p*
	No.	%	No.	%		
Gender						
Male	22	44.0	11	44.0	$\chi^2 = 0.00$	1.000
Female	28	56.0	14	56.0		
Age (years)						
Min.–max.	25.0–77.0		20.0–81.0		$t = 0.571$	0.571
Mean ± SD	50.18 ± 13.24		48.24 ± 15.06			
Median	50.0		50.0			

χ^2 Chi-square test, *t* Student's *t* test, *p p* value for comparing between the studied groups

Table 3 Levels of miR-17-3p, CEA, and CA19.9 in studied population (patients and control)

miRNA	Patients (***n*** = 50)	Control (***n*** = 25)	U	*p*
Min.–max.	1.74–32.45	0.27–3.41	5.00*	> 0.001*
Mean ± SD	9.07 ± 7.25	0.95 ± 0.63		
Median	6.85	0.88		
CEA				
Min.–max.	0.10–110.0	0.10–14.0	465.50	0.073
Mean ± SD	8.63 ± 20.83	2.94 ± 3.24		
Median	2.90	2.20		
CA19.9				
Min.–max.	0.25–700.0	5.0–30.0	302.50*	< 0.001*
Mean ± SD	39.40 ± 97.61	9.56 ± 5.20		
Median	20.45	8.0		

Using the Mann-Whitney *U* test, the microRNA 17-3P levels were found to be significantly elevated in the cell-free plasma samples of colon cancer patients compared with healthy controls ($P < 0.001$).(Table 3); also, miR-17-3p exhibited significantly different expression levels ($P < 0.001$) between stage II/III and stage VI colon cancer patients (Table 4). On the other hand, serum levels of CA19.9 were also found to be significantly higher in colon cancer patients compared to healthy controls ($P < 0.001$) (Table 3) along with significant differences between the cell-free plasma sample level of the same marker between stage II/III and stage VI colon cancer patients, yielding an assumed role in staging ($P < 0.001$) (Table 4); but on the contrary, serum level of CEA was found of no statistical significance either between colon cancer patients and control or between patients of different stages (Tables 3 and 4).

Using the ROC curve analysis to predict patients from control, the AUCs for miR-17-3p were 0.996 (95% CI

Table 4 Levels of microRNA 17-3P, CEA, and CA19.9 among group A and group B patients

miRNA	Group A (stage II + III) (***n*** = 25)	Group B (stage IV) (***n*** = 25)	U	*P*
Min.–max.	1.74–29.86	2.71–32.45	1.0	< 0.001*
Mean ± SD	7.48 ± 6.92	10.66 ± 7.37		
Median	5.28	8.69		
CA19.9				
Min.–max.	0.25–63.0	0.62–700.0	93.0	< 0.001*
Mean ± SD	19.95 ± 17.25	58.86 ± 135.5		
Median	12.0	32.0		
CEA				
Min.–max.	0.70–41.0	0.10–110.0	296.0	0.749
Mean ± SD	5.48 ± 8.09	11.78 ± 28.28		
Median	2.90	2.70		

Table 5 Agreement (sensitivity, specificity) to predict patients vs control

	AUC	p	95% CI		Cutoff	Sensitivity (CI)	Specificity (CI)	PPV (CI)	NPV (CI)
			L.L	U.L					
miRNA	**0.996***	**< 0.001***	0.989	1.003	**> 1.61**	100 (100–100)	96 (88.3–100)	96.2(94–100)	100 (100–100)
CA19.9	**0.758***	**< 0.001***	0.650	0.866	**> 9.3**	70.0(57.3–82.7)	68.0 (49.7–86.3)	81.4(69.7–93.0)	53.1 (35.8–70.4)
CEA	**0.628**	**0.073**	0.491	0.765	**> 2.29**	56 (42.3–69.7)	52 (32.4–71.5)	70 (55.8–77.3)	37.1 (43.4–65.9)

AUC area under a curve, *p* value probability value, *CI* confidence intervals, *NPV* negative predictive value, *PPV* positive predictive value
*Statistically significant at $p \leq 0.05$

0.989–1.003) and for CA19.9 was 0.785 (95% CI 0.650–0.866), respectively. At a threshold of 1.6 ng/ml for miRNA, the optimal sensitivity and specificity were 100% and 96%, respectively, in separating colon cancer patients from normal controls. At a threshold of 9.3 for CA19.9, the sensitivity and the specificity were 70% and 68%, respectively, denoting a significant role for both markers in the detection of colon cancer (Table 5) (Fig. 1).

Using the ROC curve analysis to predict patients with stage V from those with stage II/III, the AUCs for miR-17-3p were 0.713 (95% CI 0.859–0.566) and for CA19.9 was 0.682 (95% CI 0.832–0.531), respectively. At a threshold of 6.87 ng/ml for miRNA, the optimal sensitivity and specificity were 68% and 72%, respectively, in separating colon cancer patients with stage V from stage III. At a threshold of 12 ng for CA19.9, the sensitivity and the specificity were 84% and 52%, respectively, denoting a promising role for both markers for staging and prognosis of colon cancer. On the other hand, CEA was proved to be of no statistical significance in staging with AUC of 0.526 (95% CI 0.360–0.693) (Table 6, Fig. 2).

Discussion

Colon cancer should be screened and diagnosed as early as possible. Early diagnosis has a great influence on the therapeutic plan along with the outcome. Some reports have revealed the existence of non-coding (non-translational) RNAs (ncRNAs) that do not carry any genetic information concerning protein synthesis. Multiple ncRNA subtypes have been discovered. Cancer cell-derived exosomes may serve to promote both tumorigenesis and metastasis by influencing other types of cells in the tissue microenvironment [8]. Exosomes have been determined as the major carriers for miRNAs in serum [9]. They can be extracted from different body fluids such as serum, urine, milk, lymph, bile, and saliva and remain stable for long-term storage and expression profiling.

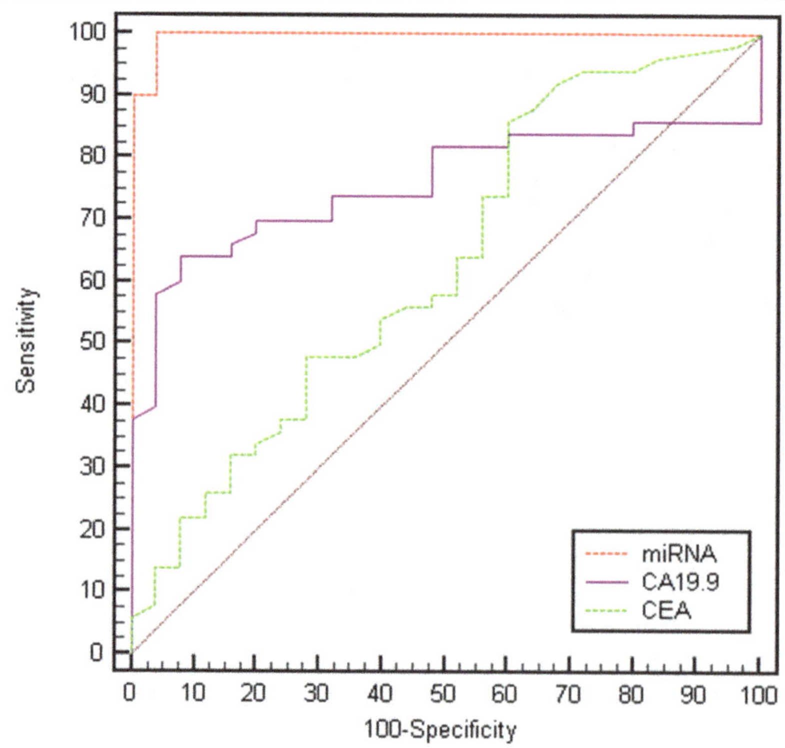

Fig. 1 ROC curve analysis to predict patients vs control

Table 6 Agreement (sensitivity, specificity) for different parameters to predict patients with stage IV from stage II + III

	AUC	*p*	95% CI		Cutoff	Sensitivity (CI)	Specificity (CI)	PPV (CI)	NPV (CI)
			L.L	U.L					
miRNA	**0.713***	**0.010***	0.566	0.859	**> 6.87**	68.0 (46.5–85.1)	72.0 (50.6–87.9)	70.8 (52.56–89.0)	69.2 (51.4–86.9)
CA19.9	**0.682***	**0.028***	0.531	0.832	**> 12**	84.0 (69.6–98.4)	52.0 (32.4–71.6)	63.6 (47.2–80.1)	76.5 (56.3–96.6)
CEA	**0.526**	**0.749**	0.360	0.693	**≤ 2.7**	52.0 (32.4–71.6)	56 (36.54–75.5)	54.2 (34.23–74.1)	53.8 (34.7–73.0)

AUC area under a curve, *p* value probability value, *CI* confidence intervals, *NPV* negative predictive value, *PPV* positive predictive value
*Statistically significant at $p \leq 0.05$

The main finding of the present results was the significant difference between the level of miRNA in patients with colon cancer and its level in healthy adults. This suggests a value of miRNA as a biomarker for colon cancer detection.

Fu et al. [10] conducted a recent study in 2018 aiming to detect candidate exosomal miRNAs that might be associated with colon cancer and its distant metastasis.

Their results revealed that 25 miRNAs had been upregulated, and 5 miRNAs had been downregulated in exosomes purified from the SW620 culture supernatant. Then, they assessed candidate miRNAs for diagnosing colon cancer using quantitative RT-PCR in colon cancer patients and proved significantly elevated expression levels of circulating both exosomal miR-17-3p and miR-92a-3p. They had a conclusion that circulating exosomal miR-17-3p and miR-92a-3p might offer a promising non-invasive diagnostic as well as a prognostic biomarker for primary and metastatic colon cancer.

The meta-analysis of Masuda and his colleagues [11] also matched our results. They studied the recently discovered types of miRNA including miR17-3p and assess its association with colon cancer. They reported that miRNAs have considerable potential as biomarkers as well as therapeutic targets. This might be explained by the fact that miRNAs can induce and modulate tumorigenesis and tumor progression in colon cancer. Nevertheless, they confirmed that the clinical importance of miRNAs as biomarkers is not conclusive yet, and independent validation studies are required for clinical application.

Many recent and even old studies have previously revealed the correlation between CEA level and colon cancer. Su et al. [12] tried to detect whether serum levels of CEA are correlated with the presence of primary colon cancer and/or recurrent colon cancer after radical resection. Nevertheless, as a result of the limited number of cases in our study, the current results in that CEA levels

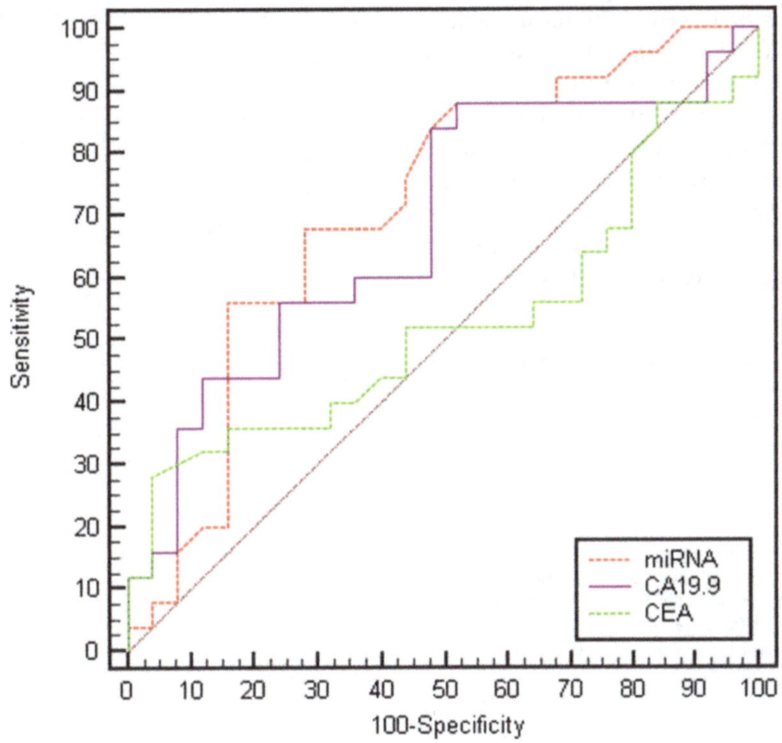

Fig. 2 ROC curve to predict stage IV from stage II + III

were not significantly higher in patients with colon cancer. Sue et al. [12] found that the overall sensitivity of CEA for the determination of primary colon cancer was 37.0%, whereas for recurrence, the sensitivity was 57%. Duffy and his colleagues [13] also reported that the CEA level was significantly higher in colon cancer patients, and that the elevated level was associated with poor prognosis.

Another essential finding of the current results was that levels of CA19.9 were significantly higher in patients with advanced colon cancer in comparison with the healthy controls. On the other hand, a significant relation was determined in advanced stages of colon cancer patients compared to the earlier stages. This was by following Vukobrat-Bijedic et al. [14] who showed that CA19.9 was a marker of advanced stages of colon cancer not for early ones. Also, Stiksma et al. [15] agreed to the current results as they reported that CA19.9 was significantly higher in colon cancer patients and ensured the possibility of using it as an additional marker to follow the disease process in colon cancer patients without increased CEA level.

Conclusion

The studied miRNA 17-3P expression was found to be a sensitive and specific biomarker for the diagnosis of cancer colon with high diagnostic accuracy. It was shown that the mean value of micro-RNA-17-3p in patients with cancer colon was significantly higher than the mean value in normal healthy control ($p < 0.001$).

The mean value of micro-RNA-17-3p in patients with cancer colon stage V was higher than the mean value in patients with cancer colon stage II/III; however, it was not statistically significant ($p < 0.\ 081$). It was also noticeable to mention that at a threshold value of 1.6 ng/ml for miRNA, the optimal sensitivity and specificity were 100% and 96%, respectively, in separating colon cancer patients from normal controls.

CA19.9 levels were found to significantly increase sensitivity and specificity in colon cancer diagnosis.

Abbreviations

AUC: Area under the ROC curve; CA19.9: Carbohydrate antigen 19.9; CEA: Carcinoembryonic antigen; CI: Confidence interval; ROC: Receiver operating characteristic

Acknowledgements

Not applicable

Authors' contributions

HH study design. EA study design and data collection. AE data collection and interpretation. MA data collection and interpretation. RA laboratory work. KS writing services. All authors have read and approved the manuscript and approved the submitted version and agreed both to be accountable for the authors own contribution.

Competing interests

The authors declare that they have no competing interests.

Author details

[1]Department of Internal Medicine, Faculty of Medicine, Alexandria University, Alexandria, Egypt. [2]Department of Clinical Pathology, Faculty of Medicine, Alexandria University, Alexandria, Egypt.

References

1. Storli KE, Sondenaa K, Bukholm IR, Nesvik I, Bru T, Furnes B et al (2011) Overall survival after resection for colon cancer in a national cohort study was adversely affected by TNM stage, lymph node ratio, gender, and old age. Int J Colon Dis 26(10):1299–1307
2. Faruq O, Vecchione A (2015) microRNA: Diagnostic perspective. Front Med (Lausanne) 2:51
3. Kara M, Yumrutas O, Ozcan O, Celik OI, Bozgeyik E, Bozgeyik I et al (2015) Differential expressions of cancer-associated genes and their regulatory miRNAs in colon carcinoma. Gene 567(1):81–86
4. Thompson JA, Grunert F, Zimmermann W (1991) Carcinoembryonic antigen gene family: molecular biology and clinical perspectives. J Clin Lab Anal 5(5):344–366
5. Fletcher RH (1986) Carcinoembryonic antigen. Ann Intern Med 104(1):66–73
6. Cen P, Walther C, Finkel KW, Amato RJ (2014) Biomarkers in oncology and nephrology. In: Cen P, Walther C, Finkel KW, Amato RJ (eds) Renal Disease in Cancer Patients. Elsevier, New York, pp 21–38
7. Locker GY, Hamilton S, Harris J, Jessup JM, Kemeny N, Macdonald JS et al (2006) ASCO 2006 update of recommendations for the use of tumor markers in gastrointestinal cancer. J Clin Oncol 24(33):5313–5327
8. Zhang L, Zhang S, Yao J, Lowery FJ, Zhang Q, Huang WC et al (2015) Microenvironment-induced PTEN loss by exosomal microRNA primes brain metastasis outgrowth. Nature 527(7576):100–104
9. Zhao K, Liang G, Sun X, Guan le L. (2016). Comparative miRNAome analysis revealed different miRNA expression profiles in bovine sera and exosomes. BMC Genomics 17(1):630.
10. Fu F, Jiang W, Zhou L, Chen Z (2018) Circulating exosomal miR-17-5p and miR-92a-3p predict pathologic stage and grade of colon cancer. Transl Oncol 11(2):221–232
11. Masuda T, Hayashi N, Kuroda Y, Ito S, Eguchi H, Mimori K (2017) MicroRNAs as biomarkers in colon cancer. Cancers 9(9):124
12. Su BB, Shi H, Wan J (2012) Role of serum carcinoembryonic antigen in the detection of colon cancer before and after surgical resection. World J Gastroenterol 18(17):2121–2126
13. Duffy MJ (2001) Carcinoembryonic antigen as a marker for colon cancer: is it clinically useful? Clin Chem 47(4):624–630
14. Vukobrat-Bijedic Z, Husic-Selimovic A, Sofic A, Bijedic N, Bjelogrlic I, Gogov B et al (2013) Cancer antigens (CEA and CA 19-9) as markers of advanced stage of colon carcinoma. Med Arch 67(6):397–401
15. Stiksma J, Grootendorst DC, van der Linden PW (2014) CA 19-9 as a marker in addition to CEA to monitor colon cancer. Clin Colon Cancer 13(4):239–244

25

Paracentesis-induced circulatory dysfunction: are there albumin alternatives?

Ayman Alsebaey*, Eman Rewisha and Imam Waked

Abstract

Background: Ascites is one of the main complications of advanced liver cirrhosis. It is defined as a pathological accumulation if free fluid in the peritoneal cavity.

Main body of the abstract: Ascites is a sign of decompensation in patients with liver cirrhosis and is associated with decreased survival. Ascites is associated with bad cosmetic figure and poor quality of life. Ascites is a predisposing factor for developing hydrothorax, hernias, diastolic dysfunction, spontaneous bacterial peritonitis, and renal impairment especially hepatorenal syndrome. The main treatment is salt restriction and diuretics. By the time the patient become non-responder and develop tense ascites, abdominal large volume paracentesis is the treatment of choice. Its advantages are rapid, cheap, and 1 day hospitalization. The main drawback is the development of paracentesis-induced circulatory dysfunction (PICD) if no volume expanding drugs are used. PICD is associated with dilutional hyponatremia, renal impairment, so it is considered the silent killer. Albumin infusion is the standard preventive measure but since costly to other alternatives such as colloids, vasoconstrictors or lowering the standard doses of the albumin was studied and is promising.

Conclusions: This review summarized the effectiveness of other alternative drugs.

Keywords: Ascites, Large volume paracentesis, Albumin, Paracentesis-induced circulatory dysfunction

Background

The ancient Egyptians identified liver disease and linked the presence of ascites to disease of the liver as early as the time of the Ebers papyrus, where paragraph 865 refers to a swelling of the abdomen with the "water going up and down" or freely moving, which is a very accurate description of ascites and how to detect it clinically [1, 2]. The recommended treatment was to pierce the abdomen with what is called a "hmmm" (supposedly a knife or sharp instrument) to drain the fluid, as in performing paracentesis. they also noted that "hardness of the liver" was a risk factor for ascites formation [3].

Hippocrates was the first one who use the term "ascites" which is derived from the Greek word (ἄσκο ; askos), i.e., a leather bag that was used to carry fluids [4].

Half of the cirrhosis patients develop ascites within 10 years. After the occurrence of ascites, the survival decreases dramatically where 50% of the patients survive for 2–5 years. The 1- and 5-year survival without transplantation is 85 and 55%, respectively [5].

Liver cirrhosis and portal hypertension account for 75% of all ascites cases [6]. Portal hypertension, arterial vasodilatation, neurohumoral activation, and renal dysfunction are the proposed pathogenesis factors [7]. Clinically, ascites can be divided into 3 grades in which the 1st and 2nd grade are treated by diuretics but the third grade is characterized by tense or marked ascites that requires large volume paracentesis (LVP) in addition to diuretics [8].

Salt restriction and diuretics (spironolactone and furosemide) are effective for ascites mobilization in 90% of

* Correspondence: aymanalsebaey@liver.menofia.edu.eg; https://orcid.org/0000-0003-3781-2312
Department of Hepatology and Gastroenterology, National Liver Institute, Menoufia University, Shebeen El-Koom 32511, Egypt

the patients. Twenty percent will become diuretic resistant, while 10% of the patients will not respond from the start [9, 10].

Main text

Refractory ascites was identified by the International Ascites Club in a consensus conference in 1996, and it was defined as "ascites that cannot be mobilized, or early recurrence of ascites which cannot be satisfactorily prevented by medical therapy" [11].

Modalities for tense ascites management

Till now, the two common tools for management of patients with tense or refractory ascites are LVP and transjugular intrahepatic portosystemic shunt (TIPS) [9, 10].

LVP is an outpatient maneuver that is highly effective for the rapid relief of ascites and related symptoms [12]. It is effective in removing ascites in one single tap using suction pump to decrease the time to 1–2 h [13]. Compared to diuretics, it is more effective in maintaining ascites-free state, shorter hospital stay, fewer complications, and mobilization of edema [14].

In fact, LVP is a known maneuver since ancient Greeks but it lost the interest with advent of diuretics but it returned back for use in mid-1980s [15]. Beethoven underwent LVP twice (11 liters and 22 liters) but the second time was infected and leaked, which resulted in his death [16]. He was excited when he saw the ascitic fluid coming out, and he shouted that it reminded him of Prophet Moses who struck the rock with his staff and made the water gush forth [17, 18].

LVP may be an indirect measure of patient compliance as regards sodium intake. About 1300 mmol sodium is removed by 10 L LVP. If the patient is consuming 88 mmol/day sodium without urinary sodium excretion and just 10 mmol/day nonurinary sodium, 10 L LVP will remove 17 days of retained sodium in a patient with no sodium excretion. As a result, if the frequency of LVP > 2 times/month, this means the patient is non-compliant with salt restriction [9, 19].

LVP is a safe maneuver, and the absolute contraindication is clinically evident fibrinolysis or clinically evident disseminated intravascular coagulation [20]. Pregnancy, severe bowel distension, and previous abdominal surgery are relative contraindication for non-ultrasound-guided (blind) paracentesis [21].

TIPS is an artificial bypass in which a shunt connects the portal vein to the hepatic vein through the liver. It was used in the past mainly for the treatment of variceal bleeding. Now, it is used for treatment of refractory ascites and hepatic hydrothorax [22]. Since the venous return increases with TIPS, the effective blood volume and the renal perfusion will improve with subsequent natriuresis. Hence, there is decreased rate of ascites formation or recurrence but unfortunately, the incidence of hepatic encephalopathy increases [23]. It was found that the nutritional status and quality of life improve markedly with TIPS [9].

Which is the better, LVP or TIPs? It is a continuous debate but generally, we should begin with LVP first but if the patient needs > 3 sessions per months, we should assess for TIPS [10].

Paracentesis-induced circulatory dysfunction:

Paracentesis-induced circulatory dysfunction (PICD) is a serious complication of performing LVP without a plasma expander. It is defined as 50% increase in the plasma renin activity (PRA) over the baseline on the sixth day after treatment, up to a value > 4 ng/mL per hour [24].

Without the use of plasma expander, the following hemodynamics were recorded. Immediately after paracentesis, there is decreased abdominal pressure and increased venous return with suppression of the renin-angiotensin-sympathetic nervous systems [25]. Unfortunately, opposite changes occur after 12 h with higher levels compared to before LVP [26]. In such case, the incidence of PICD was 75% [27], and it may persist for months [28].

PICD is an asymptomatic condition but it is associated with serious effects as rapid re-accumulation of ascites, dilutional hyponatremia, increased incidence of hepatorenal syndrome, and short survival [29, 30]. These consequences are noted if LVP is more than 5 L [27]. The development of PICD is not related to the paracentesis flow rate [31] unlike older studies [32]. Recently, β blockers were accused as a risk factor for PICD. Sersté et al. [33] performed a self-control cross-over study. Ten patients with cirrhosis and refractory ascites treated with β blockers were selected. When patients were given β blockers, the prevalence of PICD was 80%. After the withdrawal of β blockers, the prevalence of PICD dropped to 10%. Therefore, the authors concluded that the use of β blockers may be associated with a high risk of PICD in patients with cirrhosis and refractory ascites.

PICD prevention

PICD can be prevented by multiple measures as albumin infusion, synthetic colloids, extracorporeal ultrafiltration and reinfusion, vasoconstrictors (midodrine, terlipressin, and noradrenaline), and recently low-dose albumin (Fig. 1).

All the studies compared a test drug to the standard of care (standard dose albumin infusion) but our study [29] was the first head-to-head multiple drug comparison.

Synthetic colloids showed contradictory results. Gines et al. [28] did not find dextran 70 useful. The same result was reported by El-Ashry et al. [34] and Nasr et al. [35]. Other studies found dextran 40 [36] and 3.5%

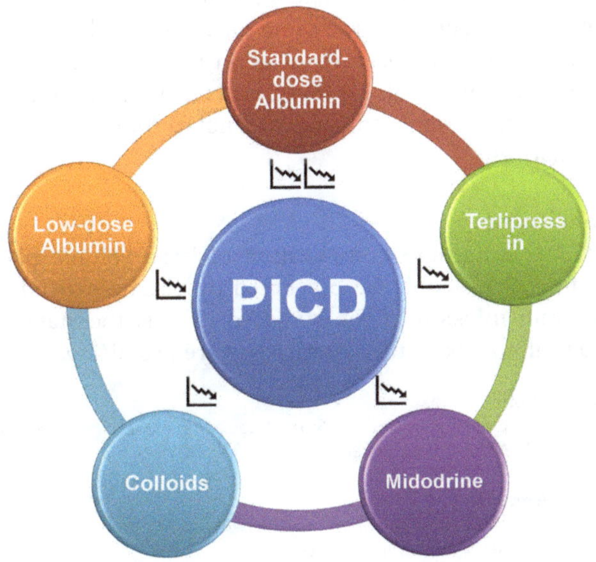

Fig. 1 Drugs used for the prevention of the paracentesis-induced circulatory dysfunction

polygeline (Haemaccel®) [37] were also ineffective drugs. Recently, hydroxy-ethyl starch (HES 6%) was found to be effective (6–8 g/L) [29, 38]. Christidis et al. [39] found that HES could increase the portal pressure as it filled the Kupffer cells (lysosomal storage), and this would increase the risk of variceal bleeding.

Terlipressin is a splanchnic vasoconstrictor. It was studied for PICD prevention [29, 40–42]. Moreau et al. [40] evaluated 20 patients with tense ascites, 10 received terlipressin (total 3 mg; 1 g IV before, 8 h, and 16 h after paracentesis) and the other 10 patients received albumin replacement (8 g/L ascites removed; 50% infused within 2 h after paracentesis and 50% after 6 h). In each group, 3 patients developed PICD. There was significant weight reduction and no renal impairment development in both groups. Singh et al. [41] assigned 40 patients with tense ascites into 2 groups as Moreau et al. [40]. In each group, 2 patients developed PICD. There was significant weight reduction, but in each group, one patient developed renal impairment [41]. Lata et al. [42] studied 49 patient but he used different doses. Twenty-four received terlipressin (1 mg every 4 h for 48 h; the first dose given immediately after paracentesis), and the other twenty five received albumin replacement (8 g/L ascites removed; 50% infused with 2 h after paracentesis and 50% after 6 h). The results in both treatment procedures suggested a similar efficacy for PICD prevention. In both groups, on the first 3 days, there was a tendency to improve hemodynamics reflected by the renin-angiotensin-aldosterone system activity. In the terlipressin group, this tendency approached statistically significant levels. All these studies found that terlipressin may be used as a measure for PICD prevention [29, 40–42].

Noradrenaline was assessed only in one study by Singh et al. [43] with promising results but no further studies.

Midodrine is an α1-agonist that increases the systemic and splanchnic blood pressure, circulating blood volume, and renal perfusion [44]. Midodrine is beneficial in hypotensive cirrhotic patients with refractory ascites [45].

Studies were contradictory as regards midodrine as a preventive measure for PICD [24, 29, 46]. Singh et al. [46] randomized 20 patients to receive midodrine (titrated dosage 5–10 mg/8 h to maintain a mean arterial pressure 10 mmHg above baseline for 72 h) and the other 20 patients to receive albumin (8 g/L ascitic fluid removed). No patient developed PICD in the midodrine group versus 2 in the albumin group. In contrast, in a study of 24 patients, Appenrodt et al. [24] randomized 11 patients to receive midodrine (12.5 mg every 8 h for 2 days) and the other 13 patients to receive albumin (8 g/L ascitic fluid removed). In the midodrine group, one patient developed HRS precipitated by pneumonia, and he was excluded as he received terlipressin as treatment and eventually died. Six patients out of 10 (60%) developed PICD in the midodrine versus 4 patients out of 9 (31%) in the albumin group. There was marked increase in the plasma renin in the midodrine group. The authors did not recommend utilization of midodrine for the prevention of PICD. Notably, they gave fixed dose of midodrine for relatively shorter period, the patients did not stop diuretics, and finally, they did not exclude the diabetic patients. Hamdy et al. [47] found that patients in the midodrine arm had more incidence of renal impairment and PICD. Seven patients died in the midodrine arm in contrast to none in the albumin group.

Being much cheaper than albumin and terlipressin and much easier to administer, midodrine may be worth more trials to assess its use instead of albumin.

Albumin infusion is the approved standard-of-care measure for PICD prevention [48, 49]. Gines et al. [27] found that albumin infusion decreased the incidence of PICD from 80 to 15–20%. A study by Tan et al. [50] had the same conclusion.

On one hand, there is some controversy regarding albumin infusion as being very expensive, causing inhibition of the endogenous albumin synthesis and increasing its degradation,[51, 52]. On the other hand, albumin has many beneficial functions that reinforce its use apart from being plasma-expanding drug. Albumin detoxifies harmful reactive oxygen, stabilizes the endothelium, prevents platelets aggregation, and can modulate the immune and inflammatory responses [53].

In 2012, a meta-analysis conducted by Bernardi et al. [54] found that albumin infusion caused 60% decrease of PICD development. Furthermore, albumin infusion decreased the hyponatremia and mortality. In 2017, Kütting et al. [55] conducted another meta-analysis with contradictory results. Kütting et al. found that albumin infusion decreased the incidence of hyponatremia and PICD development in patients without hepatocellular carcinoma. Albumin infusion in this meta-analysis unfortunately did not decrease mortality. Even in patients with hepatocellular carcinoma, the survival did not increase with albumin infusion. Their final conclusion was against albumin infusion.

The albumin dose is 6–8 g per liter of ascitic fluid removed [48, 49, 56]. It can be given once the session completed [57] or giving half the dose immediately after the paracentesis and the other half 6 h later [28, 29, 58].

Low-dose albumin infusion was studied by Alessandria et al. (4 g/L ascites removed) [59] and Alsebaey et al. (2 g/L ascites removed) [29]. Thirty-five patients were randomized by Alessandria et al. [59] for half dose albumin (4 g/L ascites) and 35 patients to full dose albumin (8 g/L ascites removed). PICD developed in 5 patients (14%) in the half dose albumin group and in 7 patients (20%) in the full dose albumin group with no significant difference. They concluded that albumin in half dose is equivalent to full dose albumin in prevention of PICD. Alsebaey et al. [29] found same finding despite lower doses.

Our study [29] was the first head-to-head comparison of different drugs for PICD prevention. It included 125 patients randomized to 5 equal groups. In the albumin group, the dose was 6 g/L. In the low-dose albumin group, the dose was 2 g/L. Hydroxyethyl starch (HES 130/0.4) was given as 8 g/L. Terlipressin dose was 1 mg IV at the onset then every 8 h for a maximum of 3 g per day. Midodrine was administered orally for 3 days (5–10 mg 8 hourly to maintain the MAP at 10 mmHg > the baseline). All groups were statistically comparable as regards the age, sex, the etiology of the liver disease, and the Child-Pugh score. Most patients had hepatitis C-related liver cirrhosis. The average volume of ascitic fluid removed was 13 ± 0.14 L. PICD occurred in two patients in both terlipressin and HES 130/0.4 groups. In each albumin group, three patients developed PICD. Five patients in the midodrine group developed PICD. Comparing all groups showed no significant difference. We concluded that low-dose albumin, terlipressin, and HES 130/0.4 were good alternatives to the standard-of-care albumin dose.

We published another new study [60] focusing on the use of low-dose albumin 2 g/L ascitic fluid removed (n = 85). The incidence of PICD development was comparable to the standard dose albumin. In the same study, we did again comparison of the new number of the low-dose albumin to the other old arms, namely, terlipressin, midodrine, HES 130/0.4, and standard dose albumin. All the groups again were the same for PICD development.

The recent European Association for the Study of the Liver guidelines [56], however, still recommend albumin (8 g/L ascites removed) and did not recommend other alternatives.

Conclusions

PICD is a harmful complication of large volume paracentesis that should be prevented by plasma expanders. Albumin infusion in the standard dose is the standard drug till now but other alternatives are promising.

Abbreviations

LVP: Large volume paracentesis; TIPS: Transjugular intrahepatic portosystemic shunt; PICD: Paracentesis induced circulatory dysfunction

Acknowledgements

The authors thank all the members of Hepatology and Gastroenterology Department, National Liver Institute, Egypt.

Authors' contributions

AA put the plan of the review article, searched the PubMed and google scholar for relevant studies, summarized them, and wrote the manuscript. ER and IW revised the manuscript. All authors have read and approved the final manuscript.

Competing interests

AA and ER declare that they have no conflict of interest.
IW: Imam Waked: investigator and/or speaker for Abbvie, Gilead Sciences, Janssen, Marcyrl, Onxio, Pharco.

References

1. Bryan CP (1931) The papyrus Ebers. D. Appleton, New York, pp 134–135
2. Ghaliounghui P (1987) The Ebers Papyrus. Academy of Scientific Research and Technology, Cairo
3. Dawson AD (1960) Historical notes on ascites. Gastroenterology 39:790–791
4. Richert A, Raines D, Lopez FA (2009) New onset ascites secondary to cirrhosis. J La State Med Soc 161(1):9–13 quiz 13, 54
5. Lee JM, Han K-H, Ahn SH (2009) Ascites and spontaneous bacterial peritonitis: An Asian perspective. J Gastroenterol Hepatol 24(9):1494–1503
6. Rochling FA, Zetterman RK (2009) Management of ascites. Drugs 69(13): 1739–1760
7. Møller S, Henriksen JH, Bendtsen F (2009) Ascites: pathogenesis and therapeutic principles. Scand J Gastroenterol 44(8):902–911
8. Zullo A, Hassan C, Lorenzetti R (2011) Rifaximin therapy in minimal hepatic encephalopathy cirrhotics. Am J Gastroenterol 106(11):2041 author reply 2041-2
9. Senousy BE, Draganov PV (2009) Evaluation and management of patients with refractory ascites. World J Gastroenterol 15(1):67–80
10. Singhal S, Baikati KK, Jabbour S II (2012) Anand, Management of refractory ascites. Am J Ther 19(2):121–132
11. Arroyo V, Ginès P, Gerbes AL, Dudley FJ, Gentilini P, Laffi G, Reynolds TB, Ring-Larsen H, Schölmerich J (1996) Definition and diagnostic criteria of refractory ascites and hepatorenal syndrome in cirrhosis. Hepatology (Baltimore, Md) 23(1):164–176
12. Grabau CM, Crago SF, Hoff LK, Simon JA, Melton CA, Ott BJ, Kamath PS (2004) Performance standards for therapeutic abdominal paracentesis. Hepatology (Baltimore, Md) 40(2):484–488
13. Kuiper JJ, De Man RA, Van Buuren HR (2007) Review article: management of ascites and associated complications in patients with cirrhosis. Aliment Pharmacol Ther 26:183–193

14. Peltekian KM, Wong F, Liu PP, Logan AG, Sherman M, Blendis LM (1997) Cardiovascular, renal, and neurohumoral responses to single large-volume paracentesis in patients with cirrhosis and diuretic-resistant ascites. Am J Gastroenterol 92(3):394–399
15. Cardenas A, Arroyo V (2005) Refractory ascites. Dig Dis 23(1):30–38
16. Kubba AK, Young M (1996) Ludwig van Beethoven: a medical biography. Lancet 347(8995):167–170
17. Reuben A (2002) Out came copious water. Hepatology (Baltimore, Md) 36(1):261–264
18. Adams PC (1987) Historical hepatology: Ludwig van Beethoven. J Gastroenterol Hepatol 2(4):375–379
19. Schouten J, Michielsen PP (2007) Treatment of cirrhotic ascites. Acta Gastroenterol Belg 70(2):217–222
20. Runyon BA (2009) Management of adult patients with ascites due to cirrhosis: an update. Hepatology (Baltimore, Md) 49(6):2087–2107
21. McGibbon A, Chen GI, Peltekian KM, van Zanten SV (2007) An evidence-based manual for abdominal paracentesis. Dig Dis Sci 52(12):3307–3315
22. Boyer TD (2003) Transjugular intrahepatic portosystemic shunt: current status. Gastroenterology 124(6):1700–1710
23. W. Hou, A.J. Sanyal, Ascites: diagnosis and management, Med Clin North Am 93(4) (2009) 801-817, vii.
24. Appenrodt B, Wolf A, Grünhage F, Trebicka J, Schepke M, Rabe C, Lammert F, Sauerbruch T, Heller J (2008) Prevention of paracentesis-induced circulatory dysfunction: midodrine vs albumin. A randomized pilot study. Liver Int 28(7):1019–1025
25. Pozzi M, Redaelli E, Ratti L, Poli G, Guidi C, Milanese M, Calchera I, Mancia G (2005) Time-course of diastolic dysfunction in different stages of chronic HCV related liver diseases. Minerva Gastroenterol Dietol 51(2):179–186
26. Ruiz-del-Arbol L, Monescillo A, Arocena C, Valer P, Ginès P, Moreira V, María Milicua J, Jiménez W, Arroyo V (2005) Circulatory function and hepatorenal syndrome in cirrhosis. Hepatology (Baltimore, Md) 42(2):439–447
27. Gines P, Tito L, Arroyo V, Planas R, Panes J, Viver J, Torres M, Humbert P, Rimola A, Llach J et al (1988) Randomized comparative study of therapeutic paracentesis with and without intravenous albumin in cirrhosis. Gastroenterology 94(6):1493–1502
28. Gines A, Fernandez-Esparrach G, Monescillo A, Vila C, Domenech E, Abecasis R, Angeli P, Ruiz-Del-Arbol L, Planas R, Sola R, Gines P, Terg R, Inglada L, Vaque P, Salerno F, Vargas V, Clemente G, Quer JC, Jimenez W, Arroyo V, Rodes J (1996) Randomized trial comparing albumin, dextran 70, and polygeline in cirrhotic patients with ascites treated by paracentesis. Gastroenterology 111(4):1002–1010
29. Alsebaey A, Abdel-Razek W, Bassuni A, Rewisha E, Khalil M, Waked I (2013) Prevention of paracentesis-induced circulatory dysfunction: could we use other albumin alternatives? Egyptian Liver Journal 3(4):118–125
30. Salerno F, Guevara M, Bernardi M, Moreau R, Wong F, Angeli P, Garcia-Tsao G, Lee SS (2010) Refractory ascites: pathogenesis, definition and therapy of a severe complication in patients with cirrhosis. Liver Int 30(7):937–947
31. Elsabaawy MM, Abdelhamid SR, Alsebaey A, Abdelsamee E, Obada MA, Salman TA, Rewisha E (2015) The impact of paracentesis flow rate in patients with liver cirrhosis on the development of paracentesis induced circulatory dysfunction. Clin Mol Hepatol 21(4):365–371
32. Coll S, Vila MC, Molina L, Gimenez MD, Guarner C, Sola R (2004) Mechanisms of early decrease in systemic vascular resistance after total paracentesis: influence of flow rate of ascites extraction. Eur J Gastroenterol Hepatol 16(3):347–353
33. Sersté T, Francoz C, Durand F, Rautou P-E, Melot C, Valla D, Moreau R, Lebrec D Beta-blockers cause paracentesis-induced circulatory dysfunction in patients with cirrhosis and refractory ascites: a cross-over study. J Hepatol 55(4):794–799
34. El-Ashry N, El-Damarawy M, Salem M, Mogawer S (2007) Large volume abdominal paracentesis effect on some humoral factors and cardiac performance in patients with liver cirrhosis and tense ascities. J Egypt Soc Parasitol 37(2):571–584
35. Nasr G, Hassan A, Ahmed S, Serwah A (2010) Predictors of large volume paracantesis induced circulatory dysfunction in patients with massive hepatic ascites. J Cardiovasc Dis Res 1(3):136–144
36. Garcia-Compean D, Blanc P, Larrey D, Daures JP, Hirtz J, Mendoza E, Maldonado H, Michel H (2002) Treatment of cirrhotic tense ascites with Dextran-40 versus albumin associated with large volume paracentesis: a randomized controlled trial. Ann Hepatol 1(1):29–35
37. Moreau R, Valla DC, Durand-Zaleski I, Bronowicki JP, Durand F, Chaput JC, Dadamessi I, Silvain C, Bonny C, Oberti F, Gournay J, Lebrec D, Grouin JM, Guemas E, Golly D, Padrazzi B, Tellier Z (2006) Comparison of outcome in patients with cirrhosis and ascites following treatment with albumin or a synthetic colloid: a randomised controlled pilot trail. Liver Int 26(1):46–54
38. Abdel-Khalek EE, Arif SE (2010) Randomized trial comparing human albumin and hydroxyethyl starch 6% as plasma expanders for treatment of patients with liver cirrhosis and tense ascites following large volume paracentesis. Arab Journal of Gastroenterology 11(1):24–29
39. Christidis C, Mal F, Ramos J, Senejoux A, Callard P, Navarro R, Trinchet JC, Larrey D, Beaugrand M, Guettier C (2001) Worsening of hepatic dysfunction as a consequence of repeated hydroxyethylstarch infusions. J Hepatol 35(6): 726–732
40. Moreau R, Asselah T, Condat B, de Kerguenec C, Pessione F, Bernard B, Poynard T, Binn M, Grangé JD, Valla D, Lebrec D (2002) Comparison of the effect of terlipressin and albumin on arterial blood volume in patients with cirrhosis and tense ascites treated by paracentesis: a randomised pilot study. Gut 50(1):90–94
41. Singh V, Kumar R, Nain CK, Singh B, Sharma AK (2006) Terlipressin versus albumin in paracentesis-induced circulatory dysfunction in cirrhosis: a randomized study. J Gastroenterol Hepatol 21(1):303–307
42. Lata J, Marecek Z, Fejfar T, Zdenek P, Bruha R, Safka V, Hulek P, Hejda V, Dolina J, Stehlik J, Tozzi I (2007) The efficacy of terlipressin in comparison with albumin in the prevention of circulatory changes after the paracentesis of tense ascites--a randomized multicentric study. Hepatogastroenterology 54(79):1930–1933
43. Singh V, Kumar B, Nain CK, Singh B, Sharma N, Bhalla A, Sharma AK (2006) Noradrenaline and albumin in paracentesis-induced circulatory dysfunction in cirrhosis: a randomized pilot study. J Intern Med 260(1):62–68
44. Tandon P, Tsuyuki RT, Mitchell L, Hoskinson M, Ma MM, Wong WW, Mason AL, Gutfreund K, Bain VG (2009) The effect of 1 month of therapy with midodrine, octreotide-LAR and albumin in refractory ascites: a pilot study. Liver Int 29(2):169–174
45. Sourianarayanane A, Barnes DS, McCullough AJ (2011) Beneficial Effect of Midodrine in Hypotensive Cirrhotic Patients with Refractory Ascites. Gastroenterol Hepatol 7(2):132–134
46. Singh V, Dheerendra PC, Singh B, Nain CK, Chawla D, Sharma N, Bhalla A, Mahi SK (2008) Midodrine versus albumin in the prevention of paracentesis-induced circulatory dysfunction in cirrhotics: a randomized pilot study. Am J Gastroenterol 103(6):1399–1405
47. Hamdy H, ElBaz AA, Hassan A, Hassanin O (2014) Comparison of midodrine and albumin in the prevention of paracentesis-induced circulatory dysfunction in cirrhotic patients: a randomized pilot study. J Clin Gastroenterol 48(2):184–188
48. European Association for the Study of the Liver EASL clinical practice guidelines on the management of ascites, spontaneous bacterial peritonitis, and hepatorenal syndrome in cirrhosis. J Hepatol 53(3):397–417
49. Runyon BA (2013) Introduction to the revised American Association for the Study of Liver Diseases Practice Guideline management of adult patients with ascites due to cirrhosis 2012. Hepatology (Baltimore, Md) 57(4):1651–1653
50. Tan HK, James PD, Wong F (2016) Albumin may prevent the morbidity of paracentesis-induced circulatory dysfunction in cirrhosis and refractory ascites: a pilot study. Dig Dis Sci 61(10):3084–3092
51. M.A. Rothschild, M. Oratz, C. Evans, S.S. Schreiber, Alterations in albumin metabolism after serum and albumin infusions, J Clin Invest 43 (1964) 1874-1880.
52. Wilkinson P, Sherlock S (1962) The effect of repeated albumin infusions in patients with cirrhosis. Lancet 2(7266):1125–1129
53. Caraceni P, Angeli P, Prati D, Bernardi M, Alessandria C, Riggio O, Salerno F, Liumbruno GM, Bennardello F, Piccoli P, Velati C, Berti P, Facco G, Fiorin F (2016) AISF-SIMTI Position Paper: The appropriate use of albumin in patients with liver cirrhosis. Dig Liver Dis 48(1):4–15
54. Bernardi M, Caraceni P, Navickis RJ, Wilkes MM (2012) Albumin infusion in patients undergoing large-volume paracentesis: a meta-analysis of randomized trials. Hepatology (Baltimore, Md) 55(4):1172–1181
55. Kutting F, Schubert J, Franklin J, Bowe A, Hoffmann V, Demir M, Pelc A, Nierhoff D, Tox U, Steffen HM (2017) Insufficient evidence of benefit regarding mortality due to albumin substitution in HCC-free cirrhotic patients undergoing large volume paracentesis. J Gastroenterol Hepatol 32(2):327–338
56. Angeli P, Bernardi M, Villanueva C, Francoz C, Mookerjee RP, Trebicka J, Krag A, Laleman W, Gines P (2018) EASL Clinical Practice Guidelines for the

management of patients with decompensated cirrhosis. J Hepatol 69(2): 406–460

57. K.P. Moore, G.P. Aithal, Guidelines on the management of ascites in cirrhosis, Gut 55 Suppl 6 (2006) vi1-v12.
58. Planas R, Gines P, Arroyo V, Llach J, Panes J, Vargas V, Salmeron JM, Gines A, Toledo C, Rimola A et al (1990) Dextran-70 versus albumin as plasma expanders in cirrhotic patients with tense ascites treated with total paracentesis. Results of a randomized study. Gastroenterology 99(6):1736–1744
59. Alessandria C, Elia C, Mezzabotta L, Risso A, Andrealli A, Spandre M, Morgando A, Marzano A, Rizzetto M (2011) Prevention of paracentesis-induced circulatory dysfunction in cirrhosis: Standard vs half albumin doses. A prospective, randomized, unblinded pilot study. Dig Liver Dis 43(11):881–886
60. Alsebaey A, Rewisha E, Waked I (2020) High efficacy of low-dose albumin infusion in the prevention of paracentesis-induced circulatory dysfunction. Egyptian Liver Journal 10(1):9

26

Impact of different anti-HCV regimens on platelet count during treatment in Egyptian patients

Sara Abd El Ghany[1], Noha M. El Husseiny[1,2*], Mohamed Roshdy[1], Heba Moustafa[1], Mohamed Taha Atallah[3], Ahmed Fathy[1,2], Heba H. El Demellawy[4], Asmaa M. Abdelhameed[1,2] and Doaa M. El Demerdash[1]

Abstract

Background: Side effects of antiviral therapies for hepatitis C, especially hematologic abnormalities, may decrease both therapeutic adherence and therapeutic success rate. Adherence to therapy is essential to achieve an early viral response (EVR), and this is vital for attaining a sustained viral response (SVR). Discontinuation of anti-viral therapy is the only way to prevent progressive thrombocytopenia; however, discontinuation of therapy may reduce the rate of viral clearance and SVR. Our aim is to study effects of antiviral therapy for HCV on platelet count. One hundred sixty eight adult patients with chronic hepatitis C were enrolled in this study and subcategorized into 3 groups: *group* (*1*) contains 56 patients receiving IFN, ribavirin and sofosbuvir (triple therapy); *group* (*2*) contains 55 patients receiving ribavirin and sofosbuvir (SOF/RBV); and *group* (*3*) contains 57 patients receiving simeprevir and sofosbuvir (SIM/SOF). HCV RNA by PCR were checked basically for all studied patients. Follow-up platelet count was done weekly during the first month then monthly till end of treatment. Follow-up of platelet count decrement was assessed at the 2nd week, 4th week and end of antiviral therapy for all studied groups.

Results: We found that in the 2nd week and 4th week, most of patients (76.2%, 71.4%) showed platelet count decrement during antiviral therapy. The decrement of platelet at the 2nd week, 4th week and at end of treatment was much noticed with the SOF/RBV antiviral therapy studied group. None of the patients developed severe thrombocytopenia; none of the patients needed to stop antiviral therapy due to thrombocytopenia, only 6 patients needed dose modification, most of them were from the triple therapy group.

Conclusion: We concluded that thrombocytopenia in chronic HCV infection has a multifactorial pathophysiology and remains a major problem. The recent change in direct-acting antiviral therapy (DAA) without IFN, as the frontline therapy for HCV, permit to avoid the dilemmas associated with initiating or maintaining IFN-based antiviral therapy. DAAs, with high SVR and few haematological adverse effects, have been shown to improve thrombocytopenia associated with HCV infection as well as advanced hepatic disease.

Keywords: HCV, Direct antiviral therapy, Thrombocytopenia

* Correspondence: Noha_el_husseiny77@yahoo.com
[1]Internal Medicine Department, Faculty of Medicine, Cairo University, Cairo, Egypt
[2]Armed Forces Faculty of Medicine (AFCM), Cairo, Egypt

Background

Egypt has the highest HCV prevalence in the world at approximately 15%, and more than 90% of cases are genotype 4 [1].

Patients with chronic hepatitis treated with antiviral therapy experience a response superior to that of therapies used in the past. However, side effects, especially haematologic abnormalities, may decrease both therapeutic adherence and therapeutic success rate. Thrombocytopenia is one of the potential hematologic abnormalities associated with peg-IFN-a-based therapy [2].

Adherence to therapy is essential to achieve an early viral response (EVR), and this is vital for attaining a sustained viral response (SVR) [3].

Discontinuation of antiviral therapy is the only way to prevent progressive thrombocytopenia; however, discontinuation of therapy may reduce the rate of viral clearance and sustained virological response (SVR) [4].

Studies to identify risk factors for antiviral therapy-induced severe thrombocytopenia are essential but are rarely conducted especially in the Egyptian population of the largest HCV epidemic in the world.

No previous studies were done on Egyptian patients to the compare effect of different antiviral therapy combinations on platelet count. Through this retrospective study, we tried to identify predictors of thrombocytopenia in HCV-treated patients on different regimens.

Methods

This research was approved by the Research Ethical Committee of Faculty of Medicine-Cairo University. It is a retrospective study. It included 168 chronic hepatitis C Egyptian patients receiving antiviral therapy. All methods were performed in accordance with the relevant guidelines and regulations. Informed consents were obtained. All were treated between 2015 and 2017 in Cairo Fatemic Hospital and Internal Medicine department of Kasr Al Aini- Faculty of Medicine. We revised all patients' files. Inclusion criteria included age > 18 years, having chronic hepatitis C and receiving antiviral therapy. Exclusion criteria included co-infection with HBV or HIV and hepatitis other than hepatitis C (eg. autoimmune) and baseline severe thrombocytopenia below 50,000/μl. Dose modification of a treatment line was done if platelet count dropped below 30,000/μl and discontinuation in case of persistent drop even with dose reduction.

Patients were subcategorized into 3 groups: *group (1)* consists of 56 patients who received IFN, ribavirin and sofosbuvir (triple therapy); *group* (2) consists of 55 patients who received ribavirin and sofosbuvir (SOF/RBV); and *group* (3) consists of 57 patients who received simeprevir and sofosbuvir (SIM/SOF). For all, the files were revised for full history and clinical examination, CBC, HCV RNA by PCR. Fibroscan was done for 61 patients, and liver biopsy was done for 22 patients. Follow-up platelet count weekly during the 1st month of therapy, rate of platelet decline (%) especially at the 2nd week of therapy, then monthly till end of therapy.

Follow-up HCV RNA by PCR was done at week 4 and at the end of therapy. FIB-4 score was calculated for all patients [5]. Child score was calculated for all patients [6].

Statistical methods

Data were coded and entered using the statistical package SPSS (Statistical Package for the Social Sciences) version 24. Data was summarized using mean, standard deviation, median, minimum and maximum in quantitative data and using frequency (count) and relative frequency (percentage) for categorical data. Comparisons between quantitative variables were done using the non-parametric Kruskal–Wallis and Mann–Whitney tests. For comparing categorical data, Chi square (χ^2) test was performed. Exact test was used instead when the expected frequency is less than 5. Correlations between quantitative variables were done using Spearman correlation coefficient. *P* values less than 0.05 were considered as statistically significant.

Results

Tables 1 and 2 demonstrate comparison of non-parametric and parametric data respectively of the three studied groups. Group 2 (SOF/RBV) showed significantly higher percentage of patients with splenomegaly and liver cirrhosis and those who received previous treatment.

Baseline haematological parameters where significantly more favourable in group 1 (triple therapy line). The baseline mean platelet count in group 2 (SOF/RBV) was lower as compared with the other 2 groups; also, the HCV load was significantly higher in this group.

Table 3 demonstrates the percentage of patients showing platelet decrement as assessed at the 2nd week, 4th week and end of antiviral therapy. Overall, most patients, 76.2% in the 2nd week and 71.4% in the 4th week, exhibited decrease in platelet count. These percentages dropped to 54.8% at the end of treatment. Highest proportion of patients with decrease in platelet count was found in group 1 (INF/SOF/RBV) 89.3%, 82.1% and 73.2% at 2nd week, 4th week and end of antiviral therapy.

Regarding the magnitude of drop of platelet count reported as mean and percent of baseline count, as presented in Table 4, group 1 showed the highest percent of drop from the baseline: 28%, 26% and 25% in the 2nd week, 4th week and end of antiviral therapy, while group 2 showed lowest level (mean count) and earliest recovery

Table 1 Non parametric parameters of the three groups on anti-HCV treatment

	SIM/SOF		SOF/RBV		Triple		*p* value
	Count	%	Count	%	Count	%	
Sex							
Male	26	45.6%	32	58.2%	38	67.9%	0.057
Female	31	54.4%	23	41.8%	18	32.1%	
Residency							
Urban	34	59.6%	42	76.4%	35	62.5%	0.138
Rural	23	40.4%	13	23.6%	21	37.5%	
History of previous ttt							
ttt naïve	54	94.7%	35	64.8%	42	75.0%	< 0.001
ttt experienced	3	5.3%	19	35.2%	14	25.0%	
Smoking							
Yes	6	10.5%	7	12.7%	11	19.6%	0.354
No	51	89.5%	48	87.3%	45	80.4%	
Comorbidities (diabetes and/or hypertension)							
Yes	21	36.8%	21	38.2%	18	32.1%	0.783
No	36	63.2%	34	61.8%	38	67.9%	
Liver by ultrasound							
Normal	0	0.0%	2	3.6%	8	14.3%	< 0.001
Cirrhotic	31	54.4%	47	85.5%	25	44.6%	
Abnormal echopattern	26	45.6%	6	10.9%	23	41.1%	
Spleen by ultrasound							
Enlarged	28	49.1%	41	74.5%	35	62.5%	0.021
Average	29	50.9%	14	25.5%	21	37.5%	
Ascites by ultrasound							
Yes	0	0.0%	1	1.8%	1	1.8%	0.549
No	57	100.0%	54	98.2%	55	98.2%	
Child score calculation							
A5	25	43.9%	26	47.3%	50	89.3%	< 0.001
A6	32	56.1%	21	38.2%	4	7.1%	
B7	0	0.0%	7	12.7%	2	3.6%	
B8	0	0.0%	1	1.8%	0	0.0%	
Stage of fibrosis							
F1	3	27.3%	1	4.0%	2	8.0%	0.003
F2	1	9.1%	1	4.0%	0	0.0%	
F3	1	9.1%	4	16.0%	14	56.0%	
F4	6	54.5%	18	72.0%	9	36.0%	
F5	0	0.0%	1	4.0%	0	0.0%	
Stage of necroinflammatory activity							
A1	1	50.0%	2	25.0%	4	33.3%	0.749
A2	1	50.0%	4	50.0%	7	58.3%	
A3	0	0.0%	1	12.5%	0	0.0%	
A7	0	0.0%	0	0.0%	1	8.3%	
A10	0	0.0%	1	12.5%	0	0.0%	
Week 4 HCV RNA by PCR							

Table 1 Non parametric parameters of the three groups on anti-HCV treatment *(Continued)*

	SIM/SOF		SOF/RBV		Triple		*p* value
	Count	%	Count	%	Count	%	
Positive	3	5.3%	7	12.7%	2	3.6%	0.183
Negative	54	94.7%	48	87.3%	54	96.4%	
Week 12 HCV RNA by PCR							
Positive	2	3.6%	1	1.8%	0	0.0%	0.325
Negative	53	96.4%	54	98.2%	56	100.0%	
HCV antiviral dose modification							
No	57	100.0%	54	98.2%	51	91.1%	0.025
Modified	0	0.0%	1	1.8%	5	8.9%	

(in the 4th week) of platelet count, considering that this group had lowest pre-treatment count.

The drop in the mean platelet count was modest as illustrated in Table 4 and Fig. 1; in all groups, according to the mean platelet count in the 2nd and 4th weeks and end of treatment, the reported thrombocytopenia is grade 1 (75,000 to 150,000/mm^3) as defined by CTCAE v3.0 [7].

The demographic data and the platelet count change through the treatment course in the 3 studied groups revealed significant positive correlation between baseline body weight and platelet count change in the 2nd week, 4th week and end of treatment in the SOF/RBV therapy only ($r = 0.27, 0.46, 0.288$; $p = 0.04, 0.001, 0.03$, respectively).

The triple therapy group demonstrated statistically significant negative correlation between FIB-4 score and the platelet count in the 2nd week ($p < 0.047$) but not at the 4th week or end of treatment, while this correlation was significant for group 2 at the 2nd and 4th weeks and for group 3 at the 4th week only ($p < 0.001$). There is no correlation between duration of illness and platelet count in the three groups (Table 5).

Table 2 Comparison of parameteric parameters of the three antiviral groups ($p > 0.0$)

	Group			
	SIM/SOF	SOF/RBV	Triple	*p* value
Age (years)	55.05 ± 8.00	53.93 ± 9.27	53.55 ± 7.56	0.764
Weight (Kg)	81.73 ± 15.29	81.35 ± 12.41	80.05 ± 13.55	0.626
Height (m)	1.64 ± .08	1.66 ± .10	1.68 ± .09	0.092
BMI (Kg/m^2)	30.36 ± 6.09	29.81 ± 4.39	28.40 ± 4.48	0.099
HCV positivity (years)	2.26 ± 2.81	6.67 ± 6.30 *	4.18 ± 5.85	< 0.001
Fib 4 calculation	5.10 ± 2.78	7.77 ± 3.79 *	3.74 ± 1.43 *#	< 0.001
Baseline platelets (*1000/mm^3)	111.84 ± 40.35	77.18 ± 18.01 *	136.89 ± 31.70 *#	< 0.001
Baseline TLC (*1000/mm^3)	4.89 ± 1.35	4.89 ± 1.52	5.97 ± 1.99 *#	0.002
Baseline ANC (*1000/mm^3)	2.64 ± .95	2.59 ± 1.01	3.11 ± 1.27 *#	0.028
Baseline Hb (g/dl)	12.63 ± 1.38	12.97 ± 1.69	13.86 ± 1.58 *#	< 0.001
Baseline Alt (IU/l)	57.35 ± 39.05	64.52 ± 37.95	75.04 ± 58.82	0.198
Baseline Ast (IU/l)	65.58 ± 36.44	78.14 ± 42.81	72.91 ± 51.74	0.106
Baseline Bil T (mg/dl)	.99 ± .39	1.18 ± .57	.99 ± .69 #	0.024
Baseline Alb (g/dl)	3.50 ± .46	3.44 ± .46	3.95 ± .44 *#	< 0.001
Baseline PC (%)	79.38 ± 12.46	75.20 ± 13.93	81.98 ± 15.38 #	0.015
Baseline Creat (mg/dl)	.74 ± .20	.80 ± .19	.83 ± .23	0.088
Creat clearance (ml/min)	120.94 ± 33.11	116.76 ± 31.33	113.68 ± 30.77	0.663
Baseline HCV RNA by PCR (IU/ml)	949,173.30 ± 1195,220.29	1,051,988.49 ± 1,824,411.25	2,473,014.05 ± 6631,407.20	0.256
TSH (μIU/ml)	1.92 ± 1.46	1.97 ± 2.05	1.67 ± 1.20	0.518
Alpha fetoprotien (IU/l)	15.66 ± 22.75	28.92 ± 29.11 *	21.00 ± 30.15	0.001

Table 3 Platelet decrement during treatment

Platelet count decrements	All studied patients		Group 1 Triple		Group 2 SOF/RBV		Group 3 SIM/SOF	
	No.	%	No.	%	No.	%	No.	%
2 Weeks								
Decrease	128	76.2%	50	89.3%	34	61.8%	44	77.2%
No decrease	40	23.8%	6	10.7%	21	38.2%	13	22.8%
4 Weeks								
Decrease	120	71.4%	46	82.1%	26	47.3%	48	84.2%
No decrease	48	28.6%	10	17.9%	29	52.7%	9	15.8%
End of treatment								
Decrease	91	54.8%	41	73.2%	16	29.1%	34	61.8%
No decrease	75	45.2%	15	26.8%	39	70.9%	21	38.2%

Least decrement% was observed in SOF/RBV

There was no statistically significant correlation between the child score calculation, ultrasonographic findings, the degree of fibrosis and necroinflammatory activity with the platelet count decrement through the course of the triple antiviral therapy, SOF/RBV and SIM/SOF antiviral therapy groups (data not shown).

The drop in PCR was significantly correlated with the improvement of platelet count ($p < 0.05$) in SOF/RBV arm in the second and fourth weeks as illustrated in Fig. 2.

During treatment, five patients (8.9%) in the INF treatment group and one patient (1.8%) in the SOF/RBV group required dose modification. None of the patients in the SIM/SOF group required dose modification. The reported response rate is 100% in the triple therapy group, 98.2% in the SOF/RBV group and 96.4% in the SIM/SOF group.

Discussion

Thrombocytopenia is frequent among patients with chronic hepatitis C virus and cirrhosis and is further aggravated by the IFN-based antiviral therapy. The development of DAA has significantly improved tolerability of treatment and cure rates. In Egypt, with the approval of sofosbuvir (SOF), different SOF-based therapies became the standard of care. We performed a retrospective study to compare the incidence of thrombocytopenia during treatment with three of the DAA regimens available for HCV treatment in Egypt. We found more noticeable lowering of mean platelet count in the 2nd week and 4th week of treatment followed by the rise of platelet count again in all the studied groups. Patients on triple therapy (group 1) showed earlier drop of platelet count (1st week) and did not return to baseline till the end of treatment.

Table 4 Mean platelet count in diffrent weeks of treatment

Platelet count ($\times10^3$ cell/mm^3)	All patients mean ± SD, mean PLT, % drop to baseline	Group 1 Triple (*n* 56), mean PLT, % drop to baseline	Group 2 SOF/RBV (*n* 55) mean PLT, % drop to baseline	Group 3 SIM/SOF (*n* 57) mean PLT, % drop to baseline	*p* value (among three groups)
Baseline PLT	108.85 ± 39.74	136.89 ± 31.70	77.18 ± 18.01	111.84 ± 40.35	< 0.001
Week 1	89.72 ± 27.93 18%	86.89 ± 23.62 37%	75.89 ± 14.09 3%	105.84 ± 33.56 6%	< 0.001
Week 2	90.87 ± 33.90 17%	99.50 ± 36.89 28%	72.58 ± 12.30 7%	100.04 ± 38.18 10%	< 0.001
Week 3	87.65 ± 25.17 20%	96.05 ± 28.4 30%	76.07 ± 13.23 2%	90.58 ± 26.68 19%	< 0.001
Week 4	88.46 ± 32.08 19%	101.71 ± 44.1 26%	77.55 ± 14.26 0%	85.98 ± 25.69 24%	< 0.001
Week 8	94.98 ± 37.93 13%	97.05 ± 39.27 29%	87.73 ± 30.95	99.93 ± 42.08 11%	0.312
Week 12	99.46 ± 41.84 9%	102.86 ± 46.37 25%	90.16 ± 30.62	105.31 ± 45.67 6%	0.17

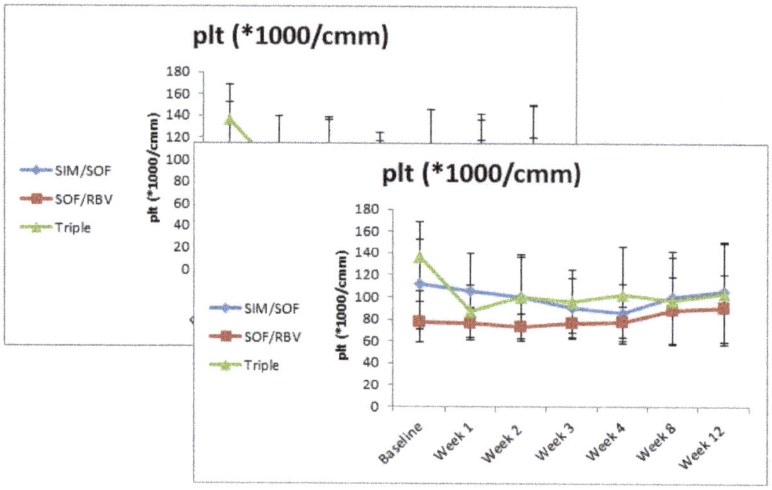

Fig. 1 Changes in mean platelet count during therapy

On the evaluation of the overall number of patients with platelet count decrement, we found that most of the enrolled patients (76.2%, 71.4%) demonstrated platelet count decrement in the 2nd and 4th weeks with mean platelet counts of $87.65 \pm 25.17 \times 10^3/\mu l$ and $88.46 \pm 32.08 \times 10^3/\mu l$, respectively, which improved towards the end of treatment: 54.8% of patients demonstrated platelet decrement with a mean platelet count of 99.46 ± 41.84.

In comparing the 3 therapeutic groups, the triple therapy group showed the highest proportion of patients with platelet decrement. While the SOF/RBV group showed the lowest mean platelet count at the 2nd week, 4th week and end of treatment. This could be explained by the lower pre-treatment platelet count in the SOF/RBV group in comparison with the other groups and the presence of more unfavourable features as higher proportion of patients with splenomegaly and those who

Table 5 Correlation between duration of illness and PLT count and between FIB-4 and PLT count in the three treatment groups

Subgroup	Parameter		Platelet count decrement		
			Week 2	Week 4	EOT
Group 1 Triple	Duration of illness	Correlation coefficient	.076	.117	.109
		p value	.578	.391	.424
		N	56		
Group 2 SOF/RBV		Correlation coefficient	.063	.071	− .125
		p value	.649	.608	.364
		N	55		
Group 3 SIM/SOF		Correlation coefficient	.129	.022	− .004
		p value	.338	.871	.974
		N	57	57	55
Group 1 Triple	FIB-4 calculation	Correlation coefficient	− .267	− .213	− .110
		p value	.047	.114	.418
		N	56		
Group 2 SOF/RBV		Correlation coefficient	-.486	− .463	− .105
		p value	< 0.001	< 0.001	.445
		N	55		
Group 3 SIM/SOF		Correlation coefficient	− .243	− .494	− .151
		p value	.069	< 0.001	.270
		N	57	57	55

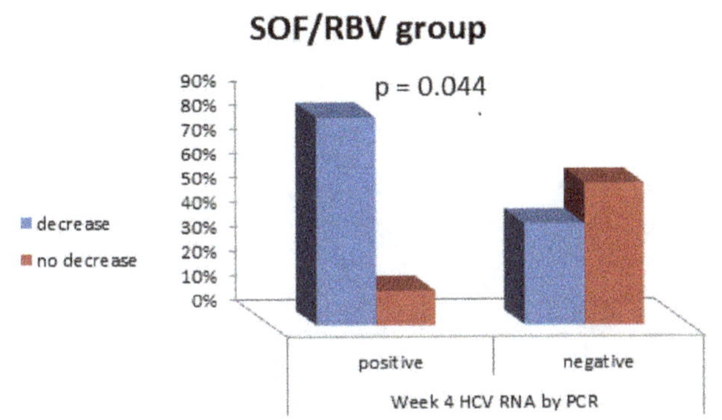

Fig. 2 Comparison between change in the platelet count in week 4 and HCV RNA by PCR

received previous treatment. It is worth mentioning that the percentage of patients affected by this significant thrombocytopenia was lower in this group compared with the other two groups in all stages of assessment.

In a large study involving 125 patients with chronic hepatitis C and baseline thrombocytopenia who received antiviral therapy with peg-IFN-a and ribavirin, it was found that platelet count was less than 100,000 before onset of treatment, and rapid early drop of platelet count on treatment are predictors of high risk of developing on-treatment severe thrombocytopenia [8, 9].

But both studies were done on peg-INF/RBV, and this arm in our study had baseline platelet count of more than 100,000/l unlike the other two arms, but still the rule of 100,000/μl could be applicable.

We compared response to therapy in the 3 subgroups of antiviral therapy and noticed that rapid virological response was in the triple antiviral therapy group, but this was not statistically significant to the other arms as well as associated with more cases that required dose modification due to thrombocytopenia in this arm. Five of six patients who required dose modification were noticed in the triple antiviral therapy group and no dose modification was needed for the SIM/SOF group.

All the three arms were associated with SVR above 95% at week 12 with no statistical difference in between. There are data that support better SVR on SOF/REB [7, 10]. Others proved less efficacy for SOF/REB vs other different combinations of DAAs or even IFN-based therapies [11–13].

On studying the demographic data of the patients, we found that the lower the baseline weight of the patients, the more the development of thrombocytopenia during SOF/RBV therapy. However, BMI did not show significant correlation in our study. This is not in agreement with Lin et al., who found that low body mass index ($p = 0.022$) was significantly correlated with the development of thrombocytopenia but they used the INF/Rib combination [8].

In our study, we found that the lower the baseline albumin of the patients, the more the development of thrombocytopenia during triple therapy. This is in agreement with Lin et al., who also found that low albumin was significantly correlated with the development of thrombocytopenia [8]. This was not applicable for the other two arms. The interpretation may be because this arm has more thrombocytopenia with lower hepatic synthetic functions from the start. But this confirms that poorer baseline liver function is a predictor of thrombocytopenia during antiviral therapy.

It was found that cirrhosis was associated with thrombocytopenia during antiviral therapy which did not show significant correlation in our study [9].

We found that the lower baseline absolute neutrophil count was not associated with significant decrement in platelet count. On the contrary, Nachnani et al., reported that lower white blood cell count was associated with thrombocytopenia during antiviral therapy [14]. The reason could be that the interferon arm patients were chosen with good CBC from the start and that the other two drug combinations have less side effects on CBC. Larger studies on patients with chronic hepatitis C and thrombocytopenia should be conducted for further studying of the suggested predicting factors and follow-up for platelet counts after end of antiviral therapy is very important with the DAAs. We also found that by the end of treatment (EOT), all patients had normalized platelet (PLT) count regardless of the initial count.

Conclusion

The recent change in direct-acting antiviral therapy (DAA) without IFN, as the frontline therapy for HCV, permits to avoid the dilemmas associated with initiating or maintaining IFN-based antiviral therapy. DAAs, with high SVR and few haematological adverse effects, have been shown to improve thrombocytopenia associated with HCV infection as well as advanced hepatic disease. The second and fourth weeks of antiviral therapy show most decrement of platelet count.

Antiviral therapy in general does not induce sever thrombocytopenia.

Triple therapy (INF/SOF/RBV) induced more thrombocytopenia rather than SOF/RBV.

Acknowledgements
We are thankful to all the patients who participated in this work.

Authors' contributions
All authors participated in the manuscript revision. SGh collected the references and prepared the data from patients' files. NH wrote the manuscript and revised the statistics. DD and MT put the research idea. AH, HD, and AF revised the data. MR revised the paper and participated in response to reviewers' comments. The authors read and approved the final manuscript.

Competing interests

The authors declare that they have no competing interests.

Author details

[1]Internal Medicine Department, Faculty of Medicine, Cairo University, Cairo, Egypt. [2]Armed Forces Faculty of Medicine (AFCM), Cairo, Egypt. [3]National Hepatology and Tropical Institute, Cairo, Egypt. [4]Internal Medicine Department, Faculty of Medicine, Beni Suef University, Beni Suef, Egypt.

References

1. Abd Elrazek AE, Bilasy SE, Elbanna AE, Elsherif AE (2014) Prior to the oral therapy, what do we know about HCV-4 in Egypt: a randomized survey of prevalence and risks using data mining computed analysis. Medicine (Baltimore) 93(28):e204
2. Fried M, Shiffman M, Reddy K et al (2002) Peginterferon alfa-2a plus ribavirin for chronic hepatitis C virus infection. N Engl J Med 347:975–982
3. McHutchison J, Manns M, Patel K et al (2002) Adherence to combination therapy enhances sustained response in genotype-1–infected patients with chronic hepatitis C. Gastroenterology 123:1061–1069
4. Shiffman M, Ghany M, Morgan T et al (2007) Impact of reducing peginterferon alfa-2a and ribavirin dose during retreatment in patients with chronic hepatitis C. Gastroenterology 132:103–112
5. Martínez S, Crespo G, Navasa M et al (2011) Noninvasive assessment of liver fibrosis. Hepatology 53:325–335
6. Cholongitas E, Papatheodoridis G, Vangeli M et al (2005) Systematic review: The model for end-stage liver disease--should it replace Child-Pugh's classification for assessing prognosis in cirrhosis? Aliment Pharmacol Ther 22:1079–1089
7. Seo K, Kim SK, Kim SR et al (2017) Comparison of Sofosbuvir Plus Ribavirin Treatment with Pegylated Interferon Plus Ribavirin Treatment for Chronic Hepatitis C Genotype 2. Dig Dis 35:541–547
8. Lin K, Ping I-H, Hsien-Chung Y et al (2012) Factors linked to severe thrombocytopenia during antiviral therapy in patients with chronic hepatitis c and pretreatment low platelet counts. BMC Gastroenterol 12:7–14
9. Roomer R, Hansen B, Janssen H et al (2010) Thrombocytopenia and the risk of bleeding during treatment with peginterferon alfa and ribavirin for chronic hepatitis C. J Hepatol 53:455–459
10. Nagaty A, Abd El-Wahab EW (2017) Real-life results of sofosbuvir based therapy in chronic hepatitis C -naïve and -experienced patients in Egypt. PLoS One 12(10):e0184654
11. Aisha Elsharkawy, Maissa El-Raziky, Wafaa El-Akel, Kadry El-Saeed, Rasha Eletreby, Mohamed Hassany, Manal Hamdy El-Sayed, Khaled Kabil, Sohier A Ismail, Magdy El-Serafy, Ashraf Omar Abdelaziz, Mohamed Kamal Shaker, Ayman Yosry, Wahid Doss, Yehia El-Shazly, Gamal Esmat, Imam Waked. Planning and Prioritizing Direct-Acting Antivirals Treatment for HCV Patients in Countries With Limited Resources: Lessons From the Egyptian Experience. J Hepatol. 2018;68(4):691-698. doi: https://doi.org/10.1016/j.jhep.2017.11.034. Epub 2017 Dec 6.
12. Elsharkawy A, Fouad R, El Akel W, El Raziky M, Hassany M, Shiha G, Said M, Motawea I, El Demerdash T, Seif S, et al. Sofosbuvir-based treatment regimens: real life results of 14 409 chronic HCV genotype 4 patients in Egypt. Aliment Pharmacol Ther. 2017;45:681–687. [PubMed] [Google Scholar]
13. El Kassas M, Alboraie M, Omran D, Salaheldin M, Wifi MN, ElBadry M, El Tahan A, Ezzat S, Moaz E, Farid AM, et al. An account of the real-life hepatitis C management in a single specialized viral hepatitis treatment centre in Egypt: results of treating 7042 patients with 7 different direct acting antiviral regimens. Expert Rev Gastroenterol Hepatol. 2018 Epub ahead of print. [PubMed] [Google Scholar]
14. Nachnani J, Rao G, Bulchandani D et al (2010) Predictors of hematological abnormalities in patients with chronic hepatitis C treated with interferon and ribavirin. Ann Hematol 89:121–125

27

Ascitic calprotectin as a useful marker in the diagnosis of spontaneous bacterial peritonitis in adults

Eman M Abdel Rahman[1], Fatma A Attia[1], Ayman Alsebaey[2*], Mohammad Abdel Khalik Elkady[3], Maha Mohammed Sayed[4], Alaa Reda Awad[5] and Eman Ahmed El-Seidi[5]

Abstract

Background: Ascitic fluid polymorphonuclear leucocyte count (PMN) is known to be the gold standard for spontaneous bacterial peritonitis (SBP) diagnosis. The aim of this work was to assess ascitic calprotectin for SBP diagnosis. Serum C-reactive protein (CRP), high sensitivity C-reactive protein (hsCRP), nitrous oxide, ascitic PMN, ascitic leucocyte esterase and ascitic calprotectin were measured.

Results: The average age of our patients was 55.25 ± 7.89 years, mostly males (n = 51, 63.8%), anti-HCV antibodies were positive in (n = 61, 76.3%). Sixty-four patients (80%) were Child-Pugh C and their average MELD was 24.29 ± 8.06. Patients with SBP had statistically significant higher median MELD score (26.5 vs. 19) and higher average Child-Pugh score (12.18 ± 1.74 vs. 10.5 ± 1.97). Forty patients had SBP and 40 patients were without SBP. Both the serum and ascitic nitrous oxide did not differ statistically between patients with and without SBP. In contrast, patients with SBP had higher median serum CRP (49 vs. 12 mg/dL), hsCRP (58,000 vs. 23,750 ng/dL) and ascitic calprotectin (7.57 vs. 1.1 ng/mL). The ascitic leucocyte esterase test was positive in 95% of SBP patients in contrast to 2.5% patients without SBP. Ascitic calprotectin >2 ng/mL had 90% sensitivity, 92.5% specificity, 92.3% positive predictive value and 90.2% negative predictive value. MELD, CRP, hsCRP and ascitic calprotectin are independent predictors of SBP.

Conclusion: Ascitic calprotectin is a useful marker for SBP diagnosis.

Keywords: Ascites, Calprotectin, hsCRP, Spontaneous bacterial peritonitis

Background

Spontaneous bacterial peritonitis (SBP) is an infection of the ascitic fluid in patients with liver cirrhosis and portal hypertension [1]. There is no obvious surgical cause as perforation or intraabdominal inflammatory focus as abscess. Up to 30% of the ascitic patients will develop SBP [2].

SBP is attributed to immune dysfunction, bacterial translocation, circulatory dysfunction and inflammatory status. SBP is diagnosed by ascitic fluid analysis [3]. SBP was defined as polymorphonuclear leucocyte count (PMN) >250/mm^3 in ascitic fluid [2, 4]. Not all cases are associated with positive ascitic fluid cultures.

There are variants of ascitic fluid infections as culture-negative neutrocytic ascites, monomicrobial non-neutrocytic bacterascites, polymicrobial bacterascites and secondary bacterial peritonitis [5].

The advent of the SBP carries a poor prognosis where the hospital mortality ranged from 10 to 50%. As a consequence, any patient with SBP should be assessed for liver transplantation. Immediate treatment with antibiotics and IV albumin should be initiated [4].

Studies were conducted on alternatives of the ascitic PMN count as high sensitivity C-reactive protein (hsCRP) [6], serum procalcitonin [7], urinary lipocalin [8], ascitic lactoferrin [9], homocysteine [10] and fecal or ascitic calprotectin [11, 12].

This study aimed to assess ascitic calprotectin as a diagnostic marker of SBP.

* Correspondence: aymanalsebaey@liver.menofia.edu.eg
[2]Department of Hepatology and Gastroenterology, National Liver Institute, Menoufia University, Shebeen El-Kom 32511, Egypt

Methods

Patients were recruited from the outpatient clinics of the Internal Medicine Department, Faculty of Medicine for Girls, El Azher University, Department of Hepatology and Gastroenterology, National Liver Institute, Menoufia University and Theodor Bilharz Research Institute, Cairo Egypt. The study was approved by the institutional review board of Faculty of Medicine for Girls, El Azhar University.

This study enrolled 80 patients out of 300 patients with decompensated liver cirrhosis with ascites who were referred for paracentesis, evaluation of abdominal pain or exclusion of ascitic fluid infection in patients with hepatic encephalopathy or gastrointestinal bleeding. Liver cirrhosis was diagnosed according to the characteristic clinical, laboratory, radiological findings that are supported by previous liver biopsy if available and not contraindicated [13].

History taking, full clinical examination, liver function tests, serum creatinine, CBC, INR, serum hsCRP, nitrous oxide, abdominal ultrasonography and ascitic fluid analysis were done on admission.

The ascitic fluid analysis parameters were PMN count, calprotectin, nitrous oxide, total protein, albumin, LDH and glucose and was tested also with leukocyte esterase dipsticks. In the case of SBP diagnosis, inoculation of bedside 10 mL of ascitic fluid into a blood culture bottle was done [2, 4]. Patients with SBP [8] underwent immediate treatment with 3rd generation cephalosporin and follow up ascitic fluid PMN 48 h after the start of treatment [4].

Sampling and methodology

Five mL blood was withdrawn by venipuncture, one ml in EDTA tube for CBC and four ml were allowed to clot. The non-hemolyzed sera were separated by centrifugation and used for determination of creatinine, uric acid, CRP, (hsCRP), nitric oxide level and liver functions (ALT, AST, total bilirubin and albumin).

The ascitic fluid sample was taken by paracentesis performed under aseptic conditions from a puncture site in the left or right lower quadrant with the patient in the supine position. All samples were immediately collected at the bedside and processed by laboratory personnel without further delay.

Immediately after the paracentesis, the ascitic fluid was tested by the use of reagent strips for the leukocyte esterase designed for rapid urine screening (Mission Expert Urinalysis Reagent Strips, Acon Laboratories, Inc, USA). Fresh ascitic fluid was collected in a clean container and the strip was immediately immersed in the ascitic fluid. We compared closely the test areas with the color chart on the bottle label after 120 s according to the manufacturer instructions. The strips have a colorimetric 4-grade scale.

Blood glucose, liver profile, and creatinine concentrations were measured on a Dimension Xpand plus chemistry analyzer (Roche Diagnostics, Basel, Switzerland) using commercially available reagents and an enzyme-based kit. Complete blood picture was measured using CELL-DYN Emerald cell counter (ABBOTT, Germany). CRP and hsCRP were measured using BIOS microwell ELISA Diagnostic Systems Kit, South San Francisco. Ascitic fluid nitric oxide level was measured using Griess Reagent Nitrite Measurement Kit, Cell Signaling Technology, USA. Ascitic fluid calprotectin was measured by using Human Calprotectin (CALPRO) ELISA kit, Assay Kit Co, USA

Statistical analysis

Data were statistically analyzed using IBM® SPSS® Statistics® version 21 for Windows (IBM Corporation, North Castle Drive, Armonk, New York, USA) and MedCalc® version 18.2.1 (Seoul, Republic of Korea). Data are expressed as mean ± standard deviation for normally distributed data, median (interquartile range) for data that lacks normal distribution and number (percentage) for nominal data. Comparisons between two groups were performed using the Student's *t* test for parametric data and Mann-Whitney test for non-parametric data. CHI-squared test ($\chi 2$) and Fisher exact test for categorical data analysis. Univariate and multivariate binary logistic regression was done for detecting the independent predictors of SBP. The receiver operating characteristic (ROC) curve analysis was used for the detection of the cutoff value of the calprotectin in the diagnosis of SBP.

Results

This study enrolled 80 patients with ascites that were divided into 2 equal groups; with and without SBP.

The average age of our patients was 55.25 ± 7.89 years, mostly males (n = 51, 63.8%), anti-HCV antibodies were positive in 76.3% of the patients. Sixty-four patients (80%) were Child-Pugh C and their average MELD was 24.29 ± 8.06.

Both groups had comparable age, sex, viral etiology of liver disease, serum AST, serum ALT, creatinine and blood hemoglobin (Table 1).

Patients with SBP had statistically significant higher median total bilirubin (4.2 vs. 2.3 mg/dL), WBCs (9800 vs. 4150 μL), INR (3.4 vs. 1.9), MELD score (26.5 vs. 19), and average CTP score (12.18 ± 1.74 vs. 10.5 ± 1.97). Both serum albumin and platelets were statistically lower in patients with SBP.

Both the serum and ascitic nitrous oxide did not differ statistically between patient with and without SBP. In contrast, patients with SBP had higher median serum

Table 1 Comparison of patients with and without SBP

	None $n = 40$	SBP $n = 40$	P	
Age (years)	54.75 ± 8.19	55.75 ± 7.64	0.574	NS
Males	25 (62.5%)	26 (65%)	0.816	NS
Females	15 (37.5%)	14 (35%)		
HCV	30 (75%)	31 (77.5%)	0.793	NS
HBV	10 (25%)	9 (22.5%)		
CTP B	12 (30%)	4 (10%)	0.025	S
CTP C	28 (70%)	36 (90%)		
Total bilirubin (mg/dL)	2.3 (1.28)	4.2 (4.9)	0.001	S
Albumin (mg/dL)	2.25 (1.1)	1.8 (0.8)	0.006	S
AST (U/L)	77.50 (28)	73 (17.25)	0.083	NS
ALT (U/L)	46.00 (26.25)	43 (21.25)	0.146	NS
Hemoglobin (g/dL)	10.10 ± 1.71	10.11 ± 1.14	0.969	NS
WBCs (μL)	4150 (5475)	9800 (4375)	0.001	S
Platelets (μL)	89,000 (22,250)	82,500 (32,750)	0.008	S
INR	1.9 (0.7)	3.4 (1.45)	0.001	S
Creatinine (mg/dL)	1.1 (0.85)	1.65 (1.4)	0.274	NS
CTP	10.5 ± 1.97	12.18 ± 1.74	0.001	S
MELD	19 (8)	26.5 (11)	0.001	S
Ascitic PMN	65 (76.75)	657.5 (652)	0.001	S
Ascitic total protein	0.41 (0.85)	0.8 (0.75)	0.004	S
Ascitic albumin	0.11 (0.35)	0.22 (0.38)	0.025	S
Ascitic glucose	126 (110)	125.5 (116.75)	0.769	NS
Ascitic LDH	20.65 (26.65)	101 (198.25)	0.001	S
Serum NO (μM)	15.5 (8.78)	17 (12.2)	0.357	NS
Ascitic NO (μM)	5.6 (6.4)	6.2 (4.5)	0.739	NS
Serum CRP (mg/dL)	12 (11.5)	49 (66.25)	0.001	S
Serum hsCRP (ng/dL)	23,750 (52,200)	58,000 (0)	0.001	S
Ascitic calprotectin (ng/mL)	1.1 (0.6)	7.57 (6.76)	0.001	S
Ascitic leucocyte esterase +ve	1 (2.5%)	38 (95%)	0.001	S

CTP Child-Pugh, *CRP* C-reactive protein, *hsCRP* High sensitivity C-reactive protein, *LDH* Lactate dehydrogenase, *MELD* Model for End-Stage Liver Disease, *NS* Non-statistically significant, *NO* Nitrous oxide, *S* Statistically significant, *PMN* Polymorphonuclear leucocyte count
Data are expressed as mean ± standard deviation for normally distributed data, median (interquartile range) for data that lacks normal distribution and number (percentage) for nominal data.

CRP (49 vs. 12 mg/dL), hsCRP (58,000 vs. 23,750 ng/dL) and ascitic calprotectin (7.57 vs. 1.1 ng/mL). The ascitic leucocyte esterase test was positive in 95% of SBP patients in contrast to 2.5% patients without SBP.

As shown in Table 2 and Fig. 1, ascitic calprotectin >2 ng/mL had 90% sensitivity, 92.5% specificity, 92.3% positive predictive value and 90.2% negative predictive value (AUC 0.963, 95% C.I 0.895–0.992, $P = 0.001$).

By univariate analysis, the independent predictors of SBP (Table 3) were MELD (odds = 1.2), serum CRP (odds = 1.1), serum hsCRP (odds = 1) and ascitic calprotectin (odds = 7.4). On multivariate analysis, only ascitic

Table 2 The receiver operating characteristic (ROC) curve analysis of ascitic calprotectin

	PCT
AUC	0.963
P	0.001
95% C.I	0.895–0.992
Cutoff	>2
Sensitivity	90%
Specificity	92.5%
PPV	92.3%
NPV	90.2%

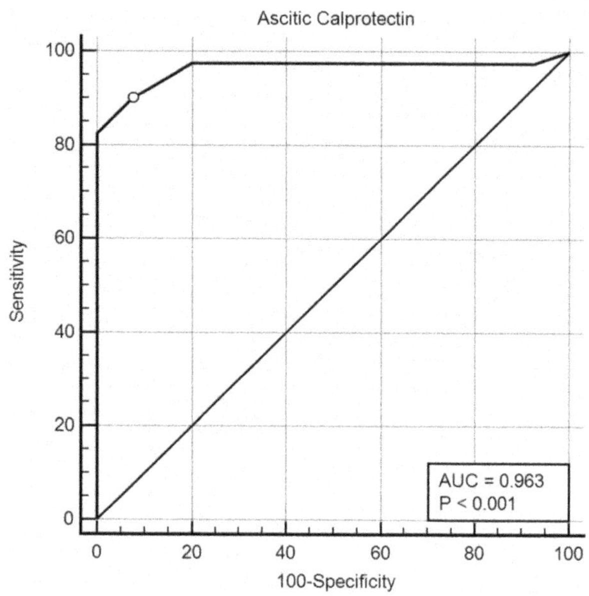

Fig. 1 The receiver operating characteristic (ROC) curve analysis of ascitic calprotectin

calprotectin (odds = 13.1) was the independent predictor of SBP.

Discussion

The gold standard test for SBP is ascitic fluid analysis with measurement of the PMN. It is useful for the diagnosis and monitoring of treatment. The culture of the ascitic fluid may be positive if was done correctly [4].

There is a variant of SBP that is called culture-negative neutrocytic ascites. It is characterized by elevated ascitic fluid PMN but the culture is negative. It is managed exactly as classic SBP. Such cases would be missed if cultures were not done [5].

The manual PMN counting is time consuming, laborious and required some experience to avoid intra- and inter-observer variability. So, a simple rapid bedside test would be useful clinically [14].

Calprotectin is acute-phase inflammatory protein that is released from the PMN. Calprotectin has anti-proliferative and antimicrobial properties [14]. Calprotectin is used clinically widespread in the diagnosis and monitoring treatment of inflammatory bowel disease [15].

In an earlier study [11], patients with liver cirrhosis had higher fecal calprotectin compared with the control. Fecal calprotectin correlated with hepatic encephalopathy grade and SBP.

Later on, studies were conducted on ascitic calprotectin [12, 14, 16–18]. Ascitic calprotectin could be measured by either enzyme-linked immunosorbent assay (ELISA) or a point-of-care (POC) lateral flow assay with the Quantum Blue® Reader [16].

Burri et al. [16] reported that patients with SBP had statistically higher values of ascitic calprotectin that was measured by two techniques namely ELISA and POC. A cutoff value (0.63 μg/mL) measured by ELISA had 94.8% sensitivity, 89.2% specificity, 60% PPV and 99% NPV. A cutoff value (0.51 μg/mL) measured by PCO had 100% sensitivity, 84.7% specificity, 100% PPV and 87.7% NPV. Both techniques were useful with excellent correlation.

Two studies assessed the ratio of ascitic calprotectin to ascitic total protein. One study [17] found that ratio was useful for SBP diagnosis unlike the other one [12].

Fernandes et al. [12] studied 88 patients of whom 41 had SBP. They were mainly males and alcoholics. Higher ascitic calprotectin was found. A cutoff value (1.57 μg/mL) measured by POC had 87.8% sensitivity, 97.9% specificity, 97.3% PPV and 90.2% NPV.

In the study conducted by Abdel-Razik et al. [18], patients with SBP had higher calprotectin, serum procalcitonin, serum and ascites TNF-α, IL-6. A cutoff value of 94 ng/mL had 94.3% sensitivity, 91.8% specificity, 93% PPV and 95% NPV.

In a recent French study [14], a 1.51 μg/mL cutoff measured by POC had 86.1% sensitivity, 92% specificity, 65.9% PPV and 97.3% NPV.

CRP is acute-phase protein that elevates in many inflammatory conditions. The hsCRP measures the low levels of CRP. The hsCRP has a higher sensitivity than CRP. Patients with SBP show elevated CRP levels that decrease with treatment [12, 14, 19]. Only one study by Guler et al. [6] assessed the role of serum hsCRP in non-neutrocytic ascites. They found that hsCRP was higher in patients with SBP and non-neutrocytic ascites

Table 3 Independent predictors of SBP

	Univariate analysis			Multivariate analysis		
	Odds	*P*	95% C.I.	Odds	*P*	95% C.I.
Age	1.0	0.569	0.961–1.075	0.9	0.285	0.701–1.110
MELD	1.2	0.001	1.103–1.319	1.1	0.438	0.843–1.486
Ascitic calprotectin	7.4	0.001	2.420–22.855	13.1	0.009	1.886–90.405
Serum CRP	1.1	0.001	1.038–1.105	1.1	0.101	0.986–1.171
Serum hsCRP	1.0	0.001	1.000–1.000	1.0	0.979	1.000–1.000

MELD Model for End-Stage Liver Disease, *CRP* C-reactive protein, *hsCRP* High sensitivity C-reactive protein

compared with the control. The levels decreased with antibiotic therapy. Leukocyte esterase is an enzyme produced by PMN in response to inflammation. It can be detected by leucocyte esterase reagent strips.

In the current study, the measurement of serum or ascitic nitrous oxide did not add a benefit in SBP diagnosis. Patients with SBP had higher serum CRP level, which is consistent with the other studies [12, 14, 19]. Furthermore, serum hsCRP was higher in SBP patients in accord with Guler et al. [6] study. Most patients had positive ascitic leucocyte esterase test (95%) in contrast few patients in the control group.

Calprotectin was significantly higher in SBP patients. Calprotectin >2 ng/mL had 90% sensitivity, 92.5% specificity, 92.3% positive predictive value and 90.2% negative predictive value. The cutoff is completely different from other studies [11, 14, 16, 18] even measured by ELISA but the sensitivity and specificity are high as reported by other studies [11, 14, 16, 18]. In fact, the methodology of measurement should be standardized in the next studies.

Limitations of the study

The number of patients is small, we did not follow the treatment measuring calprotectin and so the recurrence.

Conclusion

Ascitic calprotectin is a useful marker for spontaneous bacterial peritonitis diagnosis.

Abbreviations

CRP: C-reactive protein; CTP: Child-Pugh; hsCRP: High sensitivity C-reactive protein; LDH: Lactate dehydrogenase; MELD: Model for End-Stage Liver Disease; NO: Nitrous oxide; PMN: Polymorphonuclear leucocyte count; ROC: Receiver operating characteristic curve; SBP: Spontaneous bacterial peritonitis

Acknowledgements

None

Authors' contributions

MMS, MAE and AY contributed to data collection. EMA, AA, FAA and EAE contributed to study design. AA and EMA contributed to manuscript writing and final revision. All authors have read and approved the manuscript.

Competing interests

The authors declare that they have no competing interests.

Author details

[1]Department of Internal Medicine, Faculty of Medicine for Girls, El Azhar University, Cairo, Egypt. [2]Department of Hepatology and Gastroenterology, National Liver Institute, Menoufia University, Shebeen El-Kom 32511, Egypt. [3]Department of Hepatology and Gastroenterology, Theodor Bilharz Research Institute, Cairo, Egypt. [4]Department of Internal Medicine, Faculty of Medicine, Assiut University, Asyut, Egypt. [5]Department of Medical Microbiology and Immunology, Faculty of Medicine, Cairo University, Cairo, Egypt.

References

1. Mohamed A, Atef M, Alsebaey A, Musa Elhabshy M, Salama M (2017) Combined spontaneous bacterial empyema and peritonitis in cirrhotic patients with ascites and hepatic hydrothorax, Arab. J Gastroenterol 18(2): 104–107
2. Xiol X, Castellvi JM, Guardiola J, Sese E, Castellote J, Perello A, Cervantes X, Iborra MJ (1996) Spontaneous bacterial empyema in cirrhotic patients: a prospective study. Hepatology 23(4):719–723
3. Bernardi M (2010) Spontaneous bacterial peritonitis: from pathophysiology to prevention. Intern Emerg Med 5(Suppl 1):S37–S44
4. European Association for the Study of the Liver (2010) EASL clinical practice guidelines on the management of ascites, spontaneous bacterial peritonitis, and hepatorenal syndrome in cirrhosis. J Hepatol 53(3):397–417
5. Marciano S, Diaz JM, Dirchwolf M, Gadano A (2019) Spontaneous bacterial peritonitis in patients with cirrhosis: incidence, outcomes, and treatment strategies. Hepat Med 11:13–22
6. Guler K, Vatansever S, Kayacan SM, Salmayenli N, Akkaya V, Erk O, Palanduz A (2009) High sensitivity C-reactive protein in spontaneous bacterial peritonitis with nonneutrocytic ascites. Hepatogastroenterology 56(90):452–455
7. Wu H, Chen L, Sun Y, Meng C, Hou W (2016) The role of serum procalcitonin and C-reactive protein levels in predicting spontaneous bacterial peritonitis in patients with advanced liver cirrhosis. Pak J Med Sci 32(6):1484–1488
8. Fouad TR, Abdelsameea E, Elsabaawy M, Ashraf Eljaky M, Zaki El-Shenawy S, Omar N (2019) Urinary neutrophil gelatinase-associated lipocalin for diagnosis of spontaneous bacterial peritonitis. Trop Doct 49475519830265
9. Parsi MA, Saadeh SN, Zein NN, Davis GL, Lopez R, Boone J, Lepe MR, Guo L, Ashfaq M, Klintmalm G, McCullough AJ (2008) Ascitic fluid lactoferrin for diagnosis of spontaneous bacterial peritonitis. Gastroenterology 135(3):803–807
10. Abdel-Razik A, Eldars W, Elhelaly R, Eldeeb AA, Abdelsalam M, El-Wakeel N, Aboulmagd A (2018) Homocysteine: a new diagnostic marker in spontaneous bacterial peritonitis. Eur J Gastroenterol Hepatol 30(7):779–785
11. Gundling F, Schmidtler F, Hapfelmeier A, Schulte B, Schmidt T, Pehl C, Schepp W, Seidl H (2011) Fecal calprotectin is a useful screening parameter for hepatic encephalopathy and spontaneous bacterial peritonitis in cirrhosis. Liver Int 31(9):1406–1415
12. Fernandes SR, Santos P, Fatela N, Baldaia C, Tato Marinho R, Proença H, Ramalho F, Velosa J (2016) Ascitic calprotectin is a novel and accurate marker for spontaneous bacterial peritonitis. J Clin Lab Anal 30(6):1139–1145
13. Schuppan D, Afdhal NH (2008) Liver cirrhosis. Lancet 371(9615):838–851
14. Weil D, Heurgue-Berlot A, Monnet E, Chassagne S, Cervoni J-P, Feron T, Grandvallet C, Muel E, Bronowicki J-P, Thiefin G, Di Martino V, Bardonnet K, Thévenot T (2019) Accuracy of calprotectin using the Quantum Blue Reader for the diagnosis of spontaneous bacterial peritonitis in liver cirrhosis. Hepatol Res 49(1):72–81
15. Reenaers C, Bossuyt P, Hindryckx P, Vanpoucke H, Cremer A, Baert F (2018) Expert opinion for use of faecal calprotectin in diagnosis and monitoring of inflammatory bowel disease in daily clinical practice. United European Gastroenterol J 6(8):1117–1125
16. Burri E, Schulte F, Muser J, Meier R, Beglinger C (2013) Measurement of calprotectin in ascitic fluid to identify elevated polymorphonuclear cell count. World J Gastroenterol 19(13):2028–2036
17. Lutz P, Pfarr K, Nischalke HD, Kramer B, Goeser F, Glassner A, Wolter F, Kokordelis P, Nattermann J, Sauerbruch T, Hoerauf A, Strassburg CP, Spengler U (2015) The ratio of calprotectin to total protein as a diagnostic and prognostic marker for spontaneous bacterial peritonitis in patients with liver cirrhosis and ascites. Clin Chem Lab Med 53(12):2031–2039
18. Abdel-Razik A, Mousa N, Elhammady D, Elhelaly R, Elzehery R, Elbaz S, Eissa M, El-Wakeel N, Eldars W (2016) Ascitic fluid calprotectin and serum procalcitonin as accurate diagnostic markers for spontaneous bacterial peritonitis. Gut Liver 10(4):624–631
19. Metwally K, Fouad T, Assem M, Abdelsameea E, Yousery M (2018) Predictors of spontaneous bacterial peritonitis in patients with cirrhotic ascites. J Clin Transl Hepatol 6(4):372–376

28

Multiple biliary hamartomas "von Meyenberg complexes" in a newborn: a unique observation

Moaied A. Hassan

Abstract

Background: Biliary hamartomas are rare benign bile duct malformations consisting of multiple collections of localized duct-like structures that are lined by biliary epithelium and embedded in a fibrous stroma. In general, these malformations are asymptomatic and are usually detected incidentally during imaging, surgical exploration, or autopsy. Previously, the definitive diagnosis of these lesions was possible only with liver biopsy. The use of advanced imaging modalities made it possible to establish the diagnosis when undoubtful imaging findings are evident.

Case presentation: We present a 25-day-old male newborn who was referred to our institution with jaundice, abdominal distension, and abdominal U/S that revealed hepatomegaly and involvement of both lobes of the liver with diffuse cystic lesions of variable sizes and echogenicity without a diagnostic suggestion. We discuss the details of imaging findings that enabled to establish the diagnosis of multiple biliary hamartomas and brief the patient's status on follow-up.

Conclusion: Up to our best knowledge, the diagnosis of multiple biliary hamartomas has not been previously reported among newborns, making this report an extremely rare if not a unique observation.

Keywords: Biliary hamartomas, Liver, von Meyenburg complexes, Newborn

Background

Biliary hamartomas are rare benign bile duct malformations consisting of multiple collections of localized duct-like structures that are lined by biliary epithelium and embedded in a fibrous stroma [1]. Hanns von Meyenburg, a Swiss pathologist, was the first to describe these lesions in 1918, and because of that are referred to as von Meyenberg complexes [2]. Interrupted remodeling of the ductal plates during late embryonic development of the intrahepatic bile ducts is thought to be responsible for the development of these malformations [3]. The incidence of biliary hamartomas is very low and has been estimated at 0.69–5.6% in autopsy series, and 0.6% in needle biopsy series [4]. In general, these malformations are asymptomatic and are usually detected incidentally during imaging, surgical exploration, or autopsy [5]. The clinical significance of biliary hamartomas lies in their propensity to be easily confused with liver metastasis, Caroli's disease, microabscesses, and other cystic hepatic lesions, along with their possible malignant transformation into cholangiocarcinoma [1]. Previously, the definitive diagnosis of these lesions was possible only with liver biopsy. The use of advanced imaging modalities made it possible to establish the diagnosis when undoubtful imaging findings are evident [1]. Herein, we present the extremely rare and possibly unique occurrence of diffuse multiple biliary hamartomas in a 25-day-old newborn.

Correspondence: moaied70@yahoo.com
Pediatric Surgery Department, Basrah Children's Specialty Hospital, Basrah, Iraq

Case presentation

A 25-day-old male newborn was referred to our institution with jaundice, abdominal distension, and abdominal U/S that revealed hepatomegaly and involvement of both lobes of the liver with diffuse cystic lesions of variable sizes and echogenicity without a diagnostic suggestion (Fig. 1). Blood counts and morphology tests were within normal limits apart from hypochromic microcytic anemia. The liver function test revealed indirect hyperbilirubinemia [102 mmol/L], with elevated serum alkaline phosphatase [761 U/L] and serum glutamic-oxaloacetic transaminase [72 U/L] levels, hypoproteinemia [47 G/L], and hypoalbuminemia [24 G/L]. TORCH screen was negative, prothrombin, and partial thromboplastin times, and blood urea and serum creatinine levels were all within normal limits.

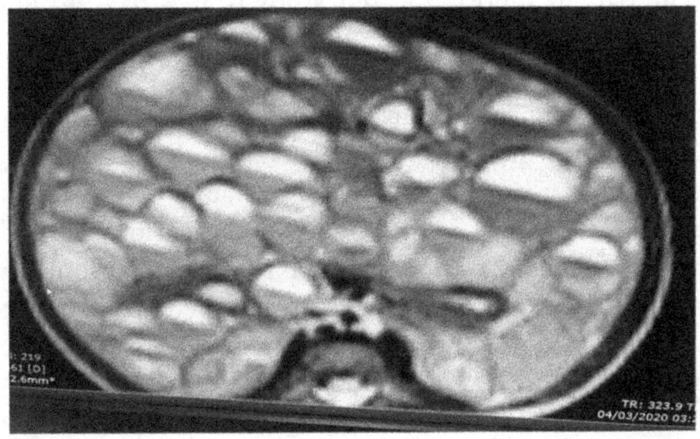

Fig. 2 Abdominal CT reveals innumerable non-enhancing cystic lesions involving both lobes of the liver

Abdominal CT revealed the presence of diffuse, innumerable, non-communicating, and non-enhancing cystic lesions involving both lobes of the liver, with the largest cyst measuring 22 × 22 mm at the left lobe segment II, with the diagnosis of multiple biliary hamartomas (Fig. 2). Abdominal MRI revealed markedly enlarged liver [liver spam=140 mm], with the liver parenchyma being replaced by non-communicating, cystic lesions of variable sizes, hyperintense at T2-weighted images giving the characteristic starry sky appearance of multiple biliary hamartomas (Fig. 3). The possibility of Caroli's disease has been excluded as these cysts shown only marginal enhancement with no significant internal enhancement.

The baby's anemia and hypoalbuminemia were corrected with blood and albumin transfusion, respectively. His general condition and vital signs were satisfactory. The family was instructed that their baby suffers an extremely rare developmental malformation of the bile ducts that mandates close clinical and imaging follow-up with special concern on the function of the liver and that surgical excision is not an option as the whole liver is replaced by these lesions considering liver transplantation in the future. So far, the baby has been followed-up closely for 4 months. The baby is now jaundice-free, liver function test is within normal limits, imaging studies reveal no significant changes, and he suffers no significant medical problems.

Discussion

Biliary hamartomas are rare benign bile duct malformations consisting of focal collections of dilated intrahepatic bile ducts embedded within a dense collagenous stroma. These lesions are usually small (< 5 mm in diameter), typically multiple and scattered throughout both lobes of the liver. Some may aggregate to appear as large solitary lesions on imaging studies [5].

Biliary hamartomas are generally asymptomatic, although abdominal enlargement, jaundice, and portal hypertension may arise as a result of mass effect [6, 7]. Being small-sized and asymptomatic, these lesions are usually detected incidentally during imaging, surgical exploration, or autopsy.

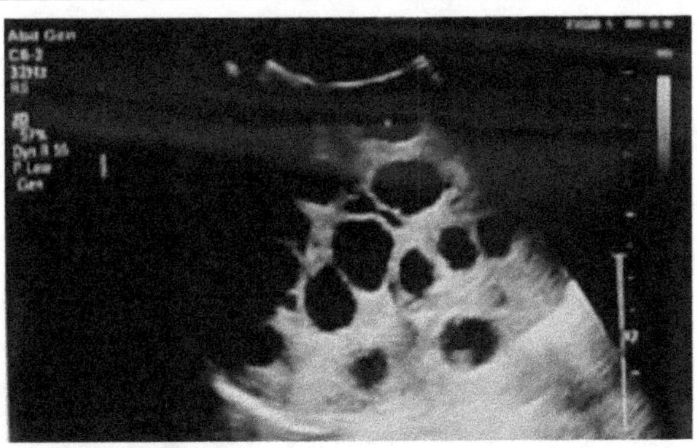

Fig. 1 Abdominal U/S reveals diffuse involvement of the liver with hypoechoic cystic lesions of variable sizes

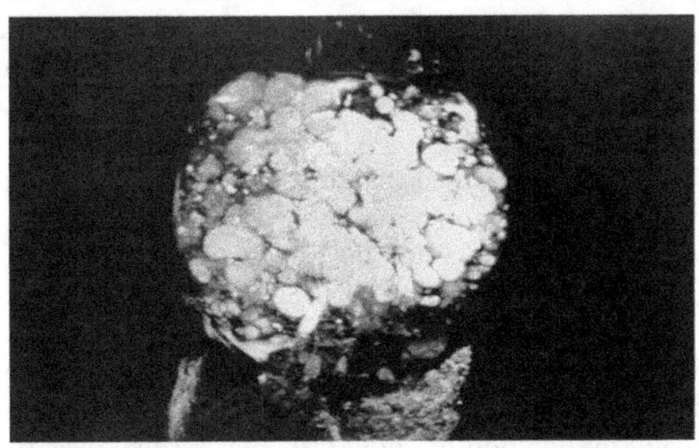

Fig. 3 Abdominal MRI reveals hyperintense cystic lesions replacing the liver parenchyma "Starry sky appearance"

The patient reported in this study is a 25-day-old newborn, and "up to our best knowledge," the diagnosis of multiple biliary hamartomas has not been previously reported among newborns, making this report an extremely rare if not a unique observation. Makhneva et al. described multiple biliary hamartomas in a 3-year-old child [7]. Jaundice and abdominal distension were the alarming sings in the reported newborn patient that brought the attention of the attending pediatrician to request an abdominal ultrasound which revealed the presence of multiple cystic lesions in the liver.

Technical advances in imaging modalities have made the detection of these malformations easy. Biliary hamartomas show characteristic features on imaging studies, and accurate diagnosis can be established when typical undoubtful features are evident obviating the need for a liver biopsy which should be performed only to confirm the diagnosis when in doubt [5, 8].

On sonography, biliary hamartomas have been described to appear as innumerable small hypoechoic or hyperechoic lesions measuring less than 10 mm and uniformly distributed throughout the liver, and may have a comet tail artifact. Variability in echogenicity reflects differences in the size of the dilated bile duct components, which, at a certain size, will show echogenicity as they behave like other microcystic structures, and below it, their complex internal structure might reflect poor echogenicity [3].

On contrast-enhanced CT, the majority of the reported cases of biliary hamartomas did not show contrast enhancement. This observation might reflect the poor vascularity of these lesions described on histology [4, 6].

On MRI, biliary hamartomas have been described to appear as hypointense lesions on T1-weighted images. On T2-weighted images, they appear hyperintense when compared with surrounding liver parenchyma giving the characteristic starry sky appearance [4, 9].

The imaging findings of the patient presented in this report were consistent with those reported in the literature; hence, the diagnosis was confirmed radiologically without the need to perform liver biopsy taking into consideration the necessity of long-term clinical and imaging follow-up.

The baby presented in this study was exclusively breastfed, and this may represent the best available explanation for the elevated liver enzymes in the presence of indirect hyperbilirubinemia. Several studies have reported elevated liver enzymes in breastfed babies with indirect hyperbilirubinemia and suggested that those findings might be the result of mild and transient hepatic dysfunction or cholestasis that resolve over time [10, 11]. Resolution of jaundice and returning of liver enzymes to their normal levels in the presented patient who is still having his pathology in place, the fact that the majority of multiple biliary hamartomas are asymptomatic along with the unavailability of previous studies that report similar pathology in newborns makes us support this explanation. Further studies and observations may provide better insight for this finding in the future.

The clinical significance of biliary hamartomas lies in their propensity to be easily confused with liver metastasis, Caroli's disease, microabscesses, and other cystic hepatic lesions, along with their possible malignant transformation into cholangiocarcinoma. The patient reported in this study is a newborn; besides, the lesions did not show enhancement on CT after the administration of IV contrast which excluded the possibility of dealing with a case of liver secondaries. Caroli's disease was excluded as the lesions did not show the "central dot" sign of central enhancement on MRI. A close and long-term clinical and imaging follow-up is required, with the possibility of performing liver biopsy when indicated to exclude other possible pathologies.

Conclusion

Biliary hamartomas are rare benign bile duct malformations resulting from the interrupted remodeling of the ductal plates during the late embryonic development of the intrahepatic bile ducts. We report the diagnosis of these rare malformations in a newborn baby, and up to our best knowledge, the diagnosis of multiple biliary hamartomas has not been previously reported among newborns, making this report an extremely rare if not a unique observation.

Acknowledgements
Not applicable.

Author's contributions
The author(s) read and approved the final manuscript.

Competing interests
The author declares that he has no competing interests.

References

1. Teng SL, Shin JS, Huang JC (2015) An unusual polynodular liver disease: multiple biliary hamartoma. Advances in Digestive Medicine 2(1):37–40
2. Singh Y, Cawich SO, Ramjit C, Naraynsingh V (2016) Rare liver tumor: symptomatic giant von Meyenburg complex. Journal of Surgical Case Reports 11:1–4
3. Markhardt BK, Rubens DJ, Huang J, Dogra VS (2006) Sonographic features of biliary hamartomas with histopathologic correlation. J Ultrasound Med 25: 1631–1633
4. Zheng RQ, Zhang B, Kudo M, Onda H, Inoue T (2005) Imaging findings of biliary hamartomas. World J Gastroenterol 11:6354–6359
5. Jáquez-Quintana JO, Reyes-Cabello EA, Bosques-Padilla FJ (2017) Multiple biliary hamartomas, the "von Meyenburg complexes". Ann Hepatol 16(5): 812–813
6. Barboi OB, Moisii LG, Albu-Soda A, Ciortescu I (2013) Drug V: biliary hamartoma. Clujul Med 86:383–384
7. Makhneva A, Aigul B, Minira B, Gauhar A (2015) Child's von Meyenburg complexes. J Histol Histopathol 2:15

8. Liu S, Zhao B, Ma J, Li J, Li X (2014) Lesions of biliary hamartoms can be diagnosed by ultrasonography, computed tomography and magnetic resonance imaging. Int J Clin Exp Med 7(10):3370–3377
9. Taguchi T, Kohsaki T (2020) "Starry sky" appearance from multiple biliary hamartomas. N Engl J Med 382(16):e33
10. Wu T-Z, Huang I-F, Chen Y-C, Chen P-H, Yang L-Y (2011) Differences in serum biochemistry between breast-fed and formula-fed infants. J Chin Med Assoc 74:511–515
11. Tazawa Y, Abukawa D, Watabe M et al (1991) Abnormal results of biochemical liver function tests in breast-fed infants with prolonged indirect hyperbilirubinaemia. Eur J Pediatr 150:310–313

29

Gallstones in Egyptian infants and children: risk factors, complications and outcome: a single center experience

A. Enayet*, R. A. Afifi, E. A. Mogahed, M. S. El-Raziky and M. A. K. Abdellatif

Abstract

Background: The widespread use of abdominal ultrasonography in children documented increased detection rate of gallstones. The aim of this study was to assess the possible risk factors of gallstones and to detect the complication rate and outcome of the disease in Egyptian infants and children from a hepatologist perspective. This prospective study included 35 cases, with ultrasound-detected gallstones, who presented to the Pediatric Hepatology Unit from July 2015 to October 2017. All patients were initially evaluated by full history, general and abdominal examination, laboratory assessment, and ultrasound findings to detect possible risk factors of gallstones. Management approach was individualized for each patient according to his/her condition, and the patients were followed up at 3 months interval.

Results: The patients' ages ranged from 3.5 months up to 17 years. The median age of gallstone detection was 2 years. Gallstones were symptomatic in 62.9% with abdominal pain in 51.4%. Complications in the form of choledocholithiasis were detected in 7 patients (20%). Laparoscopic cholecystectomy was done for 7 patients while conservative management was applied for 24 patients. Complete resolution occurred in 8.3% and partial resolution in 33.3%. Chronic hemolytic anemia was the most commonly identified risk factor for gallstones. Patients needed surgical intervention had significant higher serum cholesterol and LDL levels ($P = 0.006$ and $P = 0.002$ respectively).

Conclusion: Risk factors for gallstones could be identified in most of pediatric cases. Symptomatic presentation is common among the pediatric population. Conservative management is recommended for asymptomatic cases of gallstones in children. Laparoscopic cholecystectomy is a safe and recommended procedure for complicated and symptomatic cases of gallstones.

Keywords: Children, Complications, Gallstones, Infants, Outcome

Background

The prevalence of gallstones in the pediatric population has been reported to be uncommon with estimated overall prevalence of 0.13 to 1.9%. However, the increased use of abdominal ultrasonography (US) in recent years has led to increased rate of detection of gallstones [1].

Many etiological factors have been associated with gallstones in children. Chronic hemolytic diseases are considered the most common cause. Other risk factors include liver cirrhosis, chronic cholestasis, total parenteral nutrition, and ileal diseases such as ileal resection, ileal Crohn's disease, cystic fibrosis, prolonged use of high-dose ceftriaxone, cancer therapy, family history, obesity, and congenital anomalies in the GB [2].

Little information is available about the management of this disorder in childhood as diagnostic approach, and therapeutic strategies are extremely heterogeneous. For symptomatic cases, cholecystectomy is curative, and laparoscopic cholecystectomy has been proven to be safe and efficient [3]. Asymptomatic patients show a more difficult management dilemma. Considering the low rate

* Correspondence: afaf_enayet@hotmail.com
Department of Pediatrics, Kasr Alainy Medical School, Faculty of Medicine, Cairo University, Cairo, Egypt

of complications detected by many studies, expectant management with periodical clinical and US follow-up is recommended. Spontaneous resolution of gallstones was observed in many cases [4]. Elective cholecystectomy is recommended for children with chronic hemolytic anemia at the time of gallstone diagnosis, before symptoms, or complications develop [5].

The aim of this study was to assess the possible risk factors of gallstones and to detect the complication rate and outcome of the disease in infants and children.

Methods

This prospective study was conducted at the Pediatric Hepatology Unit during the time period from July 2015 to October 2017. All cases below 18 years of age of both sexes with US detected gallstones were enrolled in this study. The study was approved by the institutional ethical committee of the Pediatrics Department. A written informed consent was taken from patients' guardians.

Patient evaluation

Initial diagnosis

All patients were evaluated in terms of age, sex, presenting symptoms (typical biliary colic, nonspecific abdominal pain, nausea, vomiting or fatty food intolerance, and symptoms of complications as fever or jaundice), precipitating risk factor for gallstone, and other accompanying diseases.

Laboratory assessment

Complete blood count (CBC) and liver function tests, hemolytic profile (reticulocytes, osmotic fragility, quantitative glucose 6 phosphate dehydrogenase (G6PD) measurement, hemoglobin electrophoresis, direct coombs test), lipid profile (serum cholesterol (LDL-HDL-VLDL) and serum triglycerides), and sweat chloride test if cystic fibrosis was suspected (multisystem presentations: pulmonary, gastrointestinal, and others as dehydration and metabolic alkalosis), and serum amylase and lipase if pancreatitis is suspected.

Radiological assessment

Abdominal US, endoscopic retrograde cholangiopancreatography (ERCP) in cases of choledocholithiasis, magnetic resonance cholangiopancreatography (MRCP) is done when choledocholithiasis is suspected, and ERCP cannot be done for technical consideration as young age (age less than 2 years) and in cases with US documented CBD dilatation.

Management approach

Conservative management

For asymptomatic patients with no complications, it involved periodic clinical and US follow up at 3-month intervals for at least 1 year.

Medical dissolution of gallstones by Ursodeoxycholic Acid (UDCA)

A trial of oral UDCA dissolution of stones was applied at a dose of 15 mg/kg/day for those patients with symptomatic uncomplicated gallstones with periodic clinical and ultrasound follow-up for symptoms' improvement and/or stone dissolution every 3 months. Symptomatic uncomplicated gallstones were defined as the presence of biliary colic in the form of significant abdominal pain in the absence of complications as acute or chronic cholecystitis, ascending cholangitis, common bile duct stones, or pancreatitis.

ERCP

ERCP is for patients with choledocholithiasis.

Laparoscopic cholecystectomy (LC) is for (1) patients with complicated gallstones as cases with choledocholithiasis, cholecystitis, or pancreatitis, (2) patients with symptomatic gallstones not improving on UDCA, and (3) patients with chronic hemolytic anemia.

Patient follow-up

Patients who were not indicated for surgery were followed every 3 months with clinical, laboratory and ultrasound assessments. Resolution of gallstones was based on ultrasonographic evidence of absence of gallbladder and bile duct stones.

Statistical analysis

Data was analyzed by the Statistical Package of Social Science Software program, version 23. Data was presented using mean, standard deviation (SD) for homogenous quantitative variables, median and interquartile range (IQR) for quantitative variables with non-homogenous distribution, and frequency and percentage for qualitative ones. Comparison between groups was performed using Mann-Whitney test for quantitative variables and chi-square and Fisher's exact test for qualitative ones. P values less than 0.05 were considered statistically significant.

Results

Thirty-five children with gallstones were included; 54.3% were males. Their age ranged from 3.5 months to 17 years. Out of these 35 patients, 18 patients (51.4%) were below 2 years of age at the time of discovery of gallstones (infantile group), while 17 (48.6%) had their discovery onset beyond 2 years.

They were referred to hepatology clinic because of accidently detected gallstones in US done for other purposes in 25 cases (71.4%), jaundice in 7 (20%), and elevated liver enzymes in 3 (8.6%). Patients with US detected gallstones were referred from everywhere including general outpatient clinics as well as hematology and neonatology units. US was repeated in hepatology clinic for confirmation and for detailed sonographic examination. Twenty-two (62.9%) patients had symptomatic gallstones: abdominal pain as the most common presentation (51.4%), jaundice (28.6%), vomiting, nausea, and fatty food intolerance in 25.7%, 11.4%, and 14.3% respectively. Eight patients (22.9%) showed elevated total bilirubin; all with elevated direct fraction except one who had β-thalassemia major, in whom indirect bilirubin was elevated. The seven patients with direct hyperbilirubinemia included 6 patients with choledocholithiasis, and one patient had cholestasis with normal GGT.

Lipid profile showed abnormal results in 7 cases. Three patients (8.6%) had hypercholesterolemia, and 4 patients had elevated triglycerides level.

Abdominal US done by 2 operators revealed single gallstones in 17 cases (48.6%) and multiple gallstones in 18 cases (51.4%). Size of stones ranged from 0.3 to 1.6 cm with median 0.6 cm with IQR (0.4–0.8). Biliary sludge with gallstones was evident in 9 cases (25.7%) while common bile duct (CBD) stones were detected in 6 cases (17.1%); 5 (14.3%) of them showed CBD and biliary radicles dilatation.

Possible etiology could be reached in 25 patients where hemolytic anemia was the most common identified diagnosis (Fig. 1). History of dehydration and neonatal intensive care admission were more prevalent among the infantile group but with no statistical significance. Duration of NICU admission was significantly longer among patients with multiple stones ($P = 0.044$) compared to those with single stone.

The management plan was individualized for each patient (Fig. 2). For cases with complicated gallstones in the form of choledocholithiasis, cholecystectomy was performed while conservative management was planned for the other 28 cases (80%). The medical treatment was offered to non-hemolytic cases with patent cystic, and common bile duct with stone size was less than 2 cm. LC was offered for patients with hemolytic anemia, before symptoms or complications developed, but unfortunately, it was not performed except in complicated cases.

LC was done for 7 patients (20%): 6 of them had choledocholithiasis while one of the patients with choledocholithiasis dropped out of the study. A patient was indicated for LC because of attacks of agonizing abdominal pain after 3 months of conservative management with no improvement (Fig. 2).

For the 7 patients with choledocholithiasis, MRCP was done for 5 patients, and ERCP was done for 2 patients. For the 2 patients who have done ERCP, one patient was 9 years old, and ERCP showed mild dilated intrahepatic

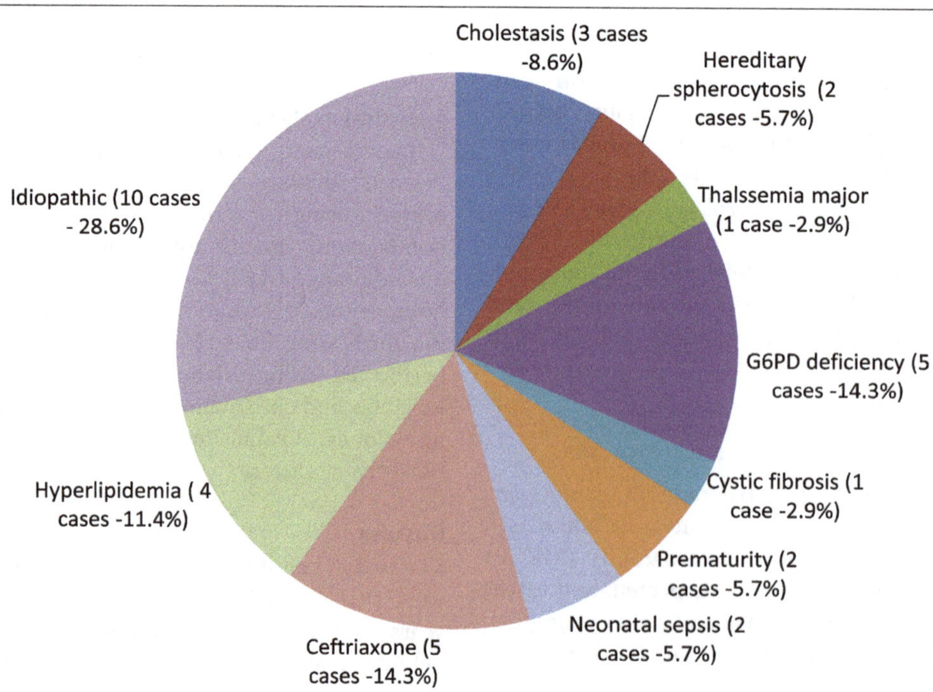

Fig. 1 Possible etiology of gallstones in the study patients

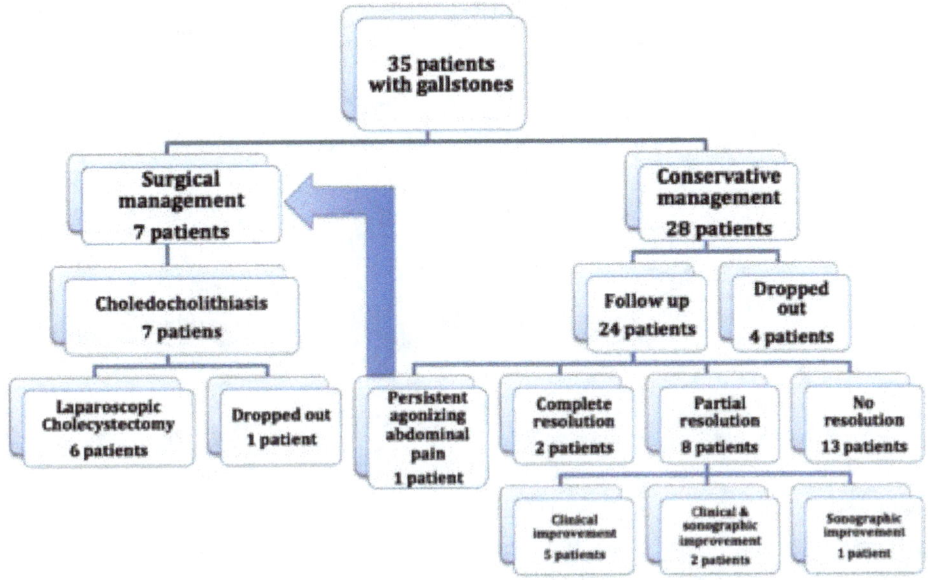

Fig. 2 The management plan of the 35 children with gallstones

biliary radicles (IHBR) and CBD, sphincterotomy with dormia basket was done, and multiple gravels were removed. The other patient was 5 years old; ERCP revealed normal CBD and IHBR with multiple stones, sphincterotomy was done, and stones were removed. Regarding the other 5 patients, one patient was dropped out, while the other 4 patients had spontaneous relief of obstructive jaundice. LC was then performed for the 6 cases. Histopathological analysis of the removed gall bladder in this study was available in 6 cases and revealed chronic cholecystitis in all of them (100%): none had papillomatosis or adenoma of the gall bladder.

For the 28 patients (80%) who were subjected to conservative management, 3 patients dropped out of follow-up, and one (an infant with cerebral palsy) died 1 month after enrollment due to septicemia. The other 24 patients were followed up for 8 to 34 months with a median of 14 months.

Twelve patients (34.3%) with symptomatic gallstones were managed conservatively with UDCA for a period ranging from 3 to 24 months and a median of 4.5 months. Follow-up showed complete resolution of gallstones in 2 patients (8.3%). One of them was a 3-year-old boy with congenital adrenal hyperplasia who showed decrease in number of stones from 2 stones to a single stone after 6 months of therapy; however, this patient showed spontaneous resolution of this remaining gallstone after another 6 months without UDCA administration. Five patients (20.8%) showed partial improvement, evident with disappearance of symptoms; one patient (4.2%) showed partial sonographic improvement while 2 patients (8.3%) showed partial clinical and sonographic improvement (Fig. 2). Sonographic improvement was based on decreased number of stones and/or disappearance of biliary sludge.

Based on their management strategy, patients were classified into two groups: medical and surgical. Those who needed LC were significantly older at the onset of stones (P = 0.005). In addition, their serum cholesterol and LDL levels were significantly higher than those who subjected to medical management (Table 1).

Patients were also divided based on symptomatology at the time of initial diagnosis into two groups: symptomatic and asymptomatic. G6PD deficiency was significantly higher in the asymptomatic group. Symptomatic cases had significant lower RBC count, hemoglobin, and hematocrit than asymptomatic cases (Table 2).

Discussion

Pediatric cholelithiasis is known to be uncommon. However, recent series documented increased detection rate of gallstones in the pediatric age group [1]. Many risk factors have been described for the development of gallstones in children as hemolytic disorders, prematurity, parenteral nutrition, chronic hepatobiliary diseases, cystic fibrosis, genetic factors, sepsis, ileal diseases, obesity, ceftriaxone use, and abdominal or cardiac surgeries [6]. Idiopathic gallstones, with no identifiable risk factors, have been reported in the literature in the range of 23.2–52.5% [2, 7, 8]. This is close to the current study where no risk factors were identified in 28.6%of cases.

Twenty to 40% of all pediatric gallstone disease can be attributed to hemolytic diseases [9]. Recent studies demonstrated hemolytic diseases in 21.6% and in 11.8% of

Table 1 Risk factors of gallstones and laboratory investigations among medical and surgical patients

	Surgical, *n* = 7 (%)	Medical, *n* = 23 (%)	*P* value
Identified risk factors	5 (71.4)	19 (82.6)	0.6
Hemolytic anemia			
Hereditary spherocytosis	1 (14.3)	1 (4.3)	0.4
Major thalassemia	0 (0)	1 (4.3)	1.0
G6PD deficiency	2 (28.6)	7 (30.4)	1.0
Dehydration	1 (14.3)	5 (21.7)	1.0
Therapy with ceftriaxone	2 (28.6)	4 (17.4)	0.6
Family history of gallstones	1 (14.3)	4 (17.4)	1.0
Hypertriglyceridemia	1 (14.3)	3 (16.7)	1.0
Cholestasis	0(0)	2 (8.7)	1.0
Prematurity	0 (0)	2 (8.7)	1.0
Cystic fibrosis	0 (0)	1(4.3)	1.0
Hemoglobin (g/dl) in mean ± SD	11.5 ± 0.95	11.7 ± 1.2	0.8
T. bilirubin (*N* < 1.5 mg/dl) median (IQR)	2.3 (1.1–5.1)	0.4 (0.2–0.8)	0.002*
D. bilirubin in median (IQR)	1.1 (0.5–3)	0.1 (0.05–0.2)	0.01*
ALT (*N* < 40 U/L) in median (IQR)	92 (32–178)	29 (20–45)	0.006*
AST (*N* < 60 U/L) in median (IQR)	55 (36–125)	37 (30–66)	0.1
GGT (*N* < 30 U/L) in median (IQR)	105 (36–114)	17 (11–64)	0.09
AP (*N* < 640 U/L) in median (IQR)	252 (180–533)	260 (192–371)	1.0
INR (*N* < 1.1) in mean ± SD	1.04 ± 0.04	1.1 ± 0.12	0.4
Cholesterol (*N* < 200 mg/dl) in mean ± SD	180 ± 47	134 ± 31	0.006*
HDL (mg/dl) in mean ± SD	38 ± 12	43 ± 9.5	0.3
LDL (mg/dl) in mean ± SD	120 ± 44	68 ± 29	0.002*
Triglyceride (*N* < 150 mg/dl) in median (IQR)	92 (62–115)	88 (62–119)	0.9

*P value is significant

ALT alanine aminotransferase, *AP* alkaline phosphatase, *AST* aspartate aminotransferase, *D* direct, *GGT* gammaglutamyl transpeptidase, *G6PD* Glucose-6-phosphate dehydrogenase, *HDL* high-density lipoproteins, *INR* international randomized ratio, *IQR* interquartile range, *LDL* low-density lipoproteins, *RBCs* red blood cells, *SD* standard deviation, *T* total

cases [10, 11]. In the current study, hemolytic anemia was identified as a risk factor in 34.3%. G6PD deficiency was identified as a risk factor in 9 cases (25.7%); this high percentage may be explained by the high prevalence of G6PD deficiency in Egypt as reported by Abo Elella et al. in 2017 who estimated an overall prevalence of G6PD deficiency of 4.3% among Egyptian neonates [12].

Therapy with ceftriaxone was identified as a risk factor in 17.1% of cases, in agreement with literature where ceftriaxone use was responsible for 6% and 27.3% of cases of gallstones [2, 13].

Chronic biliary disease in the form of cholestasis was present in 8.6% of our cases, which is close to the results of Dooki and Norouzi (2013) and Della Corte et al (2008) studies (7.5% and 5% respectively) [2, 13]. It is known that patients with chronic cholestasis especially those with progressive familial intrahepatic cholestasis (PFIC) are prone to cholelithiasis. This is attributed to impaired bile acid secretory function and supersaturation of bile with cholesterol [14]. The three cholestatic patients in this study had normal GGT cholestasis; however, the unavailable genetic analysis in Egypt limited the ability to finally diagnose their specific conditions. These patients might have had PFIC 1 or 2.

Unlike adults, children are likely to be symptomatic [8]. Our cases showed symptomatic presentation in 62.9%, which is comparable to other studies [2, 9, 10]. On the other hand, the study of Kirsaclioglu et al. [11] showed that symptomatic patients were significantly older than asymptomatic patients, and abdominal pain was the most frequent symptom [11]. Our cases also showed abdominal pain to be the most common symptom in 51.4%.

Complications were documented in 20% of our cases, which is close to the literature, where they were reported in about 7–20% of cases [6]. While some older studies reported pancreatitis as the most common complication [15, 16], recent studies reported cholecystitis and choledocholithiasis to be more common [1, 11, 17]. Our study showed choledocholithiasis to be more common; meanwhile, none of our

Table 2 Risk factors of gallstones and complications in symptomatic and asymptomatic patients

	Symptomatic, *n* = 22 (%)	Asymptomatic, *n* = 13 (%)	*P* value
Identified risk factors	14 (63.6)	13 (100)	0.01*
Hemolytic anemia			
Chronic hemolytic anemia	3 (13.6)	0 (0)	0.274
Glucose-6-phosphate dehydrogenase deficiency	3 (13.6)	6 (46.2)	0.050
Dehydration	6 (27.3)	2 (15.4)	0.680
Therapy with ceftriaxone	5 (22.7)	1 (7.7)	0.377
Family history of gallstones	2 (9.1)	4 (30.8)	0.166
Hypertriglyceridemia	1 (4.5)	3 (23.1)	0.134
Cholestasis	1 (4.5)	2 (15.4)	0.541
Prematurity	0 (0)	2 (15.4)	0.131
Cystic fibrosis	1 (4.5)	0 (0)	0.435
Choledocholithiasis	7 (31.8)	0 (0)	0.015*
RBCs (10^5 cells/mm^3) in mean ± SD	4.4 ± 0.5	5 ± 1	0.047*
Hemoglobin (g/dl) in mean ± SD	11.2 ± 1.4	12.3 ± 0.8	0.006*
Hematocrit (%) in mean ± SD	33.8 ± 3.4	37.5 ± 3.4	0.008*
T. bilirubin (N < 1.5 mg/dl) median (IQR)	0.7 (0.4–2.6)	0.3 (0.2–0.8)	0.021
ALT (N < 40 U/L) in median (IQR)	38 (27–92)	26 (17–40)	0.108
AST (N < 60 U/L) in median (IQR)	47.5 (36–75)	34 (32–71)	0.484
GGT (N < 30 U/L) in median (IQR)	37.5 (12–114)	16 (8–28)	0.147
AP (N < 640 U/L) in median (IQR)	247 (190–375)	260 (192–371)	0.905
Albumin (N > 3.5 g/dl) in mean ± SD	4.2 ± 0.8	3.9 ± 0.4	0.136
INR (N < 1.1) in mean ± SD	1.1 ± 0.1	1.1 ± 0.1	0.972

**P* value is significant

ALT alanine aminotransferase, *AP* alkaline phosphatase, *AST* aspartate aminotransferase, *GGT* gammaglutamyl transpeptidase, *INR* international randomized ratio, *IQR* interquartile range, *RBCs* red blood cells, *SD* standard deviation, *T* total

cases showed pancreatitis or acute cholecystitis. The relatively high complication rate seen in our study group could be explained by the nature of our hospital being a tertiary referral hospital. Severe and complicated cases are commonly referred to our institution, while uncomplicated cases can be managed conservatively in secondary referral centers.

In children, cholecystectomy is recommended for symptomatic and complicated gallstones. It is also recommended for asymptomatic gallstones with chronic hemolytic anemia and asymptomatic large sized gallstones (> 2 cm) for the risk of gallbladder carcinoma [4]. Otherwise, expectant management with periodic clinical and sonographic assessment appears more appropriate [4]. LC was done for 7 of our patients: 6 of them because of choledocholithiasis and one for symptomatic gallstone with agonizing typical right upper quadrant pain. Hajong et al. in 2013 reported 15 non-hemolytic cases of gallstones managed by LC; 80% were symptomatic, and 13.3% were asymptomatic while 6.7% had complicated gallstone in the form of pancreatitis [18]. Another study showed that primary indications for surgery in pediatric population were symptomatic cholelithiasis (53%), choledocholithiasis (28%), and biliary dyskinesia (16%) [9].

Histopathological analysis of the removed gall bladder (GB) in this study was available in 6 cases and revealed chronic cholecystitis in all of them (100%); none had papillomatosis or adenoma of GB. This is comparable to the results of Kim et al. study, who showed that, in 24 cases for whom cholecystectomy was performed, histopathology of most cases revealed chronic cholecystitis [19]. On the other side, the removed gallbladders in Della Corte et al. study revealed chronic cholecystitis in 84.6%, papillomatosis in 5.1%, adenoma in 2.6%, and normal GB in 7.7% [2].

Eighty percent of our cases were managed conservatively, with periodic clinical, laboratory and US follow-up for 8 to 34 months. None of them developed complications, while 2 cases showed complete spontaneous resolution of gallstones, and 8 cases showed resolution of symptoms and/or sonographic improvement. This may justify the conservative management for uncomplicated cases of gallstones in pediatric population, especially in infants. Jeanty et al., who performed their study on infantile cholelithiasis, observed complete resolution of stones in 25% of the cases [20], while Gokce et al. [21] reported spontaneous complete resolution in 50%

of infantile cases and 19.8% in older children [1]. This was higher than the resolution rate observed in the current study.

Limitations of this study include the small sample size and the short duration of follow-up in some patients. Moreover, as the study was conducted in a tertiary care unit, many uncomplicated cases may be diagnosed and managed in other centers without referral to our unit, which may explain the higher rate of complications at presentation of our cases.

The strength of this study is that it is the first study to evaluate gallstones among infants and children in Egypt. The absence of a national screening program for G6PD deficiency and other hemolytic anemias, together with high incidence of consanguineous marriages, raises the risk of childhood gallstones in Egypt.

Conclusion

Risk factors for gallstones could be identified in most of pediatric cases. Symptomatic presentation is common among the pediatric population. Conservative management is supported for asymptomatic cases. Laparoscopic cholecystectomy is a safe and recommended procedure for complicated and symptomatic cases.

Abbreviations

ALT: Alanine aminotransferase; AST: Aspartate aminotransferase; CBC: Complete blood count; CBD: Common bile duct; PFIC: Progressive familial intrahepatic cholestasis; PT: Prothrombin time; SD: Standard deviation; IHBR: Intrahepatic biliary radicles; INR: International normalized ratio; IQR: Interquartile range; LC: Laparoscopic cholecystectomy; LDL: Low-density lipoprotein cholesterol; PT: Prothrombin time; SD: Standard deviation; UDCA: Ursodeoxycholic acid; US: Ultrasonography

Acknowledgements

Not applicable

Authors' contributions

EM was responsible for constructing the research hypothesis and planning the methodology. EA was responsible for patients' inclusion and follow-up. ME collected and tabulated the data. AR was responsible for interpretation and presentation of the results. AM and EM wrote the manuscript. ME and EA revised the manuscript. All authors read and approved the final manuscript.

Competing interests

The authors declare that they have no competing interests.

References

1. Gupta SK, Shukla VK (2004) Silent gallstones: a therapeutic dilemma. Trop Gastroenterol 25:65–68
2. Della Corte C, Falchetti D, Nebbia G, Calacoci M, Pastore M, Francavilla R et al (2008) Management of cholelithiasis in Italian children: a national multicenter study. World J Gastroenterol 14:1383–1388
3. Garey CL, Laituri CA, Keckler SJ, Ostlie DJ, Stagg HW, Little DC et al (2010) Laparoscopic cholecystectomy in obese and non-obese children. J Surg Res 163:299–302
4. Dipaola F, Heubi J. Disease of gallbladder in infancy, childhood, and adolescence. In: Suchy F, Sokol R, Balistreri W, editors. Liver Disease in Children, 4th edition. Cambridge university press; 2014: 247-264.
5. Alonso M (2004) Gall bladder abnormalities in children with sickle cell disease: management with laparoscopic cholecystectomy. J Pediatr 145: 580–581
6. Svensson J, Makin E (2012) Gallstone disease in children. Semin Pediatr Surg 21:255–265
7. Wesdorp I, Bosman D, de Graaff A, Aronson D, van der Blij F, Taminiau J (2000) Clinical presentations and predisposing factors of cholelithiasis and sludge in children. J Pediatr Gastroenterol Nutr 31:411–417
8. Bogueu C, Murphy A, Gerstle J, Moineddin R, Daneman A (2010) Risk factors, complications, and outcome of gallstones in children: a single center review. J Pediatr Gastroenterol Nutr 50:303–308
9. Mehta S, Lopez M, Chumpitazi B, Mazziotti M, Brandt M, Fishman D (2012) Clinical characteristics and risk factors for symptomatic pediatric gallbladder disease. Pediatrics 129:82–88
10. Sahin Y, Sahin D, Bulut F, Turkut A, Goktepe A (2014) Gallstone in children: aretrospective study of 37 cases in southeast of Turkey. IJSR 3:398–402
11. Kirsaclioglu C, Çakır B, Bayram G, Akbıyık F, Işık P, Tunç B (2016) Risk factors, complications and outcome of cholelithiasis in children: a retrospective, single-centre review. J Paediatr Child Health 52:944–949
12. Abo Elella S, Tawfik M, Barseem N, Moustafa W (2017) Prevalence of glucose-6-phosphate dehydrogenase deficiency in neonates in Egypt. Ann Saudi Med 37:362–365
13. Dooki M, Norouzi A (2013) Cholelithiasis in childhood: a Cohort study in North of Iran. Iran J Pediatr 23:588–592
14. Suchy F, Sundaram S, Shneider B. Familial hepatocellular cholestasis. In: Suchy F, Sokol R, Balistreri W, editors. Liver Disease in Children, 4th edition. Cambridge university press; 2014:199- 215.
15. Reif S, Sloven D, Lebenthal E. Gallstones in children: characterization by age, etiology and outcome. Am J Dis Child 1991;145: 105- 108. PMID: 1898681
16. Lugo-Vicente HL (1997) Trends in management of gallbladder disorders in children. Pediatr Surg Int 12:348–352
17. Sarrami M, Ridley W, Nightingale S, Wright T, Kumar R (2019) Adolescent gallstones—need for early intervention in symptomatic idiopathic gallstones. Pediatr Surg Int 35:569–574
18. Hajong R, Tongper D, Khariong P, Mibang N (2013) Non-hemolytic childhood cholelithiasis managed laparoscopically: a report 1f 15 cases. IOSR-JDMS 7:31–34
19. Kim H, Kim S, Cho Y (2015) Pediatric cholecystectomy: clinical significance of cases unrelated to hematologic disorders. Pediatr Gastroenterol Hepatol Nutr 2:115–120
20. Jeanty C, Derderian S, Courtier J, Hirose S (2015) Clinical management of infantile cholelithiasis. J Pediatr Surg 50:1289–1292
21. Gokce S, Yıldırım M, Erdoğan D (2014) A retrospective review of children with gallstone: Single-center experience from Central Anatolia. Turk J Gastroenterol; 25:46–53.

30

Does double high-level disinfection for duodenoscopes add any value?

Osama Elbahr[1*], Amira Saleh[2], Azza Abdel Aziz[3], Samah M. Awad[3], Fatma O. Khalil[3], Sameh Afiffy[1], Ahmad Kamal[1], Ayman Alsebaey[1] and Gamal Badra[1]

Abstract

Background: Duodenoscope-emerging infection especially drug-resistant bacteria is considered a major concern nowadays. Different approaches were attempted to overcome this problem, like double high-level disinfection procedure. We performed a systematic review and meta-analysis to evaluate risk difference for positive cultures from duodenoscopes between double high-level disinfection (dHLD) and single (standard) high-level disinfection (sHLD).

Main body: A thorough literature search (in October and November 2019) for studies comparing dHLD and sHLD for duodenoscopes was performed by 3 researchers in the Web of Science, Scopus, PubMed, and Cochran databases. The search terms were "duodenoscope," "ERCP endoscope," "disinfection," "sterilization," and "reprocessing," and only randomized clinical trials with the English language were accepted.
Four trials were identified studying dHLD, and only 2 clinical trials comparing dHLD with standard sHLD were found reporting 6193 duodenoscope cultures. Overall sHLD cultures were 2972, and dHLD cultures were 3221; overall positive cultures were 140 in sHLD and 161 in dHLD.
The results of a meta-analysis using the random-effect model showed no significant risk difference (RD) between the 2 procedures for duodenoscope positive cultures (p = 0.53, RD 0.003, 95% CI "– 0.007–0.013").

Conclusions: Double HLD offered no significant difference over single HLD for duodenoscope disinfection. An alternative strategy to overcome duodenoscope-transmitted infection is a big issue to be resolved.

Keywords: Duodenoscope, ERCP, Disinfection, High-level, MDRO, CRE, Culture, Review, Meta-analysis, Bacteria

Background

Gastrointestinal (GI) endoscopy procedures are performed each year worldwide. Gastroenterologists and surgeons use flexible endoscopes for providing minimally invasive diagnostic, therapeutic, and palliative care, and the overall low rates of associated adverse events have offered such procedures optimal risk-benefit ratio [1]. The duodenoscope, a complex endoscopic instrument, is frequently utilized to accomplish the increasing demand for minimally invasive treatments of pancreatic and biliary diseases. It is, besides, the fundamental tool used to perform endoscopic retrograde cholangiopancreatography (ERCP) [2] for biliary drainage [3, 4].

Side-viewing endoscopes (duodenoscopes used for ERCP) have an additional unique feature, a cantilevered elevator mechanism at the distal tip controlled by an elevator wire (via a dedicated channel). This design is challenging to clean and disinfect and has been proposed as a contributing factor to recent outbreaks associated with duodenoscopes [5]. Severe infectious complications occur after ERCP in 2–4% of patients and include bacteremia, ascending cholangitis, cholecystitis, liver abscess, and necrotizing pancreatitis. Infection risk is higher when the biliary obstruction is present versus

* Correspondence: oelbahr@yahoo.com; osama.elbahr@liver.menofia.edu.eg
[1]Hepatology and Gastroenterology, National Liver Institute, Menoufia University, Menoufia, Egypt

absent and when an obstruction is malignant versus benign. Sepsis after ERCP has a mortality rate as high as 29% [6, 7].

Duodenoscopes undergo multistep cleaning and a high-level disinfection procedure called reprocessing so that they can be reused among patients. The complex design of duodenoscopes impedes effective cleaning [8]. Duodenoscopes require high-level disinfection (HLD) using chemical disinfectants. Glutaraldehyde, hydrogen peroxide, ortho-phthalaldehyde (OPA), peracetic acid, peracetic acid with hydrogen peroxide, and a chlorine-based system are cleared by the FDA and are dependable high-level disinfectants which provided the factors influencing that germicidal procedures are met [9].

This mini-systematic review evaluates the efficacy of double high-level disinfection (dHLD); dHLD was a possible sterilization method to overcome this problem by performing 2 cycles of the automatic standard disinfection process over standard high-level disinfection (sHLD) on the decrease of positive duodenoscope culture rates.

Main text

Search methodology

A thorough literature search (in October and November 2019) for studies comparing dHLD and sHLD for duodenoscopes was performed in the Web of Science, Scopus, PubMed, and Cochran databases. The search terms were "duodenoscope," "ERCP endoscope," "disinfection," "sterilization," and "reprocessing."

Criteria of selected studies

Types of studies

Clinical trials in the English language that study dHLD were included.

The type of participant

Humans with a hepatobiliary indication for ERCP intervention were included.

The type of intervention

dHLD means 2 cycles of automated duodenoscope sterilization while sHLD means 1 cycle of standard high-level disinfection.

Study selection

Studies were independently evaluated by five authors (E.O., A.S., S.A., AL.A., and K.A.) who screened the title, the abstract, and then the full text, with articles being removed according to the exclusion criteria at each step, and this was done by the aid of Rayyan web. To ensure that all potentially relevant studies were considered for inclusion, further evaluation by a consensus of 4 authors (B.G., AB.A., AW.S., and K.F.) was performed.

Data extraction and risk of bias assessment

By 2 authors, the following data were extracted from each study: the first author, the year of publication, the study design, the number of participants, the type of intervention, the number of positive cultures, and the presence of drug-resistant organisms.

The risk of bias was conducted on RevMan 5 software.

Primary outcome

The primary outcome is culture-positive duodenoscopes after disinfection.

The percentage of the events were used to measure the treatment effect.

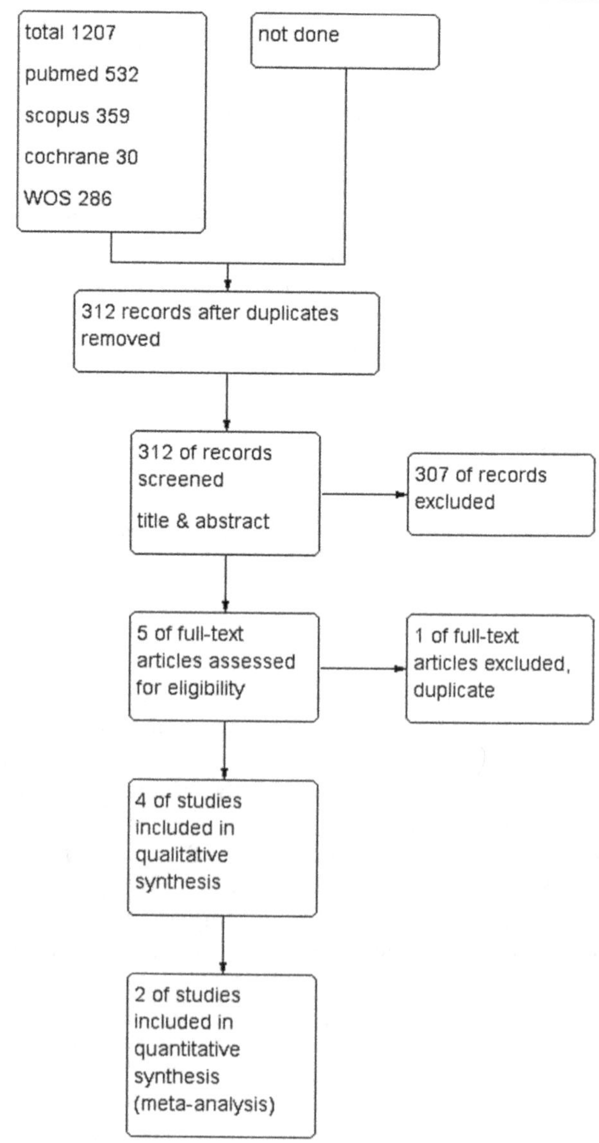

Fig. 1 Prisma flowchart for studies selection

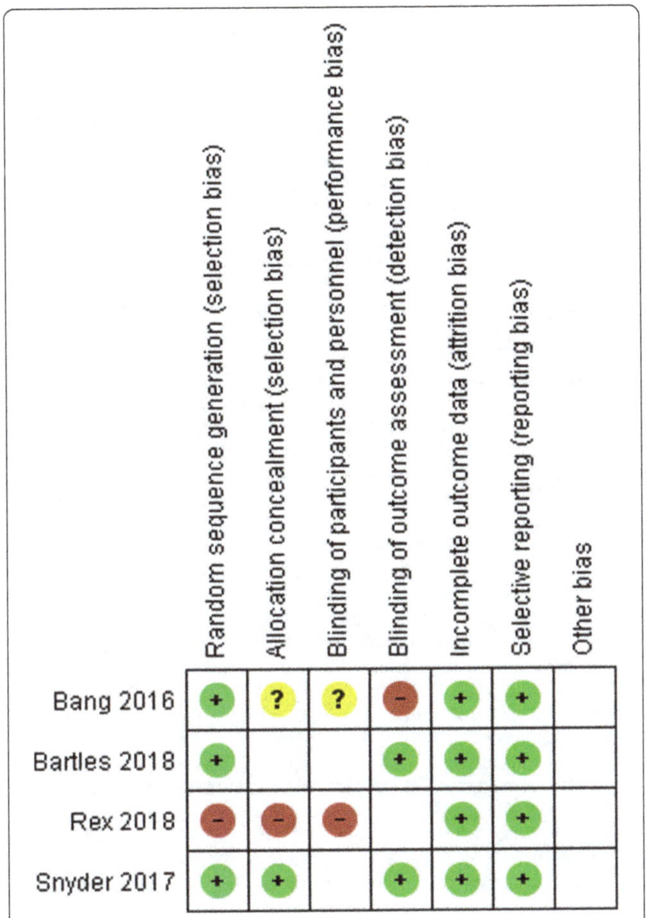

Fig. 2 Risk of bias for selected studies

Statistical analysis

All analysis was conducted on RevMan 5 software.

A meta-analysis with 95% confidence interval (CI) was performed to measure risk difference in culture-positive duodenoscopes between dHLD and sHLD for included and eligible studies, and a random-effect model was applied.

Results

χ^2 test was used to assess the presence of heterogeneity, while I^2 test was used to assess the degree of heterogeneity.

A total of 1207 records were retrieved from databases based on search criteria (Fig. 1). After reviewing the title, abstracts, and full texts, 4 studies were found to be eligible for synthetic narrative analysis while only 2 were eligible for meta-analysis (Snyder et al. [10] and Bartles et al. [11]) as they compared dHLD against sHLD. A total of 6193 duodenoscope disinfection processes were found in the 4 studies. sHLD was presented in 2 studies (Snyder et al. [10] and Bartles et al. [11]) conducted 2972 times, while dHLD was presented in 4 studies done 3221 times.

Bang et al. [12] and Rex et al. [13] were single-arm studies evaluating dHLD. Snyder et al. [10] and Bartles et al. [11] (with the highest weight in our meta-analysis 98.6%) conducted a comparative clinical trial between dHLD and sHLD. So, this is presented in the risk of bias assessment in Fig 2.

There was no significant heterogeneity between the studies (χ^2 = 0.7 and I^2 = 0%) (Fig. 3).

The primary outcome is shown in Table 1 and Fig. 3.

Positive culture rate in sHLD was 4.7% while in dHLD was 4.9%, and there is no significant risk difference (RD) between both (p = 0.53, RD 0.003, 95% CI "– 0.007–0.013").

Duodenoscope-related infections are of increasing global concern due to the emergence of multidrug-resistant bacteria such as carbapenem-resistant Enterobacteriaceae (CRE), with a bacterial biofilm production postulated as one cause of persistent infection from such virulent organisms [14]. The current standard for all flexible endoscope reprocessing includes pre-cleaning, leak testing, an additional manual cleaning step, and high-level disinfection [15]. Different disinfection alternative methods, over the standard one, were tried, such as *N*-acetylcysteine (NAC) [14], plasma-activated water (PAW) [16], and dHLD.

Our systematic review and meta-analysis tried to evaluate the efficacy of dHLD over sHLD, but we have been faced by a small number of trials on such topic. Snyder in his trial terminated the study after the follow-up period due to failure to reach the primary outcome of his study (multidrug-resistant organisms [MDRO]),

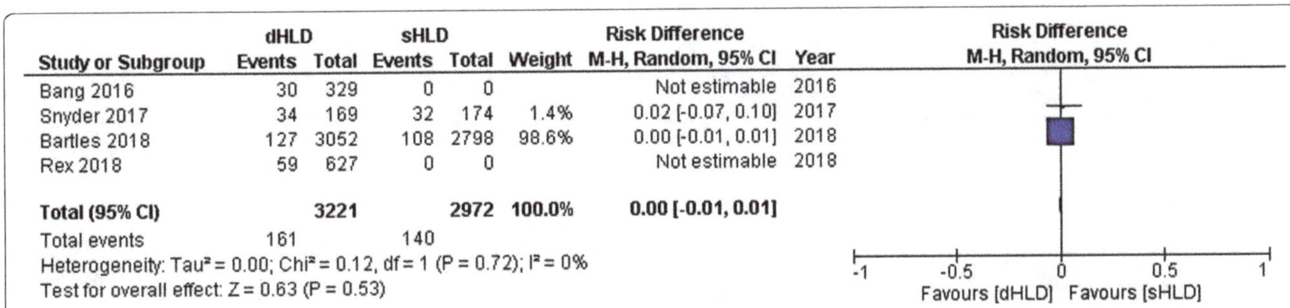

Fig. 3 Forest plot of comparison: risk difference for a positive culture

Table 1 General data

Total number of studies included	4
Total number of duodenoscopes processed	6193
sHLD positive cultures/total	140/2972
dHLD positive cultures/total	161/3221

but he concluded that dHLD did not decrease the culture-positive rate in duodenoscopes over sHLD. Bartles has conducted his study on both duodenoscopes and endoscopes and found that double HLD did not reduce culture positivity rates compared with single HLD in facilities with an already low positive culture rate.

All that was presented in our meta-analysis showed no statistically significant RD between dHLD and sHLD ($p = 0.53$, RD 0.003, 95% CI "– 0.007–0.013").

Conclusion

What are the implications of our review for the future? Our analysis showed that dHLD had no added value over the standard HLD. Therefore, another strategy should be adopted to overcome the duodenoscope-transmitted infections and quality measures should be ascertained for the following guidelines of duodenoscope disinfection.

Abbreviations

dHLD: Double high-level disinfection; sHLD: Single high-level disinfection; ERCP: Endoscopic retrograde cholangiopancreatography; MDRO: Multidrug-resistant organisms; CRE: Carbapenem-resistant Enterobacteriaceae; χ^2: Chi-square test

Acknowledgements

To all our professors

Authors' contributions

O.E: literature search, study selection, data extraction, bias assessment, review writing, and statistical analysis. A.S: literature search, study selection, review writing, data extraction, and bias assessment. S.A: literature search and study selection. A.A: literature search, study selection, and critical appraisal. A.K: literature search and study selection. G.B: resolve disagreement and critical appraisal. A.A.A: resolve disagreement and critical appraisal. S.M.A: resolve disagreement and critical appraisal. F.K: resolve disagreement and critical appraisal. All authors read and approved the final manuscript.

Competing interests

No competing interests

Author details

[1]Hepatology and Gastroenterology, National Liver Institute, Menoufia University, Menoufia, Egypt. [2]Infection Control, Student Hospital, Menoufia University, Menoufia, Egypt. [3]Medical Microbiology, and Immunology, National Liver Institute, Menoufia University, Menoufia, Egypt.

References

1. Balan GG, Sfarti CV, Chiriac SA, Stanciu C, Trifan A (2019) Duodenoscope-associated infections: a review. Eur J Clin Microbiol Infect Dis. https://doi.org/10.1007/s10096-019-03671-3
2. Higa JT (2019) Duodenoscope-related infections: overview and epidemiology. Tech Gastrointest Endosc. https://doi.org/10.1016/j.tgie.2019.150623
3. Elbahr O, Zakaria H, Zakaria HM et al (2018) Impact of preoperative endoscopic biliary drainage on postoperative outcome after pancreaticoduodenectomy. Surgery, Gastroenterol Oncol 23:3. https://doi.org/10.21614/sgo-23-2-173
4. Elbahr O (2019) Biliptysis. Egypt liver J 9. https://doi.org/10.1186/s43066-019-0005-8
5. Grein JD, Murthy RK (2018) New developments in the prevention of gastrointestinal scope-related infections. Infect Dis Clin N Am 32(4):899–913. https://doi.org/10.1016/j.idc.2018.06.008
6. Kovaleva J, Peters FTM, van der Mei Mei HC, Degener JE (2013) Transmission of infection by flexible gastrointestinal endoscopy and bronchoscopy. Clin Microbiol Rev 26(2):230–253. https://doi.org/10.1128/CMR.00085-12
7. Chandrasekhara V, Khashab MA, Muthusamy VR et al (2017) Adverse events associated with ERCP. Gastrointest Endosc 85(1):32–47. https://doi.org/10.1016/j.gie.2016.06.051
8. Chang W-K, Liu T-C, Liu T-L, Peng C-L, Wang H-P (2019) Enhanced manual cleaning efficacy of duodenoscope in endoscopy units: results of a multicenter comprehensive quality control program. Am J Infect Control 47(10):1233–1239. https://doi.org/10.1016/j.ajic.2019.03.029
9. Rutala WA, Weber DJ (2019) Reprocessing semicritical items: outbreaks and current issues. Am J Infect Control 47:A79–A89. https://doi.org/10.1016/j.ajic.2019.01.015
10. Snyder GM, Wright SB, Smithey A et al (2017) Randomized comparison of 3 high-level disinfection and sterilization procedures for duodenoscopes. Gastroenterology. 153(4):1018–1025. https://doi.org/10.1053/j.gastro.2017.06.052
11. Bartles RL, Leggett JE, Hove S et al (2018) A randomized trial of single versus double high-level disinfection of duodenoscopes and linear echoendoscopes using standard automated reprocessing. Gastrointest Endosc 88(2):306–313.e2. https://doi.org/10.1016/j.gie.2018.02.016
12. Bang JY, Rex DK, Sherman S et al (2016) Impact of implementation of double-reprocessing protocol in the prevention of duodenoscope-associated carbapenem-resistant Enterobacteriaceae (CRE) in a single tertiary referral center. Gastrointest Endosc 83(5):AB170. https://doi.org/10.1016/j.gie.2016.03.144
13. Rex DK, Sieber M, Lehman GA et al (2018) A double-reprocessing high-level disinfection protocol does not eliminate positive cultures from the elevators of duodenoscopes. Endoscopy. 50(6):588–596. https://doi.org/10.1055/s-0043-122378
14. Kwok K, Chang J, Lo S, Giap A, Lim B, Wu B (2016) A novel adjunctive cleansing method to reduce colony-forming units on duodenoscopes. Endosc Int open 4(11):E1178–E1182. https://doi.org/10.1055/s-0042-116490
15. Kim S, Muthusamy VR (2016) Current practice of duodenoscope reprocessing. Curr Gastroenterol Rep 18(10):54. https://doi.org/10.1007/s11894-016-0528-7
16. Balan GG, Rosca I, Ursu E-L et al (2018) Plasma-activated water: a new and effective alternative for duodenoscope reprocessing. Infect Drug Resist 11:727–733. https://doi.org/10.2147/IDR.S159243

31

Updates in drug-induced acute pancreatitis

Omkolsoum Alhaddad[1], Maha Elsabaawy[1*], Marwa Elfauomy[1], Dalia Elsabaawy[2] and Tarek Mansour[3]

Abstract

Background: Being infrequent, drug-induced acute pancreatitis (DIP) is an overlooked clinical entity that can be serious with significant morbidity and mortality.

Main body: A renovative review of drugs incriminated in acute pancreatitis had been presented with all relevant data and case presentations. Antibiotics, antidiabetics, antihypertensive agents, H2 blockers (H2B) and proton pump inhibitors (PPIs), anticancer therapies, and the new direct-acting antiviral therapies (DAAs) of hepatitis C virus (HCV) were discussed pertinently to DIP.

Conclusions: DIP should be suspected as a potential adverse event to every newly emerged drug. Herein, an updated review of drugs recently alleged to be implicated in DIP.

Background

Prevalence of DIP

Drug-induced pancreatitis, a potentially forgotten diagnosis that should be rigorously appreciated. In fact, the increasing number of pharmacological agents is associated with increased incidences of acute pancreatitis. Drug-induced pancreatitis represents up to 5% of all acute pancreatitis cases, hence, can be considered as the third common cause of acute pancreatitis after alcohol and gall stones are ruled out [1]. The worldwide incidence of drug-induced pancreatitis is spanning around 5–80 per 100,000 adults. DIP is reported to be higher in patients with inflammatory bowel disease, also, in children, geriatric population, and with immunosuppression [2].

Currently, more than 500 drugs have been reported in the World Health Organization database as offenders of acute pancreatitis [3].

Diagnostic concerns of DIP

Discerning a diagnosis of DIP has neither clinical nor laboratory diagnostic criteria. However, the diagnosis of acute pancreatitis is clinically persuaded through disappearance of abdominal pain and drop of pancreatic enzymes upon drug discontinuation, exclusion of other common etiologies, and recurred manifestations upon challenging the suspected drug [4]. Re-challenging the suspected drug is not feasible in critical patients; however, being applied will reduce the number of culprit medications. Exclusion of uncommon etiologies and other possible drugs than the drug of concern in multimedicated patients is always difficult.

Badalov classification system of drug-induced acute pancreatitis contains 5 classes: Ia, Ib, II, III, and IV. The number of published cases, re-challenge, and latency provides the basis of Badalov classification (Table 1) [5].

The latency between initiation of the offending drug and developing acute pancreatitis can be short (less than 24 h), intermediate (1-30 days), and long (more than 30 days). According to Badalov, the latency is described as consistent with the drug-related pancreatitis when 75% of cases were related to any of the previously mentioned groups [5].

Review of potential offenders

Propofol

Propofol introduced itself to the market about three decades ago as a safer short-acting anesthetic agent. Its use is extended as long-term hypnotic and sedative infusion in critically ill patients. Significant weight of publications and case reports mentioned a causal relationship between propofol and acute pancreatitis [6]. A recent

* Correspondence: maha.ahmed@liver.menofia.edu.eg
[1]Department of Hepatology and Gastroenterology, National Liver Institute, Menoufia University, Shebeen El-Kom, Menoufia 32511, Egypt

Table 1 Badalov classification system of drug-induced acute pancreatitis [5]

Class Ia drugs	At least 1 case report with positive re-challenge, excluding all other causes, such as alcohol, hypertriglyceridemia, gallstones, and other drugs
Class Ib drugs	At least 1 case report with positive re-challenge, however, other causes, such as alcohol, hypertriglyceridemia, gallstones, and other drugs were not ruled out
Class II drugs	At least 4 cases in the literature and consistent latency in at least 75% of cases
Class III drugs	At least 2 cases in the literature with neither consistent latency among cases nor re-challenge
Class IV drugs	Like class III drugs, but only one case report had been published, without re-challenge

systematic review specified the propofol-pancreatitis relationship as probable [7]. According to Badalov et al. classification system, propofol is a class Ia drug as acute pancreatitis is documented along with positive drug rechallenge [7]. Propofol is suspended in a lipid emulsion that can be a factor in propofol-related hypertriglyceridemia in susceptible people. Propofol-related pancreatitis has been attributed to developed hypertriglyceridemia, a traditional etiology for acute pancreatitis [8]. Hypertriglyceridemia more than 1000 mg/dl was documented at time of acute pancreatitis in reports of propofol-pancreatitis; however, in other propofol, pancreatitis was documented in absence of hypertriglyceridemia [9]. Hence, acute pancreatitis inferred to propofol could have many mechanisms. Intensive care unit (ICU) patients and prolonged high rate propofol administration are considered risk factors for propofol-pancreatitis [10]. Accordingly, monitoring serum triglycerides, amylase, and lipase is advisable in cases on prolonged propofol administration. Acute pancreatitis should be suspected in any patient developing abdominal pain after propofol infusion and the drug should be discontinued [10]. Yet, this area of propofol-associated acute pancreatitis is considered as uncertain.

Antibiotics

Minocycline is a tetracycline while tigecycline is a glycylcycline and a structural derivative of minocycline [11]. Tigecycline shares similar pharmacokinetic properties and adverse effects with tetracyclines. Acute pancreatitis tightly linked to tetracycline was not listed in FDA approval of either minocycline or tigecycline [12].

Minocycline is widely used for treatment of acne vulgaris. Also indicated for methicillin-resistant *Staphylococcus aureus* (MRSA)-related infections and rheumatoid arthritis as a disease-modifying drug [13]. A small case series described minocycline-induced pancreatitis in two cystic fibrosis patients in 2001 [14]. The inherent pancreatic insufficiency in cystic fibrosis patients could play a contribution in this serious event. In these 2 cases, neither re-challenge nor consistent latency were existing and accordingly minocycline is specified as class III drug in Badalov classification for drug-induced acute pancreatitis [14]. A newer two cases of minocycline-induced pancreatitis in non-cystic fibrosis patients had been recently published [15]. In both cases, all other etiologies of acute pancreatitis have been excluded and resolution of the condition was achieved few days after minocycline discontinuation [15]. Drug idiosyncrasy could explain minocycline pancreatitis in non-cystic fibrosis cases paralleling the explanation of minocycline-induced hepatotoxicity. Acute pancreatitis is a serious condition and clinicians should be aware of such minocycline-related adverse event. Currently, no identifiable risk factors for minocycline-induced pancreatitis.

Few case reports linked tigecycline to acute pancreatitis with variable time latency. In these cases, tigecycline was used to treat soft tissue infections except in a case of respiratory infection in a cystic fibrosis patient [16]. Tigecycline discontinuation was followed by regression of symptoms and drop of pancreatic enzymes [16]. The number of reported tigecycline pancreatitis is small and insufficient to lower its prescriptions [17]. Concerning tigecycline pancreatitis, the retrospective analyses of phases 3 and 4 clinical studies revealed mixed conclusion. In respect to seriousness of acute pancreatitis, clinicians should be aware of this potential adverse effect and should monitor patients for features of pancreatitis during treatment with tigecycline [17].

Antidiabetic drugs

In 2008 and in response to 30 post-marketing reports, FDA has ordered a warning label about a potential risk of acute pancreatitis in patients taking exenatide and sitagliptin, the first members of incretin-based therapies [18]. Afterward, the FDA adverse drug events system received a large number of spontaneously reported cases of acute pancreatitis in those taking various incretin-based therapies [18]. Further, observational studies have raised questions as to the possible association of treatment with incretin-based therapies, particularly with DPP-4 inhibitors and the risk of acute pancreatitis [19]. In 2016, in JAMA, a large multicenter and population-based study had indicated a non-significant increased risk of incretin-associated acute pancreatitis compared to other antidiabetics [20]. Also, the separate secondary analyses for glucagon-like peptide-1 (GLP1) agonists and dipeptidyl peptidase-4 (DDP4) inhibitors showed similar results.

Sodium-glucose cotransporter-2 inhibitors (SGLT2 inhibitors), a newly approved antidiabetics, have non-beta cell-dependent mechanism of action. They inhibit SGLT2 in the proximal renal tubules and thus preventing reabsorption of filtered glucose [21]. Since approval, the literature received a handful of medical articles about a link between SGLT2 inhibitors, particularly, canagliflozin and acute pancreatitis. In 2016, FDA wrote in its website that there is a safety issue but did not mention about a causal relationship between SGLT2 inhibitors and pancreatitis. In 2018, Canada Health submitted a review investigating this issue. The review concluded that there may be a link between SGLT2 inhibitors and acute pancreatitis, and physicians should be vigilant to symptoms of acute pancreatitis in patients taking these drugs [22].

Antihypertensive agents

Case reports of acute pancreatitis induced by enalapril, lisinopril, captopril, ramipril, and perindopril have been published. Some of the published reports mentioned acute pancreatitis after lisinopril re-challenge. The proposed mechanism is pancreatic angioedema with pancreatic duct obstruction [23]. A recent population-based study found that, in absence of alcohol, 7 per 10,000 attacks of acute pancreatitis/year are among users of angiotensin-converting enzyme (ACE) inhibitors [23].

Angiotensin receptor blockers (ARBs) induced pancreatitis have been introduced in a few case reports denoting a lesser risk of pancreatitis [24].

Acid-suppressing drugs

In many case reports, cimetidine and ranitidine have been associated with acute pancreatitis. Of note, acid-suppressing drugs can be prescribed for a prodrome of acute pancreatitis [25]. It was determined that hypergastrinemia induced by continuous use of proton pump inhibitors (PPIs) can stimulate pancreatic enzyme secretion eventually resulting in pancreatitis [26]. The literature contains several case reports of omeprazole-, pantoprazole-, and lansoprazole-induced pancreatitis. In more than one report, the pancreatitis was severe and necrotizing. In rats, intraperitoneal infusion of omeprazole resulted in pancreatic inflammation and elevated pancreatic enzymes. According to Badalov classification, proton pump inhibitors are specified as class I drugs based on positive re-challenge with the drug and consistent latency [27].

Anticancer therapies

Anticancer drugs almost always carry the risk of precipitation acute pancreatitis. Many of the older and recently approved anticancer therapies have been listed to cause pancreatitis. From the older agents, asparaginase used for the treatment of acute lymphoblastic leukemia is the most frequently chemotherapeutic agent-causing pancreatitis [28]. Asparaginase-related pancreatitis had been reported at an incidence of 2% to16%. Asparaginase pancreatitis is severe in up to 15% of patients and positive re-challenge is reported in up to 60% of cases [28]. Cisplatin and oxaliplatin are listed as inducing pancreatitis and discontinuation of these drugs had showed regression of symptoms and laboratory evidence of pancreatitis [29]. Everolimus and tamoxifen cause elevated serum triglycerides and hypertriglyceridemia can be the underlying mechanism of reported cases of everolimus and tamoxifen pancreatitis [30]. In many case reports and small case series, newer anticancer agents, immune check point inhibitors, tyrosine kinase inhibitors, and proteasome inhibitors have been reported to cause acute pancreatitis [31]. The proposed mechanisms of pancreatitis are immune-mediation direct toxicity or hypertriglyceridemia [31]. In concern to immune check inhibitors, nivolumab- and pembrolizumab-related pancreatitis have been recently reported in 1.8% of patients. Also, ipilimumab approved for treatment of melanoma is reported to be associated with pancreatitis in less than 1% of cases.

Pancreatitis attributed to check point inhibitors is considered as immune toxicities and in all cases, corticosteroids were the therapeutic option. The older tyrosine kinase inhibitors (TKIs), sorafenib, sunitinib, and imatinib are reported to cause pancreatitis [32]. Recent case reports have linked the newer tyrosine kinase inhibitors (TKIs), vemurafenib and ponatinib to pancreatitis and just elevated pancreatic enzymes. The famous proteasome inhibitor, bortezomib, has been repeatedly reported to cause pancreatitis [33].

Nonselective trans-arterial chemoembolization (TACE) may lead to elevated amylase in up to 40% of cases, while TACE-related pancreatitis can happen in up to 4% of cases. The larger the area infused with the chemotherapeutic agent, the greater the risk of pancreatitis [34]. Post-TACE-necrotizing pancreatitis is thought to be ischemic in nature secondary to embolic blocking of the pancreatic blood supply [35].

The new direct-acting antiviral therapies (DAAs) of hepatitis C virus (HCV)

DIP occurrence with the previously known combination of peginterferon and ribavirin had been substantiated [36]. Nevertheless, determination whether it is interferon or ribavirin-related effect is yet uncovered as all reported cases were on combination therapy. As both drugs are immune interfering, DIP might be an expected consequence.

Recently, the high safety profiles associating DAAs had denied any linkage with DIP occurrence. However, boceprevir and telaprevir were mentioned in such a fatal condition in two separate reports [37, 38]. Conversely, later generations of DAAs had been mentioned to cause DIP only in cases with ribavirin including regimens. In a 75-year-old male presenting with acute pancreatitis while on 3 weeks ombitasvir, paritaprevir, ritonavir, and dasabuvir (OTV/PTV/RTV/DSV) and ribavirin 1200 mg daily, a shift to ledipasvir/sofosbuvir regimen had improve the condition [36]. Consequently, ribavirin was principally convicted in most cases of HCV therapeutics-induced pancreatitis. Data are still limited on the potential role and pathogenic mechanisms of DAAs as DIP offenders.

Conclusion

Literature has recently liberated several reports of case reports concerning DIP with an array of newly emerged drugs like propofol infusion, antidiabetics (GLP1 agonists and DDP4 inhibitors, and SGLT2 inhibitors, particularly, canagliflozin), antibiotics (minocycline), antihypertensive agents (enalapril, lisinopril, captopril, ramipril, perindopril, and less frequently angiotensin receptor blockers), proton pump inhibitors (omeprazole, pantoprazole, and lansoprazole), anticancer drugs (nivolumab, pembrolizumab, ipilimumab), the newer TKIs (vemurafenib and ponatinib), proteasome inhibitors (bortezomib), and non-selective TACE, and direct-acting antiviral therapies (DAAs) of hepatitis C virus along with ribavirin.

DIP, which is an overlooked diagnosis in the clinical setting, must be rigorously considered whenever patients are on a set of new drugs and presenting with even, minimal symptoms and signs of acute pancreatitis. Indeed, updated vigilant clinicians and critical care medical staff can save lives.

Abbreviations

DIP: Drug-induced acute pancreatitis; ICU: Intensive care unit; FDA: Food and Drug Association; MERSA: Methicillin-resistant *Staphylococcus aureus*; DDP4: Dipeptidyl peptidase-4; GLP1: Glucagon-like peptide-1; SGLT2: Sodium-glucose cotransporter-2; ACEI: Angiotensin-converting enzyme inhibitors; ARBS: Angiotensin receptor blockers; H2B: H2 blockers; PPIs: Proton pump inhibitors; TKIs: Tyrosine kinase inhibitors; TACE: Transarterial chemoembolization; DAAs: Direct-acting antiviral therapies; HCV: Hepatitis C virus; OTV/PTV/RTV/DSV: Ombitasvir, paritaprevir, ritonavir, and dasabuvir

Acknowledgements

All respect and indebtedness to the great professor Dr. Omkolsoum Alhaddad who created this work for her unlimited, sincere, and priceless inputs complying this work to be fulfilled.

Authors' contributions

O A.: conceived and designed the study, analyzed and wrote the paper, M E.: analyzed the data and contributed in writing the paper. M E.: clinical evaluation and data collection. D E.: pharmacologic analysis of the data and revised the paper. T M.: revised and approved the paper. All authors have read and approved the manuscript.

Competing interests

The authors declare that they have no competing interests.

Author details

[1]Department of Hepatology and Gastroenterology, National Liver Institute, Menoufia University, Shebeen El-Kom, Menoufia 32511, Egypt. [2]Department of Clinical Pharmacy, National Liver Institute, Menoufia University, Menoufia 32511, Egypt. [3]Department of Internal Medicine, Faculty of Medicine, Ain Shams University, Cairo 3434, Egypt.

References

1. Scott T (2014) Drug induced acute pancreatitis: does it exist? World J Gastroenterol 20(44):16529–16534
2. Yokoe M, Takada T, Mayumi T, Yoshida M, Isaji S, Wada K et al (2015) Japanese guidelines for the management of acute pancreatitis: Japanese guidelines 2015. J Hepatobiliary Pancreat Sci 22(6):405–432
3. Rekhi B, Mannem S, Rekhi H, Mittal S, Arora S, Sathya P et al (2017) A case report on drug induced pancreatitis due to levofloxacin and methylprednisolone. Int J Case Rep Images 8(1):62–65
4. Ghatak R, Masso L, Kapadia D, Kulairi Z (2017) Medication as a cause of acute pancreatitis. Am J Case Rep 18:839–841
5. Badalov N, Baradarian R, Iswara K, Li J, Steinberg W, Tenner S (2007) Drug-induced acute pancreatitis: an evidence-based review. Clin Gastroenterol Hepatol 5:648–661
6. Jones M, Hall O, Kaye AM, Kaye AD (2015) Drug-induced acute pancreatitis: a review. Ochsner J 15:45–51
7. Asghar MU, Cheema HA, Tanveer K, Leinwand J (2019) Propofol infusion and acute pancreatitis: a review. Am J Ther 28
8. Kaur H, Nattanamai P, Qualls KE (2018) Propofol and clevidipine-induced hypertriglyceridemia. Cureus. 10(8):e3165
9. Haffar S, Kaur RJ, Garg SK et al (2019) Acute pancreatitis associated with intravenous administration of propofol: evaluation of causality in a systematic review of the literature. Gastroenterol Rep (Oxf) 7(1):13–23
10. Devlin JW, Lau AK, Tanios MA (2005 Oct) Propofol-associated hypertriglyceridemia and pancreatitis in the intensive care unit: an analysis of frequency and risk factors. Pharmacotherapy 25(10):1348–1352
11. Greer ND (2006) Tigecycline (Tygacil): the first in the glycylcycline class of antibiotics. Proc (Bayl Univ Med Cent) 19(2):155–161
12. Lin J, Wang R, Chen J (2018) Tigecycline-induced acute pancreatitis in a renal transplant patient: a case report and literature review. BMC Infect Dis 18(1):201
13. Alexis A, Del Rosso JQ, Desai SR et al (2018) BPX-01 minocycline topical gel shows promise for the treatment of moderate-to-severe inflammatory acne vulgaris. J Clin Aesthet Dermatol 11(11):25–35
14. Boyle MP (2001) Minocycline-induced pancreatitis in cystic fibrosis. Chest. 119(4):1283–1285
15. Gabriel JG, Bhogal S, Kapila A Minocycline associated pancreatitis. Am J Ther 2017; 0, 1–2.
16. Hung WY, Kogelman L, Volpe G, Iafrati M, Davidson L (2009) Tigecycline-induced acute pancreatitis: case report and literature review. Int J Antimicrob Agents 34(5):486–489
17. Akhter S, Krishnan P, Kaul P.Tigecycline-associated acute pancreatitis. Am J Ther 2018 0, 1–2.
18. U.S. Food and Drug Administration MedWatch. MedWatch safety alerts for drugs, biologics, medical devices, and dietary supplements. 2008; 8;2012.
19. Thomsen R, Pedersen L, Møller N, Kahlert J, Beck-Nielsen H, Sørensen H (2015) Incretin-based therapy and risk of acute pancreatitis: a nationwide population-based case-control study. Diabetes Care 38(6):1089–1098
20. Azoulay L, Filion KB, Platt RW et al (2016) Association between incretin-based drugs and the risk of acute pancreatitis. JAMA Intern Med 176(10): 1464–1473
21. Gutch M, Bhattacharya A, Kumar S, Pahan R, Singh R (2018) Dapagliflozin induced pancreatitis. Int J Med Public Health 8:1,45–1,47

22. Hsia DS, Grove O, Cefalu WT (2017) An update on sodium-glucose co-transporter-2 inhibitors for the treatment of diabetes mellitus. Curr Opin Endocrinol Diabetes Obes 24(1):73–79
23. Thumma S, Errico K, Manchala V, Mattana J. Lisinopril-induced acute pancreatitis. Am J Ther 2018: 0, 1–4.
24. Bexelius TS, Ljung R, Mattsson F, Lu Y, Lindblad M (2017) Angiotensin II receptor blockers and risk of acute pancreatitis - a population based case-control study in Sweden. BMC Gastroenterol 17(1):36
25. Eland IA, Alvarez CH, Stricker BH, Rodríguez LA (2000) The risk of acute pancreatitis associated with acid-suppressing drugs. Br J Clin Pharmacol 49(5):473–478
26. McCarthy DM (2020) Proton pump inhibitor use, hypergastrinemia, and gastric carcinoids-what is the relationship? Int J Mol Sci 21(2):662
27. Murtaza G, Khalid M (2018) And Nicolas a Mungo. Recurrent pantoprazole-associated pancreatitis. Am J Ther 25(4):e492–e493
28. Stefanović M, Jazbec J, Lindgren F, Bulajić M, Löhr M (2016) Acute pancreatitis as a complication of childhood cancer treatment. Cancer Med 5(5):827–836
29. Butt W, Saadati H, Saif M (2010) Oxaliplatin-induced pancreatitis: a case series. Anticancer Res December 30(12):5113–5115
30. Singh HK, Prasad MS, Kandasamy AK, Dharanipragada K (2016) Tamoxifen-induced hypertriglyceridemia causing acute pancreatitis. J Pharmacol Pharmacother 7(1):38–40. https://doi.org/10.4103/0976-500X.179365
31. Clamon G (2017) Pancreatitis associated with newer classes of antineoplastic therapies. JCSO 15(3):e135–e141
32. Bajwa R, Cheema A, Khan T et al (2019) Adverse effects of immune checkpoint inhibitors (programmed death-1 inhibitors and cytotoxic T-lymphocyte-associated protein-4 inhibitors): results of a retrospective study. J Clin Med Res 11(4):225–236
33. Brulc E, Seehaus C, Schutz N, Fantl D (2018) Management of pancreatitis related to Bortezomib treatment: report of two cases. Hematol Transfus Cell Ther 40(4):382–384
34. Krishnamurthy P, Brown M, Agrawal S, Short RF (2017) Acute pancreatitis as a complication of trans-arterial chemoembolization of hepatocellular cancer-case report and review of literature. J Gastrointest Oncol 8(1):E26–E30
35. Bae S, Yeon J, Lee J, Kim J, Lee H, Lee S et al (2012) A case of necrotizing pancreatitis subsequent to transcatheter arterial chemoembolization in a patient with hepatocellular carcinoma. Clin Mol Hepatol 18(3):321–325
36. Cristina C, Diaz A, Bolaños A et al DI-031 acute pancreatitis and hyperbilirubinaemia possibly associated with ribavirin administration and new direct antiviral agents. European journal of hospital pharmacy (2016); 23: A131. C.
37. Ventura R, Urich S, Skinner S et al (2013) First report of telaprevir-induced pancreatitis. Dig Dis Sci 58:887–888
38. Bilar J, Carvalho-Filho R, Mota C et al (2014) Acute pancreatitis associated with boceprevir: a case report. Braz J Infect Dis 18(4):454–456

Permissions

All chapters in this book were first published by Springer; hereby published with permission under the Creative Commons Attribution License or equivalent. Every chapter published in this book has been scrutinized by our experts. Their significance has been extensively debated. The topics covered herein carry significant findings which will fuel the growth of the discipline. They may even be implemented as practical applications or may be referred to as a beginning point for another development.

The contributors of this book come from diverse backgrounds, making this book a truly international effort. This book will bring forth new frontiers with its revolutionizing research information and detailed analysis of the nascent developments around the world.

We would like to thank all the contributing authors for lending their expertise to make the book truly unique. They have played a crucial role in the development of this book. Without their invaluable contributions this book wouldn't have been possible. They have made vital efforts to compile up to date information on the varied aspects of this subject to make this book a valuable addition to the collection of many professionals and students.

This book was conceptualized with the vision of imparting up-to-date information and advanced data in this field. To ensure the same, a matchless editorial board was set up. Every individual on the board went through rigorous rounds of assessment to prove their worth. After which they invested a large part of their time researching and compiling the most relevant data for our readers.

The editorial board has been involved in producing this book since its inception. They have spent rigorous hours researching and exploring the diverse topics which have resulted in the successful publishing of this book. They have passed on their knowledge of decades through this book. To expedite this challenging task, the publisher supported the team at every step. A small team of assistant editors was also appointed to further simplify the editing procedure and attain best results for the readers.

Apart from the editorial board, the designing team has also invested a significant amount of their time in understanding the subject and creating the most relevant covers. They scrutinized every image to scout for the most suitable representation of the subject and create an appropriate cover for the book.

The publishing team has been an ardent support to the editorial, designing and production team. Their endless efforts to recruit the best for this project, has resulted in the accomplishment of this book. They are a veteran in the field of academics and their pool of knowledge is as vast as their experience in printing. Their expertise and guidance has proved useful at every step. Their uncompromising quality standards have made this book an exceptional effort. Their encouragement from time to time has been an inspiration for everyone.

The publisher and the editorial board hope that this book will prove to be a valuable piece of knowledge for researchers, students, practitioners and scholars across the globe.

List of Contributors

Amir Mohammad Kazemifar
Clinical Toxicology, Metabolic Diseases Research Center, Qazvin University of Medical Sciences, Qazvin, Iran

Ali Akbar Shafikhani
Department of Occupational Health Engineering, Shahid Beheshti University of Medical Sciences, Tehran, Iran

Elaheh Haji Noormohammadi and Zahra Azarion
Department of Internal Medicine, Metabolic Disease Research Center, Qazvin University of Medical Sciences, Qazvin, Iran

Aliakbar Hajiaghamohammadi
Gastroenterologist Metabolic Diseases Research Center, Qazvin University of Medical Sciences, Qazvin, Iran

Dina M. Sweed, Zeinab A. Fayed and Mohamed Mohamady
Pathology Department, National Liver Institute, Menoufia University, Al Menoufia, Egypt

Enas M. Sweed
Radiology Department, Faculty of Medicine, Benha University, Benha, Egypt

Ahmed El-Sherif
Hepato-pancreatobiliary Surgery and Liver Transplantation, National Liver Institute, Menoufia University, Al Menoufia, Egypt

Kamala Priya M R and Priya R. Iyer
Post Graduate and Research Department of Biotechnology, Women's Christian College, College Road, Chennai 600006, India

Hany M. Elsadek
Gastroenterology & Hepatology Unit, Internal Medicine Department, Faculty of Medicine, Zagazig University, Zagazig, Egypt

Soha A. Elhawari
Tropical Medicine Department, Faculty of Medicine, Zagazig University, Zagazig, Egypt

Ahmed Mokhtar
Clinical Pathology Department, Faculty of Medicine, Zagazig University, Zagazig, Egypt

Ahmed Samir Allam and Mohamed Magdy Salama
Internal Medicine Department, Faculty of Medicine, Ain Shams University, Cairo 11211, Egypt

Haytham Mohamed Nasser
Radiology Department, Faculty of Medicine, Ain Shams University, Cairo, Egypt

Walaa Ahmed Yousry Kabiel
Clinical Pathology Department, Faculty of Medicine, Ain Shams University, Cairo 11211, Egypt

Ehab H. Elsayed
Tropical Medicine Department, National Research Center, Cairo 11211, Egypt

Eman Abdelsameea and Maha Elsabaawy
Department of Hepatology and Gastroenterology, National Liver Institute, Menoufia University, Shebeen El-Koom 32511, Egypt

Nermine Ehsan and Ahmed Elrefaey
Department of Pathology, National Liver Institute, Menoufia University, Shebeen El-Koom, Egypt

Khalid Aboelela
Department of Hepatobiliary Surgery, National Liver Institute, Menoufia University, Shebeen El-Koom, Egypt

Fabio Tuminello, Stefano Puleo and Antonio Pesce
Section of General Surgery, Department of Medical, Surgical Sciences and Advanced Technologies "G.F. Ingrassia", University Hospital "Policlinico-Vittorio Emanuele", 95123 Catania, Italy

Davide Castiglione and Antonio Basile
Radiology I Unit, Department of Medical, Surgical Sciences and Advanced Technologies "G.F. Ingrassia", University Hospital "Policlinico-Vittorio Emanuele", 95123 Catania, Italy

Giuseppe Broggi and Giada Maria Vecchio
Anatomic Pathology, Department of Medical, Surgical Sciences and Advanced Technologies "G.F. Ingrassia", University Hospital "Policlinico-Vittorio Emanuele", 95123 Catania, Italy

Ahmed Ibrahim Gad, Mohamed Rezk Elmedames and Ayman Ramadan Abdelhai
Internal Medicine Department, Faculty of Medicine, Zagazig University, Zagazig, Sharkia 44519, Egypt

Ayman Mohamed Marei
Microbiology and Immunology Department, Faculty of Medicine, Zagazig University, Zagazig, Egypt

Nguyen Thanh Xuan and Ho Huu Thien
Department of Pediatric and Abdominal Emergency Surgery, Hue Central Hospital, 16 Le Loi Street, Hue City, Vietnam

Nguyen Huu Son
Pediatric Center, Hue Central Hospital, Hue City, Vietnam

Helmy El-Shazly, El-Sayed Tharwa, Hassan Zaghla, Shrief Abass and El-Sayed Ibrahim
Hepatology and Gastroenterology Department, National Liver Institute, Menoufia University, Yassin Abdel-Ghafar street, Shebeen El-Kom, Menoufia 32511, Egypt

Mohamed El-Warraky
Radiology Department, National Liver Institute, Menoufia University, Shebeen El-Kom, Egypt

Mohamed Abdel-Samiee
National Liver Institute, Menoufia University, Shebeen El-Kom, Egypt

Phaniram Sumanam
Department of Internal Medicine, Nazareth Hospital, 2601 Holme Avenue, Philadelphia, PA 19152, USA

Sheharyar Minhas
Department of Internal Medicine, Nazareth Hospital, 2601 Holme Avenue, Philadelphia, PA 19152, USA
Rollins School of Public Health, Emory University, Atlanta, GA, USA

Ahmed Minhas and Maira Malik
Department of Internal Medicine, East Tennessee State University, Johnson City, TN, USA

Jayanta Paul
Consultant Gastroenterologist and Liver Specialist, Department of Gastroenterology, Desun Hospital and Heart Institute, Kolkata 700124, India

Hany Haroun Kaisar and Ahmed Samir Abo Halima
Gastroenterology and Hepatology Department, Faculty of Medicine, Ain Shams University, Cairo 11211, Egypt

Ramin Niknam and Nemattellah Hajizadegan
Department of Internal Medicine, School of Medicine, Gastroenterohepatology Research Center, Shiraz University of Medical Sciences, Shiraz, Iran

Vahid Mohammadkarimi
Department of Internal Medicine, School of Medicine, Shiraz University of Medical Sciences, Shiraz, Iran

Laleh Mahmoudi
Department of Clinical Pharmacy, School of Pharmacy, Shiraz University of Medical Sciences, Shiraz, Iran

Mohamed Mohei El Badry and Doaa Abdelhady Ali
Department of Tropical Medicine and Gastroenterology, Faculty of Medicine, Aswan University, Aswan, Egypt

Noha Hamdy Eltaweel
Department of Moleculer genetics, National Research Center, Cairo, Egypt

Marwa A. Abdel-Wahed
Department of Clinical Pathology, Faculty of Medicine, Ain Shams University, Cairo, Egypt

Sherif Abugamra and Aya Yassin
Department of Radiodiagnosis, Ain Shams University, Khalifa El-Maamon St, Abbasiya sq, Cairo 11566, Egypt

Asmaa Saber Mostafa Abdel-Rehim and Dina Sayed Sheha
Department of Internal Medicine, Allergy and Clinical Immunology Unit, Ain Shams University, Khalifa El-Maamon St, Abbasiya sq, Cairo 11566, Egypt

Mohamed M. Mogahed and Bahaa El Wakeel
Departments of Surgery, NHTMRI, Cairo, Egypt

Ashraf Anas Zytoon
Radiodiagnosis Department, Faculty of Medicine, Menoufia University, Menoufia, Egypt

Bassem Essa
Tropical Medicine Department, NHTMRI, Cairo, Egypt

Wessam Abdellatif
Radiology Department, NHTMRI, Cairo, Egypt

Nashwa Ghanem
Internal Medicine Department, Faculty of Medicine, Cairo University, Cairo, Egypt

Osama Aboelfotoh Aly, Wael Ahmed Yousry, Eman Mohammed Shona and Ahmed Mohamed ElGhandour
Division of Gastroenterology and Hepatology, Department of Internal Medicine, Faculty of Medicine, Ain Shams University, Cairo, Egypt

Nahla Mohamed Teama
Division of Nephrology, Department of Internal Medicine, Faculty of Medicine, Ain Shams University, Ramsis street 38, Abbasia, Cairo 11566, Egypt

Gabriel Perri Esteves, Camila Sanches Manca, Paula Payão Ovidio, Héric Holland and Alceu Afonso Jordao
Department of Health Sciences, Ribeirao Preto Medical School, University of Sao Paulo, São Paulo, Brazil

Hellen Paraguassú Veida-Silva
Department of Physiology, Ribeirao Preto Medical School, University of Sao Paulo, São Paulo, Brazil

Flávia Sayuri Matsuo and Mariana Kiomy Osako
Department of Cell and Molecular Biology and Pathogenic Bioagents, Ribeirao Preto Medical School, University of Sao Paulo, São Paulo, Brazil

Reza Javadrashid, Abolhassan Shakeri Bavil Olyaei, Mohammad Kazem Tarzamni, Roghayeh Razzaghi and Javad Jalili
Radiology Department, Medical Radiation Sciences Research Group, Imam Reza Hospital, Tabriz University of Medical Sciences, Tabriz, Iran

Shahryar Hashemzadeh
General and Vascular Surgery Department, Imam Reza Hospital, Tabriz University of Medical Sciences, Tabriz, Iran

Mohammad Mirza-Aghazadeh-Attari
Aging Research Institute, Tabriz University of Medical Sciences, Tabriz, Iran

Ali Kiani Nazarlou and Armin Zarrintan
Department of Radiology, Imam Reza Hospital, Tabriz University of Medical Sciences, Tabriz, Iran

Hossam El-Din A. Mahmoud, Wael A. Yousry and Shereen A. Saleh
Internal Medicine Department, Gastroenterology and Hepatology Unit, Faculty of Medicine, Ain Shams University, Abbassia, Cairo 11341, Egypt

Mohamed El Badry
Tropical Medicine and Gastroenterology Department, Faculty of Medicine, Aswan University, Aswan, Egypt

Ahmed Hussein
Diagnostic and Interventional Radiology Department, Faculty of Medicine, Ain Shams University, Cairo, Egypt

Mostafa Hassan Ali
Internal Medicine Department, Nephrology Unit, Ahmed Maher Hospital, Ministry of Health, Cairo, Egypt

Hazem M. El-Hariri
Department of Community medicine, National Research Centre, Dokki, Egypt

Mohamad-Sherif Mogawer, Amany Abdel-Maqsod, Ahmed Abdel-Ghani and Abeer Awad Abdellatif
Internal medicine department, Hepatogastroenterology and liver transplantation unit, Kasr Al-Ainy Hospital, faculty of medicine, Cairo University, Cairo University, Cairo, Egypt

Mostafa EL-Shazly and Ayman Salah
General surgery department and liver transplantation unit, Kasr Al-Ainy Hospital, faculty of medicine, Cairo University, Cairo, Egypt, Cairo University, Cairo, Egypt

Omar Abdelaziz
Diagnostic and intervention Radiology department, Kasr Al-Ainy Hospital, Faculty of Medicine, Cairo University, Egypt, Cairo university, Cairo, Egypt

Mahmoud Essam
Tropical Medicine Department, and liver transplantation unit, Kasr Al-Ainy Hospital, Faculty of Medicine, Cairo University, Cairo, Egypt

Mohamed Ahmed Abdel Aziz, Ezzat Ali Ahmed, Amany Ahmed Elbanna, Khloud Salahuddin Afifi and Hanan Hosny Nouh
Department of Internal Medicine, Faculty of Medicine, Alexandria University, Alexandria, Egypt

Reham Abdel Halim
Department of Clinical Pathology, Faculty of Medicine, Alexandria University, Alexandria, Egypt

Eman Rewisha and Imam Waked
Department of Hepatology and Gastroenterology, National Liver Institute, Menoufia University, Shebeen El-Koom 32511, Egypt

Sara Abd El Ghany, Mohamed Roshdy, Heba Moustafa and Doaa M. El Demerdash
Internal Medicine Department, Faculty of Medicine, Cairo University, Cairo, Egypt

Noha M. El Husseiny, Ahmed Fathy and Asmaa M. Abdelhameed
Internal Medicine Department, Faculty of Medicine, Cairo University, Cairo, Egypt
Armed Forces Faculty of Medicine (AFCM), Cairo, Egypt

Mohamed Taha Atallah
National Hepatology and Tropical Insssstitute, Cairo, Egypt

Heba H. El Demellawy
Internal Medicine Department, Faculty of Medicine, Beni Suef University, Beni Suef, Egypt

Eman M Abdel Rahman and Fatma A Attia
Department of Internal Medicine, Faculty of Medicine for Girls, El Azhar University, Cairo, Egypt

Ayman Alsebaey
Department of Hepatology and Gastroenterology, National Liver Institute, Menoufia University, Shebeen El-Kom 32511, Egypt

Mohammad Abdel Khalik Elkady
Department of Hepatology and Gastroenterology, Theodor Bilharz Research Institute, Cairo, Egypt

Maha Mohammed Sayed
Department of Internal Medicine, Faculty of Medicine, Assiut University, Asyut, Egypt

Alaa Reda Awad and Eman Ahmed El-Seidi
Department of Medical Microbiology and Immunology, Faculty of Medicine, Cairo University, Cairo, Egypt

Moaied A. Hassan
Pediatric Surgery Department, Basrah Children's Specialty Hospital, Basrah, Iraq

A. Enayet, R. A. Afifi, E. A. Mogahed, M. S. El-Raziky and M. A. K. Abdellatif
Department of Pediatrics, Kasr Alainy Medical School, Faculty of Medicine, Cairo University, Cairo, Egypt

Osama Elbahr, Sameh Afiffy, Ahmad Kamal and Gamal Badra
Hepatology and Gastroenterology, National Liver Institute, Menoufia University, Menoufia, Egypt

Amira Saleh
Infection Control, Student Hospital, Menoufia University, Menoufia, Egypt

Azza Abdel Aziz, Samah M. Awad and Fatma O. Khalil
Medical Microbiology, and Immunology, National Liver Institute, Menoufia University, Menoufia, Egypt

Omkolsoum Alhaddad and Marwa Elfauomy
Department of Hepatology and Gastroenterology, National Liver Institute, Menoufia University, Shebeen El-Kom, Menoufia 32511, Egypt

Dalia Elsabaawy
Department of Clinical Pharmacy, National Liver Institute, Menoufia University, Menoufia 32511, Egypt

Tarek Mansour
Department of Internal Medicine, Faculty of Medicine, Ain Shams University, Cairo 3434, Egypt

Index

www.ingramcontent.com/pod-product-compliance
Lightning Source LLC
LaVergne TN
LVHW060554210926
848485LV00005B/1311
* 9 7 8 1 6 4 6 4 6 5 9 5 8 *